1994

Methods in Neurosciences

Volume 20

Pulsatility in Neuroendocrine Systems

Methods in Neurosciences

Editor-in-Chief

P. Michael Conn

Methods in Neurosciences

Volume 20
Pulsatility in Neuroendocrine Systems

Edited by
Jon E. Levine

Department of Neurobiology and Physiology
Northwestern University
Evanston, Illinois

College of St. Francis Library
Joliet, Illinois

ACADEMIC PRESS
A Division of Harcourt Brace & Company
San Diego   New York   Boston   London   Sydney   Tokyo   Toronto

Front cover photograph: In situ hybridization of luteinizing hormone-releasing hormone (LHRH) mRNA-expressing cells in the basal forebrain of the female rat. A large proportion of all LHRH neurons project to the zona externa of the median eminence, where neurosecretion of the decapeptide is governed by a neuroendocrine "LHRH pulse generator."

Academic Press, Inc.
A Division of Harcourt Brace & Company
525 B Street, Suite 1900, San Diego, California 92101-4495

United Kingdom Edition published by
Academic Press Limited
24–28 Oval Road, London NW1 7DX

International Standard Serial Number: 1043-9471

International Standard Book Number: 0-12-185289-X

PRINTED IN THE UNITED STATES OF AMERICA
94 95 96 97 98 99   E B   9 8 7 6 5 4 3 2 1

Table of Contents

Section III Central and Peripheral Sampling of Pulses *in Vivo*

Section IV Mathematical Procedures for Pulse Analysis

Contributors to Volume 20

Article numbers are in parentheses following the names of contributors. Affiliations listed are current.

JACQUELINE F. ACKLAND (22), Department of Neurobiology and Physiology, Northwestern University, Evanston, Illinois 60208

EDE M. APOSTOLAKIS (12), Division of Perinatal Biology, Loma Linda University School of Medicine, Loma Linda, California 92350

GEORG BRABANT (18), Department of Klinische Endokrinologie, Medizinische Hochschule Hannover, 30625 Hannover, Germany

ALAIN CARATY (9), Station de Physiologie de la Reproduction, Institut National de la Recherche Agronomique, Nouzilly 37380, France

KEVIN J. CATT (4), Endocrine and Reproductive Research Branch, National Institute of Child Health and Human Development, Bethesda, Maryland 20892

ADRIA A. ELSKUS (22), Department of Neurobiology and Physiology, Northwestern University, Evanston, Illinois 60208

WILLIAM C. ENGELAND (13), Department of Surgery, University of Minnesota, Minneapolis, Minnesota 55455

GONZALA MARTINEZ DE LA ESCALERA (1), Departmento de Fisiologia, Instituto de Investigaciones Biomedicas, Universidad Nacional Autonoma de Mexico, 04510 Mexico City DF, Mexico

PATRICIA C. FALLEST (22), Division of Endocrinology, University of Virginia Medical Center, Charlottesville, Virginia 22908

LINDSAY M. FAUNT (17), Division of Endocrinology and Metabolism, Departments of Pharmacology and Internal Medicine, University of Virginia Health Sciences Center, National Science Foundation Center for Biological Timing, Charlottesville, Virginia 22908

CHARLES J. GOODNER (11), Division of Metabolism, Endocrinology, and Nutrition, University of Washington School of Medicine, Seattle, Washington 98195

EVE S. HIATT (22), Department of Obstetrics and Gynecology, Universiy of Louisville School of Medicine, Louisville, Kentucky 40292

BERTIL HILLE (5), Department of Physiology and Biophysics, University of Washington, School of Medicine, Seattle, Washington 98195

MICHAEL S. JASPER (13), GI Unit, Massachusetts General Hospital, Boston, Massachusetts 02114

MICHAEL L. JOHNSON (15, 17), Division of Endocrinology and Metabolism, Departments of Pharmacology and Internal Medicine, University of Virginia Health Sciences Center, National Science Foundation for Biological Timing, Charlottesville, Virginia 22908

FRED J. KARSCH (9), Reproductive Sciences Program, University of Michigan, Ann Arbor, Michigan 48109

MARTIN J. KELLY (3), Department of Physiology, School of Medicine, Oregon Health Sciences University, Portland, Oregon 97201

ERNST KNOBIL (6), Laboratory for Neuroendocrinology, University of Texas Houston Medical School, Houston, Texas 77225

KERRY L. KNOX (22), Department of Neurobiology and Physiology, Northwestern University, Evanston, Illinois 60208

LAZAR Z. KRSMANOVIC (4), Endocrine and Reproductive Research Branch, National Institute of Child Health and Human Development, Bethesda, Maryland 20892

PIERRE J. LEFÈBVRE (23), Division of Diabetes, Nutrition, and Metabolic Disorders, C.H.U. Sart Tilman (B35), Department of Medicine, University of Liège, B-4000 Liège 1, Belgium

JON E. LEVINE (8), Department of Neurobiology and Physiology, Northwestern University, Evanston, Illinois 60208

ALAIN LOCATELLI (9), Station de Physiologie de la Reproduction, Institut National de la Recherche Agronomique, Nouzilly 37380, France

JAMES EDWARD ALISTER MCINTOSH (20), Department of Obstetrics and Gynecology, Wellington School of Medicine, University of Otago, Wellington 2, New Zealand

JOHN M. MEREDITH (8), Department of Neurobiology and Physiology, Northwestern University, Evanston, Illinois 60208

GEORGE R. MERRIAM (16), Division of Metabolism, Endocrinology, and Nutrition, Department of Medicine, and Department of Obstetrics and Gynecology, and Research Service (151), American Lake Veterans Administration Medical Center, University of Washington School of Medicine, Seattle, Washington 98195

SUZANNE M. MOENTER (9), Reproductive Sciences Program, University of Michigan, Ann Arbor, Michigan 48109

JOHN MOORMAN (15), Departments of Internal Medicine and Pharmacology and, National Science Foundation Center for Biological Timing, University of Virginia Health Sciences Center, Charlottesville, Virginia 22908

YUJI MORI (7), Department of Veterinary Ethology, Veterinary Medical Science, The University of Tokyo, Tokyo 113, Japan

ERIK MOSEKILDE (19), Physics Department, Technical University of Denmark, DK-2800 Lyngby, Denmark

ROSALIND P. MURRAY-MCINTOSH (20), Department of Medicine, Wellington School of Medicine, University of Otago, Wellington 2, New Zealand

MASUGI NISHIHARA (7), Department of Veterinary Physiology, Veterinary Medical Science, The University of Tokyo, Tokyo 113, Japan

JEFFREY R. NORGLE (8), Department of Neurobiology and Physiology, Northwestern University, Evanston, Illinois 60208

KEVIN T. O'BYRNE (6), Laboratory for Neuroendocrinology, University of Texas Houston Medical School, Houston, Texas 77225

GIUSEPPE PAOLISSO (23), Istituto di Gerontologia e Geriatria, Università di Napoli, Naples, Italy

TARJA PORKKA-HEISKANEN (8), Department of Physiology, University of Helsinki, Helsinki SF-00170, Finland

KLAUS PRANK (18), Department of Klinische Endokrinologie, Medizinische Hochschule Hannover, 30625 Hannover, Germany

OLINE K. RØNNEKLEIV (3), Department of Physiology, School of Medicine, Oregon Health Sciences University, Portland, Oregon 97201

ANDRÉ J. SCHEEN (23), Division of Diabetes, Nutrition and Metabolic Disorders, C.H.U. Sart Tilman (B35), Department of Medicine, University of Liège, B-4000 Liège 1, Belgium

NEENA B. SCHWARTZ (22), Department of Neurobiology and Physiology, Northwestern University, Evanston, Illinois 60208

EUGENE SENETA (17), School of Mathematics and Statistics, University of Sydney, Sydney, New South Wales 2006, Australia

MARGARET A. SHUPNIK (21), Departments of Internal Medicine and Physiology, University of Virginia Health Sciences Center, Charlottesville, Virginia 22908

DANIEL J. SPERGEL (4), Endocrine and Reproductive Research Branch, National Institute of Child Health and Human Development, Bethesda, Maryland 20892

STANKO S. STOJILKOVIC (4), Endocrine and Reproductive Research Branch, National Institute of Child Health and Human Development, Bethesda, Maryland 20892

JEPPE STURIS (19), Department of Medicine, Pritzker School of Medicine, University of Chicago, Chicago, Illinois 60637

MICHIO TAKAHASHI (7), Department of Veterinary Physiology, The University of Tokyo, Tokyo 113, Japan

EI TERASAWA (10), Wisconsin Regional Primate Research Center, University of Wisconsin–Madison, Madison, Wisconsin 53715

MELANIJA TOMIC (4), Endocrine and Reproductive Research Branch, National Institute of Child Health and Human Development, Bethesda, Maryland 20892

AMY TSE (5), Department of Pharmacology, University of Alberta, Edmonton, Alberta, Canada T6G 2H7

FRED W. TUREK (8), Department of Neurobiology and Physiology, Northwestern University, Evanston, Illinois 60208

RANDALL J. URBAN (14), Department of Internal Medicine, University of Texas Medical Branch, Galveston, Texas 77555

EVE VAN CAUTER (19), Department of Medicine, Pritzker School of Medicine, University of Chicago, Chicago, Illinois 60637, and Institute of Interdisciplinary Research, School of Medicine, Université Libre de Bruxelles, B-1070 Brussels, Belgium

JOHANNES D. VELDHUIS (15, 17), Division of Endocrinology and Metabolism, Department of Internal Medicine, University of Virginia Health Sciences Center, National Science Foundation Center for Biological Timing, Charlottesville, Virginia 22908

KENNETH W. WACHTER (16), Departments of Demography and Statistics, University of California, Berkeley, Berkeley, California 94720

JILL T. WALWORTH (13), Department of Surgery, University of Minnesota, Minneapolis, Minnesota 55455

RICHARD I. WEINER (1), Reproductive Endocrinology Center, Departments of Obstetrics and Gynecology, and Reproductive Sciences, University of California School of Medicine, San Francisco, California 94143

ANDREW M. WOLFE (8), Department of Neurobiology and Physiology, Northwestern University, Evanston, Illinois 60208

SUSAN WRAY (2), Laboratory of Neurochemistry, National Institute of Neurological Disorders and Stroke, National Institutes of Health, Bethesda, Maryland 20892

STEVEN M. YELLON (12), Division of Perinatal Biology, Loma Linda University School of Medicine, Loma Linda, California 92350

MI-JEONG YOO (7), Department of Veterinary Physiology, The University of Tokyo, Tokyo 113, Japan

Preface

Pulsatility in neuroendocrine systems has been recognized for more than twenty years, and yet it is only now that we are gaining a foothold in understanding the cellular basis of this phenomenon. One fact has become increasingly clear—pulsatility is a critically important operating characteristic of virtually all neurosecretory cells. It may ultimately be found that this mode of intercellular communication is not limited to neuroendocrine systems, but may additionally be utilized by central neurotransmitter cell groups as well as by many peripheral endocrine cells. Indeed, it is so early in the study of this process that we have yet to determine if one basic, stereotypical pulse-generating mechanism among all cells exists, or if several different types of pulse generators, each with a distinct cellular mode of operation, exist. Many such fundamental questions about pulsatility remain unanswered. For example: Are the neural mechanisms governing pulse generation closer in nature to those which control circadian rhythmicity? Are they perhaps more directly related to the cellular events which drive bursting activity? Or, are these mechanisms comprised of some hybrid of the cellular processes which controls rhythmicity in these respective time domains, or perhaps even totally unrelated? A corollary question also remains largely unanswered: How do target cells recognize and respond appropriately to pulsatile, as opposed to nonpulsatile, signals? The good news is that recent technical developments, such as those described in this volume, have brought the field of neuroendocrinology to the threshold of a fundamental understanding of pulse generation, regulation *of* pulsatility, and regulation *by* pulsatility.

In the past, studies of ultradian biological rhythmicity have been avoided by many neuroendocrinologists, given the well-known technical "should-nots" and "cannots" in these types of experiments: *In vivo,* one should not try to monitor pulsatility in anesthetized animals; one should not try to analyze pulsatility in subjects that experience (uncontrolled) stress; one cannot find and perform electrophysiological recordings from identified pulsing neurons. *In vitro,* one cannot study single, identified peptidergic cells and/or circuits because they are so diffuse and heterogeneous; one cannot measure ionic fluxes or secretory activity of single neuroendocrine cells; one cannot hope to see synchronized pulsatile secretion by identified peptidergic cells in culture. At long last, these methodological barriers are beginning to be both skirted and hurdled. In part, this has happened in recent years through the refinement and adaptation of established technologies, such as portal blood collection procedures, remote multiunit activity measurements, and intracellular recording, *in situ* hybridization, and dye injection in hypothalamic slice preparations. In other areas, methodological transfers from other disciplines have opened new avenues of research, examples of these being patch-clamping, intracellular calcium imaging, microdialysis, or deconvolution analysis. In some instances, the birth of completely new paradigms, such as superfusion of transformed neuronal cell lines or capacitance measurements in single endocrine cells, appears to have literally "jump-started" new lines of study in neuroendocrine pulsatility.

The goal of this volume is to provide a practical, working guide for the use of these molecular, cellular, physiological, and mathematical approaches. Chapters are written by those who have specially developed and used their own versions of these methods in their studies of neuroendocrine pulsatility. In most cases, of course, the methodologies are equally important and powerful in the investigation of nonpulsatile biological phenomena, and in this respect the volume should be useful as a general benchtop reference for neuroendocrinologists as well as for those in other areas of neuroscience or endocrinology. This book will also avail current neuroendocrine investigative tools to biomedical scientists working on extra-neuroendocrine systems in which pulse generation may operate, but as yet has not been discovered. Use of these approaches, and methods that they will likely spawn in the future, will undoubtedly reveal that nature makes more widespread use of pulsatile signaling systems than is currently imagined.

Thanks are due the staff of Academic Press for their help in generating this volume and to the contributing authors for their enthusiasm, attention to detail, and willingness to impart all of their "tricks of the trade." I would also like to acknowledge the inspiration provided by Will Cryer Levine, who has shown that one can ultimately find a method to accomplish just about anything.

JON E. LEVINE

Methods in Neurosciences

Section I

Molecular and Cellular Assessment of Pulsatility

[1] Analysis of Pulsatility in Immortalized GnRH Cell Lines

Gonzalo Martinez de la Escalera and Richard I. Weiner

Introduction

Reproduction in mammals is regulated by endocrine interactions between the hypothalamus, anterior pituitary, and gonads. The transmission of these descending and ascending signals is encoded in the amplitude and frequency of secretion of various neuropeptides and hormones. Gonadotropin-releasing hormone (GnRH) neurons play a central role in this process. These neurons comprise the final common pathway that receives neuronal and hormonal afferent inputs and in turn controls the episodic release of pituitary gonadotropins and the preovulatory luteinizing hormone (LH) surge during the estrous cycle. Extensive data support the idea that GnRH is released into the portal vessels in a pulsatile ultradian pattern. The precise cellular mechanisms and organization of the so-called GnRH pulse generator remain to be elucidated.

In both the rat (1) and monkey (2) surgical isolation of the mediobasal hypothalamus does not interfere with GnRH pulses. Lesions of the acruate nuclei in primates which destroy many of the GnRH neurons abolish the ultradian pattern of release. Neural activity within this region also has been correlated with LH pulses (3, 4). Furthermore, superfused hypothalamic fragments *in vitro* release GnRH in a pulsatile fashion (5). Altogether, these results suggested that the oscillator responsible for this intermittent neurosecretion is localized within the mediobasal hypothalamic-anterior hypothalamic-preoptic area. However, the cellular elements comprising the pulse generator were not addressed by these experiments. Potentially GnRH neurons individually or as a component of a neuronal circuit could constitute the pulse generator. The circuitry could include GnRH/GnRH neuronal interactions, GnRH neurons interacting with an unknown neuron, or glia/neuronal interactions. Obtaining synchronized pulses of GnRH secretion from multiple GnRH neurons requires (i) the timing of release of GnRH, i.e., a clock, and (ii) the synchronization of the timing mechanisms between multiple GnRH neurons. Potentially each GnRH neuron could function as a biological clock; however, networks of cells must be involved to achieve coordinated release.

General Strategy and Rationale

Addressing these fundamental questions as well as the biochemical mechanisms involved in the operation of the pulse generator was experimentally hampered by the paucity of GnRH neurons, their diffuse localization, and the complexity of the neuroanatomy of the hypothalamus (6). The total number of GnRH neurons identified by immunocytochemistry was estimated between two and three thousand cells. Furthermore, the cells were not localized in defined nuclei but scattered throughout an extensive area within the mediobasal, anterior hypothalamus and the preoptic area. Therefore, it was difficult to directly record electrical activity of identified GnRH neurons or measure peptide secretion from isolated GnRH neurons. The availability of the immortalized GT1 GnRH neuronal cell lines (7) has made it possible to analyze peptide secretion from a homogeneous population of GnRH neurons. In this chapter we describe methodology to continuously monitor spontaneous GnRH secretion of cultured immortalized GnRH neurons. A precise study of the temporal pattern of secretion was performed with the aid of a perifusion system of cells cultured on plastic coverslips (8).

Experimental Procedures

Cells

GT1 cell lines (GT1-1, GT1-3, and GT1-7) are developed from a tumor induced in a transgenic mouse by the expression of the potent oncogene, SV40 T antigen, targeted to GnRH neurons by the promoter/enhancer regions of the rat GnRH gene (7). These cells appear to be highly differentiated neurosecretory neurons. GT1 cells have a characteristic neuronal phenotype, express a number of neuronal markers, and express and process the GnRH gene at high levels (7).

Secretion of GnRH from GT1 cells is coupled to depolarization (7). Large increases in GnRH secretion occur in response to opening Na^+ channels with veratridine or opening voltage-dependent Ca^{2+} channels with high K^+. Treatment of the cells with tetrodotoxin, a specific blocker of fast Na^+ channels, prevents the action of veratridine but not the effect of high K^+. Furthermore, treatment with tetrodotoxin significantly inhibits 60% of basal GnRH release, suggesting that GT1 cells are capable of generating spontaneous, propagated action potentials which result in hormone secretion.

To obtain synchronized episodic release of GnRH a mechanism must be present for synchronization of release from neighboring cells. GT1 cells in culture form numerous interconnections with neighboring cells by neuretic processes which in some areas are consistent ultrastructurally with synaptic connections (7, 9). Approximately 15% of the cells are coupled by gap junctions (10). A similar network of GnRH neurons is found in rodents (11) and primates (12). Therefore release may be synchronized via electrotonic coupling of cells via gap junctions or via a synaptic mechanism.

In addition, GT1 cells express a number of receptors and signaling pathways that could potentially participate in mediating afferent inputs to the cells. GT1 cells express β_1-adrenergic (13) and D_1-dopaminergic (14) receptors, both of which are positively coupled to adenylate cyclase. GABA exerts a biphasic effect on GnRH secretion whereas arginine vasopressin and prolactin inhibit secretion (15, 16).

Cell Culture

GT1-1 cells between passages 5 and 25 are cultured in Dulbecco's modified Eagle's medium (DMEM) supplemented with 10% fetal bovine serum, 4.5 mg/ml glucose, nonessential amino acids, and 10 μg/ml of penicillin/streptomycin. A mixture of 5% equine and 5% fetal bovine serum can be used instead of 10% fetal bovine serum. Cells are plated on 25-mm plastic coverslips (Thermanox, Miles Laboratories, Naperville, IL), coated with a 20% solution of Matrigel (Collaborative Research, Bedford, MA) placed in 35-mm plastic petri dishes (Falcon Labware, Oxnard, CA). The use of the reconstituted basement membrane preparation, Matrigel, on coverslips results in cells adhering to the coverslips throughout the perifusion. The cultures are maintained at 37°C in a water-saturated atmosphere of 95% O_2 and 5% CO_2. Cells are cultured until they reach 50–70% confluency at which time medium is replaced by a defined medium (Opti-MEM, Gibco, Grand Island, NY) without serum for 2 days. Cells should not be allowed to grow to higher densities. Our experience is that regulated GnRH release is difficult to see in overgrown cultures. Cells are removed from serum for 2 days prior to experiments to inhibit cell growth and to synchronize cells in a nondividing state. Furthermore in the absence of serum, GT1 cells extend more extensive networks of neurites and take on a more characteristic neuronal phenotype. An advantage of culturing the cells on coverslips is that cells can be maintained until a given cell density is obtained. Furthermore, the effect of neurotrophic factors on neurite outgrowth, etc., can be assessed on the coverslips prior to performing the experiment. Coverslips can be photographed under phase-contrast microscopy and morphology assessed quantitatively relative to function.

Superfusion

The development, characterization, and utilization of this superfusion technique with anterior pituitary cells has been thoroughly described in a previous paper (16). Accordingly, in this chapter we focus on the adaptation and characterization of this method as used with the GT1 cells. The spontaneous release of the GnRH over time is characterized using Sykes–Moore chambers (Bellco Glass, Inc., Vineland, NJ) in which two coverslips separated by a gasket comprise the superfusion chamber. The volume of the chamber is 200 μl. Two superfusion configurations can be used with the chamber, with either one coverslip containing cells or both coverslips containing cells. Multiple cell types, e.g., astroglia and GnRH neurons, can be cocultured either on the same coverslip or separately on opposing coverslips comprising the chamber. Thereby cell-to-cell and paracrine interactions can be differentiated. For example, when one cell-coated coverslip comprises the chamber both cell-to-cell contacts and paracrine interactions with neighboring cells can be evaluated. The degree of interactions should vary with the density of cell cultures. When opposing coverslips contain cultured cells the two sides of the chamber can only communicate by a diffusable factor.

A second approach in which cells have been cultured on Cytodex beads has been used successfully to study GnRH secretion from GT1 cells (10, 18). However, it is more difficult to evaluate cell-to-cell interactions and bead-to-bead contacts in perifused Cytodex beads placed in a column.

Media used for superfusion are (a) Locke's medium (mM): NaCl 154; KCl 5.6; CaCl$_2$ 2.2; MgCl$_2$ 1; NaHCO$_3$ 6; glucose 10; HEPES 2; (b) the same without CaCl$_2$; or (c) Opti-MEM (Gibco), a defined medium. All media are supplemented with 20 μM bacitracin (Sigma Chemical Co., St. Louis, MO) to prevent proteolytic degradation of GnRH(19). Cells are superfused at a flow rate of 0.08–0.15 ml/min. We chose Locke's medium for the perifusion media since basal secretion is low resulting in larger relative changes with various treatments. This is most likely related to the low level of K$^+$ in the media. Furthermore this medium was used successfully for studies of the release of GnRH from hypothalamic fragments (19). Using defined media is also essential for studying the effect of various transmitters and neuromodulators on the biology of the cells. A disadvantage of using Opti-MEM is that the full composition of the medium is proprietorial. After an equilibration period (usually 60 min is sufficient for the stabilization of the secretion levels), samples are frequently collected (usually every 4 min) for up to 180 min. Samples are boiled for 3 min (to inactivate proteolytic enzymes) and stored at $-20°C$ until radioimmunoassay (RIA).

Experimental Considerations

The flow rate of the superfusion is critical for the resolution of the time-dependent release of GnRH. It is desirable to use a fast flow rate to obtain well-defined and sharp peaks when the peptide is released in pulses. However, there are a number of parameters that limit the rate of flow. At high flow rates mechanical changes in pressure and detachment of cells from the coverslip are problematic. Furthermore the sensitivity of the GnRH assay also limits the ability to detect a signal. Additionally, the number of cells in the chamber and the amount of GnRH released by the particular subclone of GT1 cells all influence the amount of GnRH per sample. We have found an optimal balance between these parameters is a flow rate of 0.15 ml/min, sampling time of 4 min, cell density of 0.8–1 million GT1-1 cells/chamber, and RIA sensitivity of 2 pg/ml. We have found it difficult to perform perifusion experiments with GT1-3 and GT1-7 cells because of the lower levels of GnRH released by them, approximately 10 and 30% that released by GT1-1 cells.

GnRH Determination

GnRH in the superfusate is determined by RIA in duplicates using the rabbit polyclonal antibody R1245, obtained from T. Nett, which is specific for the decapeptide (20). It is essential to use a well-characterized antibody to GnRH for the RIA. Various other peptides formed from the GnRH precursor molecule are secreted by the cells. Changes in peptide processing will influence the observed results with an antibody recognizing various metabolites (10). All samples from an experiment are analyzed in the same assay to decrease variability. The limit of detection is 2 pg/ml and the intraassay coefficient of variation 4.3%. Samples are not stored for longer than 1 month prior to assay.

Pulse Analysis

GnRH pulses can be identified and their parameters determined by the computer algorithm cluster analysis developed by Veldhuis and Johnson (21). Individual point standard deviations are calculated using a power function variance model from the experimental duplicates. A 2×2 cluster configuration and a t-statistic of two for the upstroke and downstroke are used to maintain false-positive and false-negative error rates below 10%. The statistical significance of the pulse parameters are tested with one-way analysis of variance (ANOVA) followed by Fisher's multiple comparison test at the 0.05 level of significance.

Results

Validation of the Method

To eliminate the possibility of pulses being aberrantly generated by the experimental conditions, in six control experiments synthetic GnRH (Sigma Chemical Co.) was continuously perfused through the perfusion system. Under these conditions, no pulses are detected.

Spontaneous Release of GnRH by GT1 Cells

Release of GnRH from GT1 cells is clearly pulsatile when data are analyzed by cluster analysis (8). In the experiments where only one coverslip contains cells, the analysis with the pulse-detection algorithm revealed that cells spontaneously released GnRH with a frequency of approximately one pulse every 25 min. This frequency was observed irrespective of the cells being superfused with Locke's medium or Opti-MEM. A rhythmic pattern with identical frequency was obtained from chambers composed of two cell-coated coverslips. Comparison of pulse parameters (mean interval between peaks, mean peak width, mean peak height, and mean valley width) between experiments with one or two cell-coated coverslips and Locke's or defined medium, revealed no significant differences when analyzed by ANOVA. Overall the results show that GT1 cells spontaneously secrete GnRH in pulses at intervals of 25.8 ± 1.58 min, with an average peak width of 18.83 ± 1.46 min and an average height of $150.5 \pm 6.01\%$ above the preceding nadir, while the average valley length between pulses is 7.25 ± 0.27 min. These findings have been confirmed by experiments with perifused GT1 cells cultured on Cytodex beads (10, 22).

Ca^{2+} Dependency of GnRH Pulses

No significant GnRH pulses were identified by cluster analysis when GT1 cells were cultured in Ca^{2+}-free Locke's medium (8). This effect was reversible, since return of Ca^{2+} to the superfusion medium after a period of 4 hr in Ca^{2+}-free Locke's medium resulted in significant spontaneous pulses of

GnRH. No significant differences in the parameters of the pulses were observed between this latter treatment and the control cells superfused with complete Locke's medium. The Ca^{2+} dependency of pulsatile GnRH release from GT1 cells has been shown to be dependent on voltage-sensitive Ca^{2+} influx (22).

Conclusions

Cultures of GT1 cells secrete GnRH in a calcium-dependent rhythmic pattern of discrete pulses (8). Since GT1-1 cells are a clonal cell line, this finding demonstrates that the ability to generate rhythmic pulses is an inherent property of GnRH neurons or networks of GnRH neurons. At this time it is impossible to state whether isolated GT1 cells are a single-cell oscillator (23). Experiments using whole-cell patch-clamping or Ca^{2+} flourescent-imaging techniques may be able to answer this fundamental question. To observe pulsatile release from the large number of neurons cultured on a coverslip a mechanism for synchronization of the release of GnRH must exist. A model of cell-to-cell communication via intercellular contacts could explain synchronization of pulses in the experiments performed with a perifusion chamber containing a single cell-coated coverslip. However, only approximately 10% of GT1 cells in culture appear to be coupled by gap junctions (10). Synchronization could also be mediated by synaptic mechanisms. Synaptic-like profiles have been observed also (7, 9). Synapses between GnRH-containing processes have been seen in both the rat (24) and the monkey hypothalamus (25). However, such contacts do not adequately explain how cells on opposing coverslips become synchronized. Our finding that chambers composed of two coverslips both containing cells release GnRH in a pulsatile fashion suggests that a diffusable mediator may be involved. Whether these paracrine-like interactions observed with GT1 cells actually occur *in vivo* is unclear. Paracrine effects in our experiment could be an artifact of the proximity of large numbers of GnRH cells in the chambers. A putative mediator of synchronization could reach concentrations normally only seen in a synaptic cleft. However these observations suggest that a diffusable substance released from the GT1 cells is involved in synchronization of the cells.

One candidate for the mediator of synaptic or paracrine regulation is GnRH. Previous work suggested that GnRH was involved in an ultrashort loop feedback (26). The mouse GnRH receptor was recently cloned and the mRNA for the receptor was found to be expressed by GT1 cells (27). Other likely candidates as mediators are the peptides processed from the pro-GnRH molecule, including GnRH-associated peptide. However, the possibility of a factor not related to GnRH cannot be excluded. A small percentage of rat GnRH neurons in the brain has been reported to contain galanin (28) and delta sleep-inducing peptide (29). Whether these or other putative neuromediator(s) are expressed in GT1 cells is unknown.

The pattern of GnRH pulses varies among species, physiological state, and method of determination. No data are available on the pattern of GnRH pulses in the mouse. However, the pattern of GnRH pulses from perifused GT1 cells resembles very closely that measured by push–pull perifusion of ovariectomized rats (30). It should be remembered that the shape of the pulses in the present experiments is dependent on the perifusion rate of the chambers, a parameter set by the practical considerations of assay sensitivity and sample frequency. At the flow rate at which sampling was done, it takes 80–160 sec to completely exchange the media in the chambers. Therefore, even if GnRH was released over a short period of time, the pulses would appear more prolonged. Another possibility is that the broad width of the pulse reflects the time it takes for cells at some distance on the coverslips to coordinate their release. The mean pulse frequency observed with the GT1-1 cells of one pulse every 25.8 ± 1.5 min is in close agreement with the interpulse interval observed in castrated rats (30) and mice (personal communication, R. Steiner).

Future Directions

The data presented demonstrate that the pulsatile release of GnRH is an inherent property of cultures of GnRH neurons. The following fundamental questions must now be answered: (i) Is a single GnRH neuron the oscillator or is pulse generation dependent on networks of GnRH neurons? (ii) How is synchronization of the activity of neighboring GnRH neurons mediated? (iii) What is the biochemical basis of the timing of the pulse frequency, i.e., The biological clock? This final question will be difficult to pursue without elucidation of biochemical markers which are proximal to the timing mechanisms. For example, a periodicity gene (PER) has been described in *Drosophila*. Single point mutations in the PER gene were described which increase or decrease the periodicity of diurnal behavioral activities (32). Unfortunately a homologue of this gene has not been observed in mammals. Simply following GnRH secretion to study the biological clock could be misleading, since it is easy to imagine that peptide secretion could be uncoupled while the cellular timing mechanism is unaffected.

Acknowledgments

We thank Steven Zippin for his technical assistance with RIA. This work was supported by NIH Grants HD08924 and HD11979 (to R.I.W.) and Rockefeller Foundation Biotechnology Career Fellowship (to G.M.E).

References

1. C. A. Blake and C. H. Sawyer, *Endocrinology (Baltimore)* **94,** 730 (1974).
2. L. Krey, W. Butler, and E. Knobil, *Endocrinology (Baltimore)* **96,** 1073 (1975).
3. R. C. Wilson, J. S. Kesner, J. Kaufman, T. Uemura, T. Akema, and E. Knobil, *Neuroendocrinology* **39,** 256 (1984).
4. T. M. Plant, L. C. Krey, J. Moossy, J. T. McCormack, D. L. Hess, and E. Knobil, *Endocrinology (Baltimore)* **102,** 52–56 (1978).
5. J. P. Bourguignon and P. Franchimont, *C.R. Soc. Biol. (Paris)* **175,** 389 (1981).
6. A. J. Silverman, *in* "The Physiology of Reproduction" (E. Knobil and J. D. Neill, eds.), pp. 1283–1304. Raven Press, New York, 1988.
7. P. L. Mellon, J. J. Windle, P. C. Goldsmith, C. A. Padula, J. L. Roberts, and R. I. Weiner, *Neuron* **5,** 1 (1990).
8. G. Martinez de la Escalera, A. L. H. Choi, and R. I. Weiner, *Proc. Natl. Acad. Sci. U.S.A.* **89,** 1852 (1992).
9. Z. Liposits, I. Merchenthaler, W. Wetsel, J. Reid, P. Mellon, R. Weiner, and A. Negro-Vilar, *Endocrinology (Baltimore)* **129,** 1575 (1991).
10. W. Wetsel, M. Valenca, I. Merchenthaler, Z. Liposits, F. Lopez, R. Weiner, P. Mellon, and A. Negro-Vilar, *Proc. Natl. Acad. Sci. U.S.A.* **89,** 4149 (1992).
11. C. Leranth, L. M. G. Segura, M. Palkovits, N. J. MacLusky, M. Shanabrough, and F. Naftolin, *Brain Res.* **345,** 332 (1985).
12. K. K. Thind and P. Goldsmith, *Neuroendocrinology* **47,** 203 (1988).
13. G. Martinez de la Escalera, A. L. H. Choi, and R. I. Weiner, *Endocrinology (Baltimore)* **131,** 1397 (1992).
14. G. Martinez de la Escalera, F. Gallo, A. L. H. Choi, and R. I. Weiner, *Endocrinology (Baltimore)* **131,** 2965 (1992).
15. R. I. Weiner and G. Martinez de la Escalera, *Soc. Neurosci. Abstr.* **18,** 928 (1992).
16. L. Milenkovic, G. D'Angelo, and R. Weiner, *Soc. Neurosci. Abstr.* **18,** 929 (1992).
17. G. Martinez de la Escalera, K. C. Swearingen, and R. I. Weiner, *in* "Methods in Enzymology" (P. M. Conn, ed.), Vol. 168, pp. 254–263. Academic Press, San Diego, 1989.
18. L. Krsmanovic, S. Stojilkovic, T. Balla, S. Al-Damluji, R. Weiner, and K. Catt, *Proc. Natl. Acad. Sci. U.S.A.* **88,** 11,124 (1991).
19. S. Drouva, J. Epelbaum, M. Hery, L. Tapiaa-Arancibia, E. Laplante, and C. Kordon, *Neuroendocrinology* **32,** 155 (1981).
20. T. M. Nett, A. M. Akbar, G. D. Niswender, M. T. Hedlund, and W. F. White, *J. Clin. Endocrinol. Metab.* **36,** 880 (1973).

21. J. Veldhuis and M. Johnson, *Am. J. Physiol.* **250**, E486 (1986).
22. L. Krsmanovic, S. Stojilkovic, F. Merelli, S. Dufour, M. Virmani, and K. Catt, *Proc. Natl. Acad. Sci. U.S.A.* **89**, 8462 (1992).
23. R. R. Llinas, *Science* **242**, 1654 (1988).
24. C. Leranth, L. Segura, M. Palkovits, N. Maclusky, M. Shanabrough, and F. Naftolin, *Brain Res.* **345**, 332 (1985).
25. P. Marschall and P. Goldsmith, *Brain Res.* **193**, 353 (1980).
26. D. K. Sarkar, *Neuroendocrinology* **45**, 510 (1987).
27. L. Krsmanovic, S. Stojilkovic, L. Mertz, M. Tomic, and K. Catt, *Proc. Natl. Acad. Sci. U.S.A.* **90**, 3908 (1993).
28. I. Merchenthaler, F. Lopez, and A. Negro-Vilar, *Proc. Natl. Acad. Sci. U.S.A.* **87**, 6326 (1990).
29. P. G. Vallet, Y. Charnay, C. Boura, and J. Z. Kiss, *Neuroendocrinology* **53**, 103 (1991).
30. J. E. Levine and V. D. Ramirez, *Endocrinology (Baltimore)* **111**, 1439 (1982).
31. C. Masotto and A. Negro-Vilar, *Endocrinology (Baltimore)* **123**, 747 (1988).
32. W. Zehring, D. Wheeler, P. Reddy, R. Konopka, C. Kyriacou, M. Rosbash, and J. Hall, *Cell (Cambridge, Mass.)* **39**, 369 (1984).

[2] Use of Organotypic Cultures for the Study of Neuroendocrine Cells

Susan Wray

Introduction

Neuroendocrine cells have long been used as models to study neurosecretion. The ubiquity of pulsatile release of hormones has become clear through extremely difficult *in vivo* studies which measured small amounts of the released peptides in portal blood and/or discharges of nuclear organized neuroendocrine cells (for reviews see 1–8). Although these studies have beautifully documented the pulsatility of numerous neuroendocrine systems, the intrinsic properties of the cells which generate and regulate this pulsatile response remain poorly understood. Within the past decade, organ cultures have reemerged as an important complement to *in vivo* studies for examining regulatory mechanisms in various neuroendocrine systems. The principle behind organ cultures is to maintain tissue in a state which is as close as possible to that found *in vivo*, i.e., to preserve some characteristics of the spatial, structural, and/or synaptic organization of the original tissue. As a result, such cultures are termed *organotypic* and are valuable tools to study organized, yet relatively isolated, neuronal systems either acutely or long term.

In organ cultures, the regulation of biological events in neuroendocrine cell types can be compared in slices (a) obtained from different brain regions, (b) generated from different aged animals, and (c) with the same cells but obtained from a different anatomic orientation (sagittal, coronal, etc.). In this way, one can systematically control the anatomically defined population of neuroendocrine cells under study as well as their environment. Various developmental aspects of neuroendocrine systems can also be studied since the tissue used in these cultures can be derived from either embryonic animals or postnatal animals (starting material which is already substantially differentiated). For example, one can compare cultures of neuronal areas prior to synaptic innervation to cultures derived from tissue in which synapses are already established. In such an investigation, morphologic, cellular, molecular, and neurosecretory changes associated with neuronal circuit development can be addressed. Hence, by combining different technical assays with different slice parameters, one can achieve enormous experimental flexibility. These features make organ cultures a viable and attractive model

Methods in Neurosciences, Volume 20

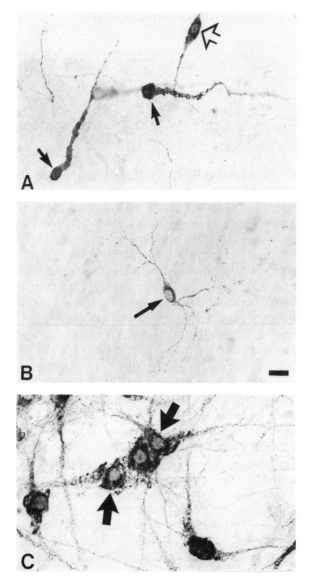

FIG. 1   Neuroendocrine cell types maintained in organotypic explant slice cultures. All cultures were derived from Postnatal Day 4 rats and maintained for 17–21 days *in vitro*. (A) LHRH-immunopositive cells located in a slice derived from the preoptic area. LHRH-positive cells in slice explant cultures generally possessed a simple, bipolar morphology (open arrow), but as observed *in vivo* (45), unipolar irregular LHRH cell types are also present *in vitro* (solid arrows). (B) A multipolar corticotropin-releasing hormone-immunopositive cell (arrow) with many branching processes

system for addressing questions on the development and regulation of neuro-endocrine cells.

Slice Explant Roller-Tube Cultures

Of the organ culturing methods available, the slice explant roller-tube culture technique (9–15) allows long-term culturing of tissues and facilitates thinning, while maintaining organotypic intercellular relationships. A variety of neuronal and nonneuronal tissue types has been studied using slice explant cultures (9–13; for review see 14 and 15). Particularly relevant for the study of neuroendocrine cells is the fact that slice explant cultures have been routinely obtained from the preoptic area/hypothalamus of postnatal rat (9–15). Several laboratories have found slice explant roller-tube cultures highly effective in maintaining differentiated, postnatal neuroendocrine cells in long-term organ cultures including luteinizing hormone-releasing hormone (LHRH) cells (15, 19, 21–23), oxytocin (OT) cells (15–17, 19, 22, 24), and corticotropin-releasing hormone (CRH) cells (19, 25) (Fig. 1). These roller-tube cultures retain or reexpress many organotypic features of the neuroendocrine cells being cultured, such as axonal plexi, nuclear organization, cell morphology, and synaptic relations (Figs. 1 and 2; 14, 15, 19, 25).

Visualization of Individual Neuroendocrine Cells

In optimal slice explant roller-tube cultures, the tissue thins to a quasi-monolayer, one to three cells thick. The thinning process takes place within the first few days and is due to cell death and cell movement. The thinness of these slice explant cultures is one of the most important and useful features of this culture technique. It permits single-cell analysis of neuroendocrine cells in *fixed* cultures using (i) light and electron microscopic immunocytochemical and immunohistochemical methods (17, 19–22, 32–35); (ii) receptor autoradiography (9); and (iii) *in situ* hybridization histochemistry (15, 21–24, 31, 33). These methods provide valuable data concerning survival of neuroendocrine cell types (16, 17, 19, 20, 32),

---

maintained in slice culture in the periventricular region. (C) Culture from the level of the paraventricular nucleus immunocytochemically stained for neurophysin (NP). Immunopositive magnocellular NP cells (arrows) were usually found in clusters (averaging 20–30 μm in diameter). Scale bar = 25 μm for all panels.

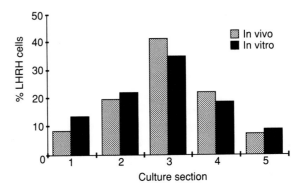

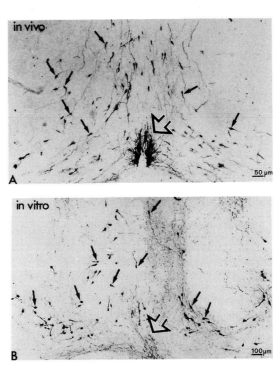

FIG. 2   Maintenance of topographic distribution *in vitro* of a dispersed neuroendo-crine population: LHRH cells. LHRH cells form a continuum *in vivo* (45) which spans the forebrain. The relative distribution of LHRH cells *in vivo* is maintained *in vitro* (after 18 days) in five consecutive forebrain slice cultures (histogram, for anatom-ical location of five regions see Fig. 5 and Ref. 19). An example of slice 3 and its original *in vivo* counterpart is shown in A and B. (A) Fifty-micrometer vibratome

organotypic organization of the slices (17, 19, 26), afferent connections (17, 27, 30, 36), efferent projections (19), functional activity (16, 19), and gene transcription (21–24, 31). The compatibility of slice explant roller-tube cultures and *in situ* hybridization histochemistry (21–24) enables one to examine (i) developmental onset of phenotypic expression; (ii) receptor-mediated changes in transcription and translation of specific neuronal genes in differentiated cells; (iii) second messenger systems which directly influence gene expression; (iv) regulation of gene expression in embryonic and/or nonsynaptically associated cells; and (v) the sequence of genes activated which lead to the final event, e.g., secretion of a product. Thus, together, these histochemical and immunocytochemical techniques yield data with high anatomic resolution which can be used to determine how individual neurons and/or organized neuronal circuits, albeit "simplified," respond to specific stimuli, both internally and externally located.

Due to thinning, *living* cells can be visualized in slice explant cultures using phase-contrast microscopy or Nomarski optics. In addition, single cells can be identified from specific brain regions based on morphologic features (magnocellular neuroendocrine cells in the supraoptic nucleus; 26) and microinjections of dyes and/or electrophysiological recordings performed (12, 14, 22, 26–31). We have succeeded in obtaining patch-clamp electrophysiological recordings from identified LHRH cells in fetal explants (unpublished data) and believe that this strategy is compatible with differentiated neuroendocrine cells in postnatal slice explant cultures. In addition, roller-tube slice explant cultures have been examined by optical methods (14, 32). Optical recordings and image analysis of differentiated, primary neuroendocrine cells should provide information pertinent to the temporal and spatial aspects of information processing and communication in these specialized cells and thereby increase our understanding of the intrinsic versus extrinsic (transsynaptic) mechanism(s) underlying

---

section from a 4-day-old rat immunocytochemically stained for LHRH. This section is at the level of the organum vasculosum lamina terminalis (OVLT), a region known to contain a large portion of the LHRH neuronal population *in vivo* (45). (B) Culture section derived from a 4-day-old animal, from the same anatomic level as that shown in A, immunocytochemically stained for LHRH after 18 days *in vitro*. Solid arrows point to a few of the immunopositive LHRH cells (A and B). Open arrows indicate the ventral fiber plexus around the OVLT (A and B). Note that the LHRH neuronal distribution is similar *in vivo* and *in vitro*, with the LHRH cells forming an inverted V around the midline, but that the *in vitro* tissue has spread to almost twice the surface area originally present *in vivo* (see scale lines).

pulsatility. Such studies are currently being undertaken in our laboratory on preoptic area/hypothalamic slice explant cultures containing LHRH and OT cells.

Organotypic Organization, Ingrowth, and Neurosecretion

In a single slice these cultures contain relatively normal interneuronal and glial interactions and anatomic distribution of various cell types (10, 14, 19–21, 32). If one has several slices through a given neuronal region, then the organotypic nature of these cultures expands to include relative neuronal topography. This means that cell populations found in several neuronal regions may maintain the same relationship *in vitro*, i.e., occurring in particular slice cultures in a manner proportional to that seen *in vivo* (Fig. 2; 19).

Having the ability to change the synaptic environment via slice orientation and age of initial animals can yield important information about the cells studied. In addition, the ability to reintroduce specific inputs experimentally by coculturing in the presence of tissue containing afferent systems opens up a variety of investigations concerning axonal choice and mechanisms of ingrowth of neuroendocrine cells (14, 15, 19). Finally, slice explant roller-tube cocultures seem well suited for studies on neurosecretion. These organotypic cultures permit coculture of neuroendocrine cells with specific target systems (16–19). Pituitary tissue survives well in these cultures (Fig. 3; 16–19) and our laboratory has been able to maintain nonneuronal tissues in slice explant cultures including neonatal ovaries (Fig. 4) and testes. Since the entire slice explant culture is maintained in a small volume of media (which can be removed), release of neurohormones can be monitored directly or via bioassays. For the latter situation, cocultures can be used to determine whether *indirect* interactions between tissues occur (via secretion into the media; 14–17, 19, 23). Thus, cocultures of neuroendocrine systems, e.g., the hypothalamohypophyseal system, enable analysis to be made of the effects of neuroendocrine cell types on the release of a variety of pituitary hormones, thereby facilitating investigations of neurosecretion in synaptically organized, yet relatively isolated, neuronal systems, without systemic complications.

Due to its thinness, maintenance of organotypic features, and coculture properties, the slice explant roller culture system is an *in vitro* model system particularly appropriate for examining the intrinsic properties of identifiable single neuroendocrine cells, neuroendocrine subpopulations, and total populations (monitoring cellular activity, gene, and gene products) and the ways in which these neuroendocrine subtypes respond to extrinsic factors (both humoral and synaptic). As such, slice explant cultures provide a model

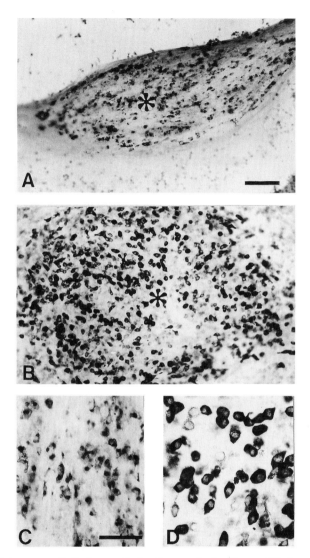

FIG. 3   Maintenance of pituitary cells in slice explant cultures. Pituitary tissue from
Postnatal Day 4 rats survives for long periods *in vitro* and several cell types maintain
expression of their appropriate pituitary hormone. Pituitaries maintained for 18 days
in slice explant cultures in the presence of horse serum were immunocytochemically
stained for prolactin (A and C) or luteinizing hormone (B and D). Numerous hormone-
expressing cells were detected. *Pituitary tissue. Scale bar = 100 μm in A and B;
50 μm in C and D.

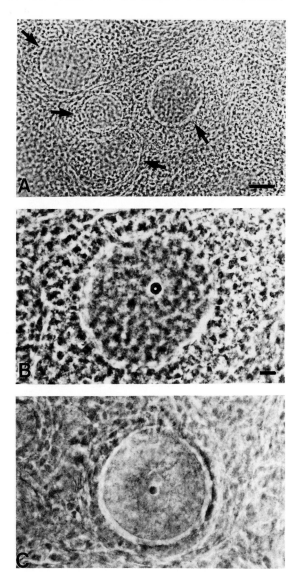

FIG. 4 Gonadal tissue in slice explant cultures. Neonatal gonadal tissue can be cocultured with brain and/or pituitary tissues in slice explant cultures. (A) Neonatal ovary tissue maintained for 18 days *in vitro* with hypothalamic slices (not shown). Immature follicles can be seen (arrows) using phase microscopy. Scale bar = 50 μm in A. Higher magnification of center follicle is shown in B. (C) High magnification of follicle maintained in coculture containing ovary, pituitary, and hypothalamic tissues. Scale bar = 10 μm in B and C.

system for the study of specific neuroendocrine subtypes in which the cascade of events, starting with receptor-mediated stimulation, through transcription, precursor processing, and ending with neurosecretion, can be readily studied in a controlled environment.

Slice Explant Protocol

The success of slice explant cultures depends greatly on treating the initial tissue as *gently* as possible. Many factors can contribute to culture death: contamination, poor media quality, condition of donor animals, and/or the adhering substrate used. While these variables affect culture survival, treatment of the tissue prior to culturing (handling by the investigator) is often a variable which is overlooked and is critical to tissue survival. Thus, it is important to perfect the dissecting technique before evaluating the reasons for success or failure of the culture procedure.

General Setup for Culturing

Culture Area
The area where the initial dissections, cutting, and plating of the slice cultures are performed should be as "sterile" as possible. In our laboratory, these procedures are done in a tissue enclosure hood in an area of limited traffic. [Note: a laminar flow hood is used only when the cultures are inserted into the test tubes (before rotation) and during feeding (see below).]

Instruments and Materials Used for Generation of Slice Explant Cultures
The following instruments are routinely used during the dissection and plating procedures: dissecting microscope, fiber optic lighting, tissue chopper, repeating Eppendorf pipettes, small oven, large surgical scissors (decapitation), small scissors (to remove the brain from the calvarium), fine-tipped forceps (removal of the pia, blood vessels, etc., and manipulation of the tissue slices), polished flat-surfaced small spatulas (transfer of the blocked tissue and tissue slices), razor blade holders and breakable blades (to dissect out the area of interest), and aclar film (plastic disks used on tissue chopper, which can be sterilized and discarded after using).

Cleaning Procedures
All tools, with the exception of the fine forceps and small scissors, are heat-sterilized in a small oven before culturing. All tools are resterilized throughout the plating procedure by rinsing in a series of alcohol washes (water, 50, 95,

and 100%). Aclar disks are used on the tissue chopper as disposable, sterile cutting surfaces. They are cut from aclar film* (Allied Fibers and Plastics), washed several times in alcohol, air-dried, and placed in packages which are then gas-sterilized and set aside for at least 2 weeks (to remove any harmful components of gases). The tissue chopper and surface of the tissue enclosure hood are wiped down with alcohol before culturing, throughout the culture procedure, and after the last tissue sections are generated. It is important to remove all "dirty" solutions and material from the culture area prior to plating the tissue slices onto the coverslips. Glass coverslips, on which the cultures are plated, are cleaned by rinsing 3 × 1 hr with 95% alcohol and then put into fresh alcohol, covered, and left overnight. The following day the alcohol is replaced by deionized, distilled water, and the coverslips are boiled for 20–30 min. After cooling, the water is replaced by several alcohol rinses. The coverslips are stored in fresh alcohol until the day of use. On the morning of culturing, the coverslips are placed in a glass petri dish and heated in a small oven (Fisher, Isotemp 500 series) at ~200°C for 1 hr and then cooled.

Experimental Animals

Successful slice explant cultures are obtained from either postnatal or embryonic animals. However, the age of the animal from which the tissue is obtained can critically affect the survival, thinness, and/or organotypic characteristics of the final culture. Hence, the age of the initial animal should be chosen carefully while taking into account the neuronal area, neuroendocrine cell type, etc., to be studied. In general, "immature" tissue shows greater distortion of the original cytoarchitecture than older tissue. The term immature here can apply to either embryonic or postnatal tissue and relates to when the structure studied develops (cell differentiation, synapse formation, etc.). Such distortion is most likely due to enhanced cell migration, proliferation of undifferentiated cell types (both glial and neuronal), and lack of synaptic input. In either case, the age of the tissue from which long-term cultures are generated is an extremely important variable. In general, good cultures are obtained from tissues taken from 4- to 6-day-old pups (for procedures used on embryonic animals see Ref. 15). This postnatal age group thins and maintains organotypic characteristics from a variety of brain regions, including hippocampus, anterior hypothalamus, cerebellum, and brain stem as well as survival of phenotypically different cell types (14, 15). The oldest animals used in our laboratory are 9–10 days of age. While robust fiber outgrowth and survival of neuroendocrine cells are seen in material from 9- to 10-day-

*See Table I for a list of products and suppliers.

TABLE I Products and Suppliers[a]

Product	Supplier	Catalog No.
Aclar film (gauge 7.80 mils)	Allied Corporation, Engineer Plastics Department	
Albumin, bovine	Sigma	A-0281
Anocell	Anotec	
Basal Media Eagle	Gibco Laboratories	320-1010 or 1017
Blade breaker/blades	Surgimed-MLB, Inc.	
Chicken plasma	CoCalico Biologicals, Inc.	30-0390
Collagen type 1	Sigmal Chemical	C7661
Earle's BSS	Gibco Laboratories	310-4010 or 4015
F-12 nutrient mix	Gibco Laboratories	320-1765AG
Geys's BSS	Gibco Laboratories	310-4260 (for slides)
Glass coverslips	Fisher Scientific	3312 Gold Seal (12 × 24)
Horse serum	Source varies	
Insulin, bovine	Sigma Chemical	I-5500
L-Glutamine	Gibco Laboratories	320-5030AG (200 mM)
McIlwain tissue chopper	Brinkmann	
PSN antibiotic mix	Gibco Laboratories	600-5640
Putrescine	Sigmal Chemical	P-7505
Roller drum	Bellco Glass Biotechnology	7736
Sodium selenite	Sigma Chemical	S-1382
Thrombin	Sigma Chemical	T-4265
Tissue culture water	Source varies	
Tissue enclosure hood	Labconco	
Transferrin, bovine	Sigma Chemical	T-5761

Supplier	Phone No.
Allied Corporation, Engineer Plastics Department P.O. Box 1205, Pottsville, PA 17901	(800)233–0251
Anotec 226 East 54th St., New York, NY 10022	(212)751–3770
Bellco Glass Biotechnology 340 Edrudo Rd., P.O. Box B, Vineland, NJ 08360	(800)257–7043
Brinkmann Cantiague Rd., Westbury, NY 11590	(800)645–3050
CoCalico Biologicals, Inc. 449 Stevens Rd., P.O. Box 265, Reamstown, PA 17567	(215)267–7548
Fisher Scientific P.O. Box 1768, Pittsburgh, PA 15230	(412)562–8300
Gibco Laboratories 3175 Staley Rd., Grand Island, NY 14072	(800)828–6686
Sigma Chemical P.O. Box 14508, St. Louis, MO 63160	(800)325–3010
Surgimed-MLB, Inc. 22 S. State St., Newtown, PA 18940	(215)968–3186

[a] Note: Most of these products are available from many different sources.

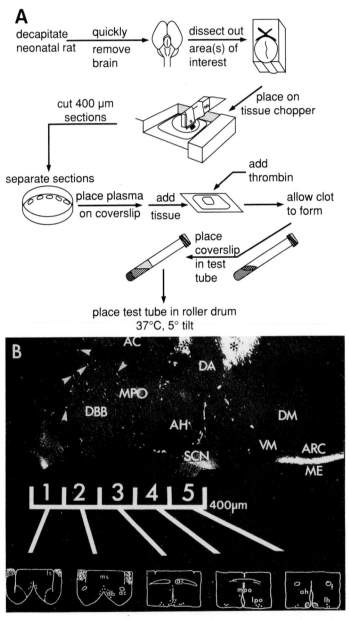

FIG. 5   Generation of slice explant roller-tube cultures. (A) Schematic of protocol, outlined in text, for generating slice explant cultures from brain tissues. (B) Parasagittal view of the preoptic/hypothalamic areas from a Postnatal Day 4 brain, illustrating the positions of the 400-μm coronal sections taken for culturing. Rostral is to the

old rats, this tissue consistently becomes more necrotic after 13 days in culture than tissue generated from younger animals. Our observations agree with previous accounts (13): the older the animal, the less the tissue survives, or the greater cell death. It is also important to remember that the health of the pups from which the cultures are made can greatly influence the survival of the cultured material; poor cultures are obtained when rat pups appeared to be in less than optimal health. With this in mind, animals received from an outside facility should be allowed to recover for 2–3 days to regain a nutritionally healthy condition.

Generating Brain Slice Explant Cultures from Postnatal Animals

Dissection and Slice Preparation (Fig. 5)

To gain access to the brain, neonatal rats are quickly decapitated using large scissors, under aseptic conditions, in a tissue enclosure hood (Labconco). Small scissors are placed in the spinal opening and a cut is made toward the ear, keeping the scissors pulled outward so as not to damage the tissue with too deep a cut. A second cut is made toward the eyes and a third cut is then made directly across the skull. At this point the scissors are removed and replaced in the spinal opening and a single cut is made in the skull, on the opposite side of the first cut, toward the ear. The scissors are removed and the flap of the skull is lifted up, exposing the dorsal aspect of the brain. The brain is gently lifted upward, the optic nerves are carefully cut, and the brain stem is freed from the surrounding skull. The brain is removed from the skull and placed in a petri dish containing Geys balanced salt solution (GBS, Gibco) enriched with glucose (5 mg/ml). The tissue to be cultured must be kept moist (GBS + glucose) at all times.

---

left. The photomicrograph is a composite of two consecutive 100-μm vibratome sections (midline) which were immunocytochemically stained either for neurophysin [NP, the caudal aspect (right of slice 3)] or LHRH (the rostral aspect). This procedure enabled specific anatomical boundaries to be delineated. The areas contained within the 400-μm culture sections at plating are indicated below the photomicrograph (dots indicate areas containing LHRH perikarya). AC, anterior commissure; AH, anterior hypothalamus (hypo); ARC, arcuate nucleus; DA, dorsal area of the hypo; DBB, diagonal band of Broca; DM, dorsomedial nucleus of the hypo; f, fornix; lh, lateral hypo; lpo, lateral preoptic area; ME, median eminence; MPO, medial preoptic area; SCN, suprachiasmatic nucleus; VM, ventromedial nucleus of the hypo; asterisk, NP staining in the paraventricular nucleus of the hypo; arrowheads, LHRH staining.

Using forceps, the pia, meninges, and blood vessels are quickly *but gently* removed from those areas surrounding the tissue of interest, e.g., the ventral surface of the preoptic area/hypothalamus. Neuronal tissue blocks, as small as possible, containing the area of interest, are quickly cut using homemade razor scapels made from breakable blades. It is important that these cuts are sharp and clean. The blade should pass through the tissue in a single stroke. Leaving this blade in place, a second razor scapel is passed across the back side of the first blade. This technique ensures clean cuts between the tissue block and discarded brain tissue. Twenty microliters of chicken plasma (Cocalico, Reamstown, PA) is placed on the aclar disk on the tissue chopper and the tissue block is gently transferred to this drop using a spatula. [Note: Prior to dissecting brain tissue from each animal, an aclar disk is placed on the cutting disk of the tissue chopper (McIlwain tissue slicer, Brinkmann). However, the chicken plasma is added just before the tissue block is transferred from the petri dish to the tissue chopper]. Thrombin (20 μl, Sigma) is then added to the tissue/plasma drop and allowed to coagulate (a few seconds). The tissue is sectioned at 400 μm. (No apparent benefits are seen when thinner or thicker sections are used and often the end result is less advantageous.) After the tissue block has been sliced, the aclar disk with tissue is removed from the tissue chopper, excess plasma/thrombin clot cleaned away from the tissue, and the sliced tissue block gently pushed off the aclar (take care to keep the block intact, so as not to lose the order of the slices) into a drop of GBS + glucose in a clean petri dish. Using a spatula and forcep, the individual slices containing the specific area(s) to be investigated are separated, placed in fresh GBS + glucose in a new petri dish, and refrigerated. The entire process from decapitation to refrigeration for each brain should take about 5–10 min.

Pituitary

Access to the pituitary is relatively easy, once the brain has been removed. Using fine forceps the membrane surrounding the pituitary is gently removed and the pituitary is lifted from the sella turcica with a spatula and placed in GBS + glucose. When working with a small piece of tissue, such as the pituitary, it can be manually dissected rather than sliced on the tissue chopper.

Plating and Incubation of the Tissue Slices

After all the tissue sections have been collected, the dissection area is cleaned with alcohol. Precleaned coverslips (Gold seal, 12 × 24 mm, cleaning procedure described above) are arranged in a sterile petri dish and 20 μl of chicken plasma (Cocalico, Reamstown, PA) is spread over the coverslip surface.

(The plasma/thrombin used for plating is made fresh on the day of culturing. The plasma/thrombin clot used to adhere the tissue block while cutting may be frozen from the fresh material used on previous culture days.) Tissue slices are transferred to the plasma-coated coverslips using a spatula and thrombin (0.4 NIH U/20 μl GBS + glucose, Sigma) is added to the coverslip. Coagulation should start immediately, adhering the explant to the coverslip. At this point, the petri dishes are covered and placed in a sterile hood for ~20 min. The coverslips are then placed in 15-ml plastic tubes (Falcon) containing 1.0 ml of media (media recipe below), tightly capped, and placed in a test tube rack where they are left upright for ~1 hr. (The tissue slices should not change position on the coverslip; if movement occurs, then the plasma/thrombin clot is not working.) After 1 hr, the test tubes are inserted in a roller drum (Bellco) and rotated at approximately 10 revolutions/hr at 37°C.

Coculture Preparation

Two types of cocultures can be used. The first type involves placing tissues on the same surface of a single coverslip; the second places tissues on separate coverslips, back-to-back, in the same tube. The latter procedure does not allow direct contact between the different tissues to occur, but allows for humoral interactions. For both coculturing paradigms, the procedure used is similar to that described above for single cultures.

Materials Used for Plating Cultures

Glass coverslips have most often been used as substrate surfaces for slice explant cultures. The only requirement for these coverslips is that they fit snuggly into the roller tubes. Nonglass and porous coverslips are potentially attractive alternatives to glass coverslips because they allow penetration of oxygen and nutrients from both surfaces and enable the cultures to attach directly to the growth surface. Such products are available and many of these are compatible with histochemical procedures (15, 37; Millicell from Millipore and Anocell from Anotek, Fig. 6). Although many of these products may provide a good alternative to the glass coverslips routinely used, tissue types can exhibit ''surface preference'' and many of these membranes may be incompatible with the desired end assay such as electrophysiological recordings. The exact mechanism behind surface preference is unclear and presently one must determine for each tissue which support surface is appropriate.

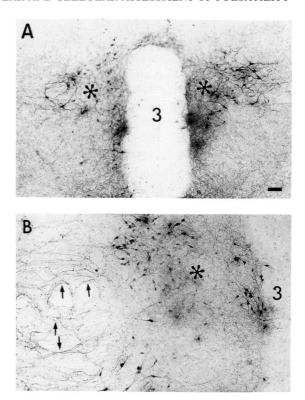

FIG. 6 Example of a slice explant culture grown on nonglass coverslip (Anocell). These cultures were derived from Postnatal Day 5 rat pups and cultured for 13 days. Both explants are from the hypothalamus at the level of the paraventricular nucleus (PVN) and were immunocytochemically stained for oxytocin (OT), a neuroendocrine neuron known to be located in this area *in vivo*. These cultures thinned to different extents. The culture in (A) remained relatively thick. However, due to the porous nature of the coverslip, numerous cells survived. Postfixation immunocytochemical analysis revealed bilateral PVNs (asterisk), containing numerous OT-positive cells. In contrast, (B) shows a culture grown on the same type of coverslip as that in A, but which thinned dramatically. The extent to which the culture spread is emphasized by the fact that only one side of the culture is seen in this panel, i.e., two PVNs are seen in A while only one PVN (asterisk) is seen in B. 3, third ventricle. Numerous oxytocin cells and fibers (small arrows) are visible in both cultures. Scale bar = 100 μm in A and B.

Substances Used as Culture Substratum

The substance used to adhere the tissue slice to the support surface must (i) be strong enough to maintain the culture relatively stable through continual rolling, (ii) permit thinning, and (iii) allow survival of neural tissue and potentially promote fiber outgrowth. Of all the adherents tried by our lab, cultures grown in the presence of chicken plasma/thrombin clots thin most readily while maintaining an organotypic nature.

Plasma/Thrombin Clot

While many commercial sources of chicken plasma are available, most have been unsuitable; one problem is the anticoagulant used. Heparin appears to be the most compatible anticoagulant for tissue survival, but the concentration used during plasma preparation is critical (see Ref. 38 for review of plasma preparation). We have established a commercial source, Cocalico (Reamstown, PA), to produce a plasma that is well suited to our roller-tube explant-culturing needs. Cocalico chicken plasma is received frozen, lyophilized, and stored at −20°C. On the day of culturing, the plasma is reconstituted with distilled water. Both plasma and thrombin are centrifuged at 6000 rpm for ~20 min before use.

The plasma obtained from Cocalico maintains healthy cultures for at least 2 weeks. Longer growth periods may result in some thickening and reorganization of the tissue, but this effect is tissue dependent. We have found that this plasma maintains a variety of tissue types, including hypothalamus, preoptic areas and pituitary from postnatal rats, as well as brain and nasal areas from embryonic mice (15).

The source of thrombin is less of a problem due to standardization; 0.4–0.5 units of thrombin is applied in a volume equal to that of plasma. In our laboratory, thrombin (Sigma, 100 units) is reconstituted with 5 ml of GBS + glucose and centrifuged (see above), and 20–25 μl is applied to an equal volume of plasma.

Other Adherents

Slice explant cultures have been successfully maintained on polyornithine, polylysine, or collagen-coated coverslips (see Ref. 15 for preparation; unpublished data). Slice explants cultured on polyornithine- or polylysine-coated coverslips rarely thin substantially. However, slice explants maintained on collagen-coated coverslips thin depending on the tissue type and concentration of collagen used (unpublished data). Collagen is available from many commercial sources or can be made by the investigator (38–40). We have had some success using commercially obtained collagen (Sigma, rat tail type

I; between 2–6 mg/ml). The collagen is diluted in 0.01–0.05 M acetic acid, placed on the coverslips, and allowed to dry.

After plating, treatment of the tissue slices depends on the adherent used. If the adherent bonds the tissue to the coverslip quickly, e.g., plasma/thrombin clot, the slides are placed in test tubes and rotated within 1 hr. If the adherent takes time to bond the tissue to the coverslip, as with polyornithine and/or collagen, the coverslips are set in sterile humid petri dishes, 40–50 μl of media is added on top of the tissue, and the dishes are placed flat in humid incubators. The cultures are maintained in this manner until the tissue has adhered (~24 hr) and then inserted in test tubes and rotated as indicated above.

Media

We have found that the presence of horse serum is important for thinning of slice explant cultures. We have not had preoptic area/hypothalamic cultures thin consistently, to the extent required for single-cell analysis, if grown from onset in non-serum-containing media. If extensive thinning is not required, then serum-free media (see below) can be used throughout culturing. Alteratively, after thinning, cultures can be transferred into defined media, allowing one to work in a controlled environment.

Serum-Containing Medium

The medium outlined below is used by many investigators (10, 15, 19, 41) and supports a variety of tissues including preoptic area/hypothalamus, brain stem, pituitary, and gonadal.

The serum-containing medium used consists of 25% inactivated horse serum (heat at 56°C for 30 min in a water bath), 50% Eagle's basal medium, and 25% Earles' balanced salt solution. The medium is supplemented with 5.0 mg/ml glucose, 2 mM glutamine, and 25 μg/ml penicillin, 25 μg/ml streptomycin, and 50 μg/ml neomycin (PSN antibiotic mixture).

Although contamination of short-term cultures is not a problem, the PSN antibiotic mixture ensures long-term culture survival. Since we have not seen any deleterious effects of this antibiotic mixture on the cultures, the PSN antibiotic mixture is routinely used for all our cultures. In our laboratory, cultures have been successfully grown for as long as 53 days. Most experiments in our laboratory, however, are performed on explants cultured for 17–21 days. Serum-containing medium is changed one to two times a week depending on the type and amount of tissue being cultured.

Defined Media (Serum-Free)

Cellular properties of neurons should preferentially be studied in cultures maintained in defined media, thereby eliminating unknown factors present in serum. However, we have found that for optimal thinning to occur, cultures are best grown first in the presence of serum and then changed into a serum-free medium. Our cultures survive well in serum-free media for at least 6 days (Fig. 7). The present feeding schedule used in our laboratory is that, for the first 11–12 days, the cultures are grown in serum-containing media (see above), followed by defined (serum-free) media for a maximum of 6 days (22). If changing to defined media, we recommend at least two changes, separated by 1–2 days, be done, in order to assure removal of the original serum. Thus, all experimental manipulations are done only after two changes in defined media.

Our defined medium recipe is based on previous formulations (40). It is composed of 50% Eagle's basal media (Gibco); 50% Ham's F-12 nutrient mixture (Gibco); 10 mg/ml bovine serum albumin (Sigma); $1 \times 10^{-4} M$ putrescine (Sigma); 5 μg/ml insulin (Sigma); 100 μg/ml transferrin (Sigma); 2 mM glutamine (Gibco); 5 μl/ml PSN antibiotic mixture (Gibco); $3 \times 10^{-8} M$ selenium (Sigma); 5.0 mg/ml glucose (Sigma); and 38 μM ascorbic acid. Defined medium is changed at least every 2–3 days.

Antimitotics

For slice explant cultures derived from postnatal animals, antimitotics can be used to reduce the number of nonneuronal cells. However, we have not found overgrowth to occur in these cultures and thus do not routinely use antimitotics. When slice explant cultures are derived from embryonic tissue, antimitotics are often necessary because of the large number of proliferating cells. If antimitotics are required, we have used fluorodeoxyuridine ($8 \times 10^{-5} M$, Sigma). The antimitotic is added a few days after the cultures are plated; the length of exposure is dependent on the tissue being cultured.

Culture Maintenance

The cultures should be fed in a sterile environment, i.e., in a laminar flow hood. The media should be allowed to warm to room temperature. Test tubes are gently removed from the roller drum and placed in a test tube rack. To change the media, simply remove test tube cap, turn test tube upside down, and pour old media into a beaker. Add 1 ml fresh media, recap test tube tightly, and replace in roller drum.

Slice Explant Cultures: A Model System for Examination of Neuroendocrine-Expressing Cells

This section describes several examples of organotypic slice explant cultures of neuroendocrine cells. For exact experimental details, it is recommended

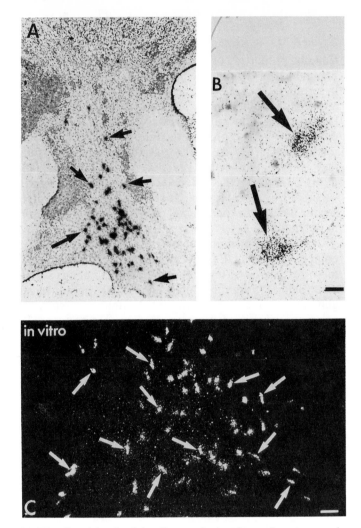

FIG. 7 LHRH cells maintained in slice explant cultures in serum and serum-free media. (A) Low-magnification, brightfield photomicrograph of a slice 3 culture which was maintained in serum-containing media for 18 days. Following fixation, this culture was labeled for cells containing LHRH mRNA using *in situ* hybridization histochemistry. Note that the pattern of labeled cells is similar to that seen *in vivo* (see Fig. 2). (B) High magnification of cell expressing LHRH mRNA. As reported by several groups, isotopic labeling is seen in the cell soma and initial process. Unlike cut sections, the entire cell body is present in these cultures. Thus, the isotopic signal often appears to fill the cell soma with some labeling appearing over the area of the nucleus. Scale bar = 10 μm. (C) Culture section as in A, but this section was maintained for the last 6 (of 18) days in defined media. Scale bar = 100 μm. Arrows point to a few of the cells expressing LHRH mRNA.

that the reader refer to the original papers. It should be emphasized that, as this field progresses, various combinations of techniques will yield a greater amount of information from any one culture. Briefly described in the Appendix are protocols for immunocytochemistry and *in situ* hybridization histochemistry on slice explant cultures.

Neuroendocrine cells are extremely diverse, and even cells expressing the same neuropeptide gene and gene products can be composed of functionally distinct subpopulations based on the heterogeneity of (i) projections, (ii) afferents, (iii) coexistence with other neurotransmitter and/or neuropeptide products, (iv) receptors, and (v) access to humoral environment. This enormous complexity has made examination of molecular and functional properties of neuroendocrine cells *in vivo* extremely difficult. Our laboratory has chosen to examine the regulation of these cell types in slice explant roller-tube cultures.

Determination of the Electrophysiological Properties of Postnatal, Differentiated Neuroendocrine Cells

It is often possible in slice explant cultures to identify a cell type by its morphologic features, e.g., cell shape, size, and/or location in neuronal region (magnocellular neuroendocrine cells in the supraoptic nucleus; 26). In addition, detailed morphologic aspects of individual living cells have been obtained using injections of various dyes, such as Lucifer Yellow (28), once the culture has thinned. Often these dyes can be used to identify neuronal pathways (cocultures) as well as cellular morphology. We have used DiI (42) and fluorescent latex microspheres (43) to retrogradely label cells already in culture (unpublished results). Once a cell type has been idenitifed as indicated above, cellular activity (both ionic and receptor mediated) can be monitored using various electrophysiologic techniques, including extracellular (14, 16, 27, 30), intracellular (14, 28), and patch-clamp recordings (22, 31, 41). Neuronal activity has been characterized in a number of different hypothalamic cell types maintained in slice explant cultures (14, 29, 32, 44 also Refs. above). However, without appropriate markers, one is often recording from nonneuroendocrine cells located in regions containing the neuroendocrine cells of interest.

An alternative approach which our laboratory is currently pursuing is to label neuroendocrine cells prior to culturing. We have developed a strategy (see Fig. 8) which allows for the identification of neuroendocrine cells *in vivo* by retrograde transport of fast blue (31). This fluorescent marker is maintained in the neuroendocrine cell soma *in vitro*, and allows for "identification" of the living neurons which can then be patch-clamped for electro-

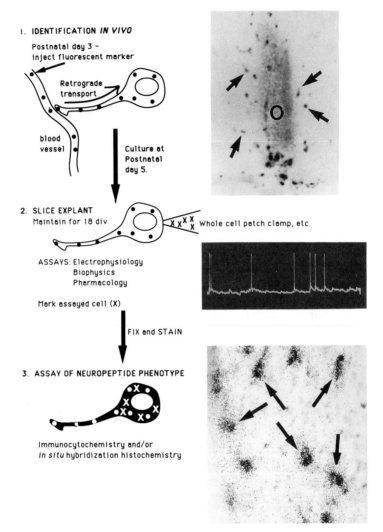

FIG. 8   Strategy for the analysis of intrinsic properties in identified neuroendocrine cells in slice explant cultures. Neuroendocrine cells are marked *in vivo* (1) by an intraperitoneal injection of Fast Blue (0.07 cc, 5 mg/ml into 2- to 3-day-old rat pups). Two days later slice explant cultures are made and slices quickly examined under fluorescence microscopy [upper right panel shows fluorescent cells (arrows) around the OVLT (O)]. After 18 days *in vitro*, fluorescent cells in the thinned slice cultures are patch-clamped (2) and studied. Middle right panel shows spontaneous action potentials recorded from an hypothalamic neuron (31). After recording, the cell is

physiological recording, remarked, and retrospectively phenotypically identified. To date, we have been able to label neuroendocrine hypothalamic cells using intraperitoneal injections of Fast Blue into 2- to 3-day-old pups (31). In these experiments Fast Blue is taken up by nerve terminals which project to circumventricular organs (outside the blood–brain barrier, e.g., neuroendocrine cells). Tissues from these animals are cultured 2–3 days later (as described above). On plating, the slices are viewed under a fluorescent microscope and numerous labeled cells can be detected. Using extremely sterile techniques, these cells can be monitored during culturing (31). Labeling cells, prior to culturing, with nontoxic markers not only gives information on morphology and circuitry, but also enhances the probability of recording directly from the cells of interest. Thus, this strategy should facilitate analysis of putative intrinsic pulse generator properties of known neuroendocrine cell types.

Determination of Neuroendocrine Phenotype, Transsynaptic Relations, Regulation of Gene Expression, and Neurosecretion

Oxytocin Neurons in Slice Explant Cultures (Figs. 9 and 10)

Neuroendocrine-expressing cells can be located in relatively discrete nuclei but intermingled with numerous other cell types. The OT neurons in the paraventricular nucleus are an example of such a neuroendocrine population (24). We have reported (15, 19, 24) that hypothalamic OT neurons (i) can be maintained organotypically for 13–21 days in slice explant cultures (Fig. 9) and (ii) respond to depolarization by a twofold increase in OT mRNA levels (Fig. 10; 24). In contrast to dispersed neuroendocrine systems, such as the LHRH system (see below), the OT system can be quantitatively analyzed by both single-cell (Fig. 9) or X-ray film image analysis to monitor changes in mRNA levels (Fig. 10; 24). Currently, we are investigating the effects of second messengers on OT gene expression and neurosecretion.

---

marked using a dye, such as Lucifer Yellow, which can be placed in the electrode prior to recording and does not interfere with patch-clamp measurements. Following marking, the neuroendocrine cell is evaluated (3) by immunocytochemistry or *in situ* hybridization histochemistry (lower right panel shows cells expressing LHRH mRNA) and thus intrinsic electrophysiologic properties of *identified* neuroendocrine cell types can be evaluated in a controllable environment.

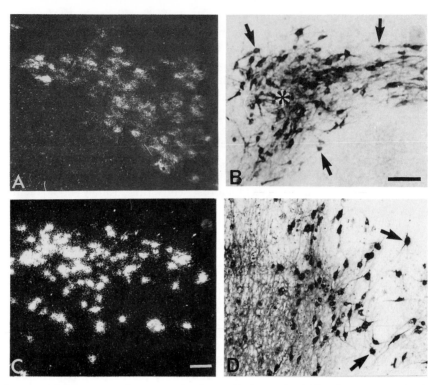

FIG. 9   Maintenance of neuroendocrine cells located within discrete nuclei: OT neurons. The paraventricular nucleus (PVN) is a discrete nucleus, containing numerous neuroendocrine cells, including oxytocin (OT) neurons *in vivo* (B). After 18 days in slice explant cultures (A, C, and D), although the surface area of the nucleus increases and is slightly distorted in shape, the OT cells are found in regions, similar to that seen *in vivo*. (B) A 100-μm vibratome section, at the level of the PVN (asterisk), from a 4-day-old rat immunocytochemically stained for NP. Right half of bilateral PVN is shown. (A, C and D) Culture sections derived from 4-day-old animals, from the same anatomic level as that shown in B, maintained for 18 days *in vitro*. (A and C) Darkfield photomicrographs of left halves of PVNs in slice explant cultures which were evaluated for the presence of cells expressing OT mRNA using *in situ* hybridization histochemistry. Note: Isotopic signal appears as white grains. (D) Right half of a PVN in slice explant culture immunocytochemically stained for OT. Large numbers of OT-positive cells remained grouped proximal to the lateral border of the 3rd ventricle (midline) comparable to their position *in vivo*. Scale bar = 100 μm for panels A and C. Scale bar = 100 μm for panels B and D.

A. CONTROL   B. K⁺ STIMULATION

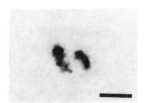 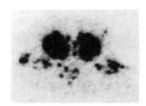

FIG. 10 OT mRNA in slice cultures of rat PVN after potassium depolarization. The images shown are X-ray film autoradiographs of slice explant cultures, at the level of the PVN, which were hybridized with an antisense ^{35}S-labeled synthetic deoxynucleotide for OT mRNA (24). Note the bilateral film image reminiscent of the PVN *in vivo* and the dramatic increase in the level of OT mRNA expression after 4 hr of 40 mM K⁺ depolarization (24). Scale bar = 50 μm in both panels.

The Luteinizing Hormone-Releasing Hormone System in Slice Cultures (Figs. 2, 7, and 11)

In rats, the LHRH system is composed of ~1300 cells, which are distributed in a continuum throughout the forebrain (45). The anatomy of this system makes studying the entire LHRH population *in vivo* extremely difficult. We have reported (19, 21) that 20–30% of LHRH neurons survive, exhibit robust fiber growth, express their appropriate gene and gene products, and maintain an organotypic distribution for long periods of time *in vitro* in slice explant cultures (Figs. 2 and 7). Importantly, the majority of LHRH neurons is contained in three slices, making regulatory studies on this system *in vitro* much more feasible than that *in vivo* (Fig. 2). In determining intrinsic neuroendocrine properties versus extrinsic (transsynaptic) influences we have used tetrodotoxin (TTX), which inhibits sodium channels, axon conductance, and synaptic interactions, to study the effects of various pharmacological agents on LHRH gene expression in slice explant cultures (Fig. 11; 22). Using this paradigm, LHRH neurons maintained in slice explant cultures responded to estradiol, a stimulus known to affect the system *in vivo* (2–6). *In situ* hybridization histochemistry and single-cell analysis procedures, to monitor mRNA level changes in individual cells, revealed that a specific population of LHRH cells responded to estradiol (46). Thus, in slice explant cultures, LHRH cells are maintained in a dispersed, yet anatomically correct, distribution pattern and respond appropriately to a humoral agent. For the LHRH system and other neuroendocrine systems which are anatomically dispersed, slice explant cultures offer a unique opportunity to examine large numbers of cells from distinct anatomic regions, under controllable environmental conditions.

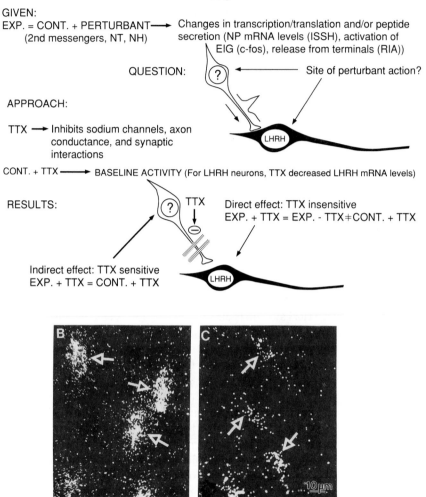

A

TTX Paradigm

GIVEN:
EXP. = CONT. + PERTURBANT ⟶ Changes in transcription/translation and/or peptide
(2nd messengers, NT, NH)   secretion (NP mRNA levels (ISSH), activation of
                               EIG (c-fos), release from terminals (RIA))

QUESTION: ? ⟵ Site of perturbant action?

APPROACH:

TTX ⟶ Inhibits sodium channels, axon
        conductance, and synaptic
        interactions

CONT. + TTX ⟶ BASELINE ACTIVITY (For LHRH neurons, TTX decreased LHRH mRNA levels)

RESULTS: TTX   Direct effect: TTX insensitive
          ?   ↓   EXP. + TTX = EXP. - TTX ≠ CONT. + TTX

Indirect effect: TTX sensitive
EXP. + TTX = CONT. + TTX

FIG. 11 Strategy for the analysis of the regulation of neuropeptide gene expression
in identified neuroendocrine cells in slice explant cultures. To determine if a perturbant
acts directly on the neuroendocrine cell of interest, we are conducting our experiments
in defined media in the presence and absence of tetrodotoxin (TTX). If an effect is
seen in the absence and presence of TTX, then it is likely that the action of the agent
was directly on the cell of interest. If, however, the effect is blocked by the presence
of TTX, then the action of the agent was probably via an interneuron. This strategy
is outlined in the upper part of this figure (A). (B and C) The level of LHRH mRNA
in cells maintained in cultures grown in serum-free media (B) or serum-free media
plus 2 days of TTX (C). Note: 2 days of exposure to 10^{-6} M TTX reduced LHRH
mRNA levels (see Ref. 22 for details). NT, neurotransmitters; NH, neurohormones;
NP, neuropeptide; EIG, early intermediate genes.

As mentioned earlier, cocultures using the slice explant roller-tube method offer a unique opportunity to compare direct interactions between tissue types and humoral interactions (16, 17, 19). Such questions can be addressed by simply plating the tissue onto two rather than one coverslip. Slice explant cocultures of preoptic area/hypothalamus-containing LHRH neurons and pituitary or brain stem have been useful in studying LHRH fiber ingrowth and axonal target selection (14, 19) as well as synaptic formation and induction of morphologic changes, e.g., LHRH dendritic spine formation (19).

To determine whether the LHRH cells in our cultures are functional (certainly the presence of gene and gene products is helpful, but not conclusive), we wanted to show secretion of LHRH. Most explant studies on neuronal secretion involve the use of acute or short-term cultures (18, 47). However, the few secretion studies performed using long-term roller-tube cultures indicate the usefulness of this technique in studying (i) neuropeptide release (bursts, pulsatile, etc.) and (ii) localization of synthesis site (14–17, 19). These studies involved measurement of secreted product in the media using standard radioimmunoassay methods or bioassays. In our laboratory we used the latter approach to demonstrate LHRH secretion from slice explant cultures (Fig. 12). Since LHRH cells normally influence gonadotropes, we cocultured forebrain-containing LHRH cells with pituitary pieces. These cocultures include both tissues on the same coverslip as well as each tissue on a separate coverslip, back-to-back, in the same test tube. We found that in either case, gonadotropes were detectable in the pituitary tissue. However, when an LHRH antagonist was added to the media, the number of gonadotropes dramatically decreased. These results strongly suggest that LHRH cells are, in fact, secreting processed peptide in a physiological manner (19).

Summary

The important aspects to consider when thinking about the uses of slice explant roller-tube cultures are (i) the ability to use either embryonic or differentiated, postnatal tissue containing neuroendocrine cells, (ii) the retention of structural and connective organization, (iii) the ability to visualize and monitor individual cells, (iv) the capability of measuring neurosecretion, and (v) the ability to control the experimental environment. These five features make slice explant cultures appropriate for examination of the intrinsic properties of neuroendocrine cell function, as well as the extrinsic factors (transsynaptic and humoral) which influence these properties. Thus, this model system, due to its organotypic nature, may identify the developmental

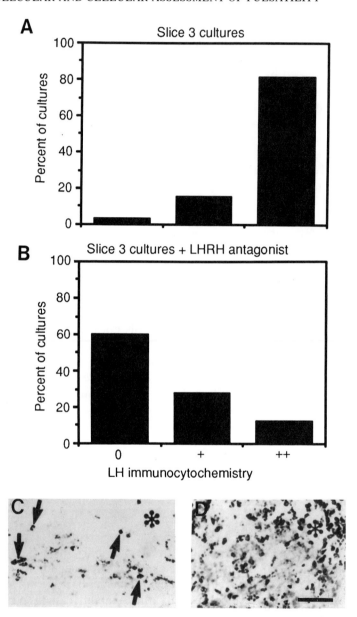

FIG. 12   Cocultures as a bioassay: Evidence for LHRH secretion *in vitro*. Effect of preoptic/hypothalamic tissues on luteinizing hormone (LH) cell staining in cocultured anterior pituitary tissue. (A) Hypothalamus-anterior pituitary coculture (*n* = 32). (B) Coculture in the presence of an LHRH antagonist in the culture media (*n* = 25).

and homeostatic mechanisms which regulate gene expression, neuronal circuitry, and pulsatile secretion in neuroendocrine cells.

Appendix

Protocol for Immunocytochemistry on Slice Explant Cultures

For immunocytochemical assays, we made only a few changes from the protocol used in our laboratory to process tissue sections (19). In general, we found that slice cultures tend to have a slightly higher background than tissue sections. Thus, the signal-to-noise ratio must be critically evaluated for each antibody used.

Cultures are fixed (4% paraformaldehyde–0.2% picric acid for 1–2 hr), rinsed in phosphate-buffered saline (PBS) (2 × 10 min) to remove excess fixative, and blocked in 10% normal goat serum with detergent (0.2% Triton X-100) for 1 hr. Cultures are rinsed in 10% normal goat serum (2 × 30 min) and then incubated in primary antiserum overnight at 4°C. The next day, the cultures are processed using standard immunocytochemical methods. We have obtained sensitive staining using the avidin–biotin–horseradish peroxidase complex (Vector Laboratories, CA; see Figs. 1–3). Double-label immunocytochemistry (19), as well as fluorescent procedures, are also compatible with slice explant roller-tube cultures.

X-axis, the pituitary LH-staining pattern was classified as follows: 0 = no LH-positive cells; + = <30 cells, lightly stained (example shown in C); ++ = >30 cells, heavily stained (example shown in D). Scale bar = 100 μm in C and D. Y-axis, percentage of anterior pituitary cocultures found in 0, +, ++ category. Eighty percent of the pituitary tissues were heavily stained when cocultured with preoptic/hypothalamic tissue containing LHRH cells. The hypothalamus did not have to be in contact with the anterior pituitary (back-to-back coverslips in the same test tube) for LH cells to be detected. LH cell detectability in these cocultures was abolished by the addition of a highly specific LHRH antagonist to the culture media (B, see Ref. 19 for details). This study suggests that LHRH was secreted into the media in a physiologically relevant manner, capable of effecting gonadotropes. This indicates that an aspect of the *in vivo* relationship, between releasing hormone- and hormone-producing cells was maintained in these slice explant cocultures.

Protocol for in Situ Hybridization Histochemistry on Slice Explant Cultures

We have found that a good signal is achieved using synthetic deoxynucleotide probes, approximately 50 nucleotides in length, or ribonucleotide probes on slice-cultured material (Figs. 8–11). Explant cultures are processed for *in situ* hybridization histochemistry by a modified procedure previously used on tissue sections (21). Briefly, cultures are fixed with 4% formaldehyde (15–20 min), rinsed in PBS (2 × 5 min), placed in 0.25% acetic acid/0.1 M triethanolamine hydrochloride–0.9% NaCl (10 min), rinsed in 2 × SSC (2 × 1.5 min), dehydrated [70, 80, 95, and 100% ethanol (2 min/wash)], delipidated in chloroform (7 min), rehydrated (1 min each in 100, 95, 80, and 70% ethanol), rinsed in 2 × SSC, and hybridized.

Synthetic 48- to 50-base deoxynucleotide probes (5 pmol) are 3′ end labeled with [^{35}S]dATP to a specific activity of 7,000–15,000 Ci/mmol. Labeled probe is applied to individual cultures in 25 μl (500,000 cpm) of hybridization buffer. The cultures are hybridized overnight at 37°C in humid chambers. The following day, cultures are rinsed in 2× SSC, washed in 2× SSC/50% formamide at 40°C (4 × 15 min), rinsed in 2× SSC at room temperature (2 × 1 hr), and then allowed to air-dry. After drying, the coverslips are dipped in NTB3 (Eastman Kodak) and exposed. The emulsion-covered cultures are developed, counterstained, dried, and then mounted culture-side up onto microscope slides.

Quantification of *in situ* hybridization histocytochemistry can be done when a radioisotope-labeled probe is used. Integrated densities of areas of silver grains over individual labeled cells and the cell areas enclosing these grains are measured using an image analysis system (21). This density/cell value reflects the level of mRNA/cell. Hence, the direction of change in mRNA levels and the statistical significance of these changes can be determined (21, 22).

Acknowledgments

I thank Sharon Key for her expert technical assistance and Drs. H. Gainer and K. Kusano for their collaborative efforts in this research program.

References

1. D. Lincoln, *in* "Pulsatility in Neuroendocrine Systems" (G. Leng, ed.), p. 36. CRC Press, Boca Raton, FL, 1988.
2. D. L. Foster, *in* "The Physiology of Reproduction" (E. Knobil and J. D. Neill, eds.), p. 1739. Raven Press, New York, 1988.

3. J. B. Wakerley, G. Clarke, and A. J. S. Summerlee, *in* "The Physiology of Reproduction" (E. Knobil and J. D Neill, eds.), p. 2283. Raven Press, New York, 1988.

4. E. Knobil and J. Hotchkiss, *in* "The Physiology of Reproduction" (E. Knobil and J. D. Neill, eds.), p. 1971. Raven Press, New York, 1988.

5. T. M. Plant, *in* "The Physiology of Reproduction" (E. Knobil and J. D. Neill, eds.), p. 1763. Raven Press, New York, 1988.

6. E. Knobil and J. D. Neill "The Physiology of Reproduction," Vol 2. Raven Press, New York, 1988.

7. G. Leng, *in* "Pulsatility in Neuroendocrine Systems" (G. Leng, ed.), p. 3. CRC Press, Boca Raton, FL, 1981.

8. G. Leng "Pulsatility in Neuroendocrine Systems." CRC Press, Boca Raton, FL, 1988.

9. C. D. Toran-Allerand, *Colloq. Int. CNRS* **280,** 759 (1978).

10. B. H. Gähwiler, *J. Neurosci. Methods* **4,** 329 (1981).

11. B. H. Gähwiler, *Experientia* **40,** 235 (1984).

12. F. Baldino, Jr., and H. M. Geller, *in* "Modern Methods in Pharmacology." Vol. 3. "Electrophysiological Techniques in Pharmacology" (H. M. Geller, ed.), p. 103. Alan R. Liss, New York, 1986.

13. B. H. Gähwiler, *Trends Neurosci.* **11,** 484 (1988).

14. B. H. Gähwiler, T. Knopfel, P. Marbach, M. Muller, L. Rietschin, M. Scanziani, C. Staub, I. Vranesic, and S. M. Thompson, *in* "The Brain in Bits and Pieces" (G. Zbinden, ed.), p. 153. Verlag, Switzerland, 1992.

15. S. Wray, *in* "Neuromethods." Vol. 23. "Practical Cell Culture Technique" (A. A. Boulton, G. B. Baker and W. Walz, eds.), p. 201. Humana Press, New Jersey, 1992.

16. A. J. Baertschi, J-L Beny, and B. H. Gähwiler, *Nature (London)* **295,** 145 (1982).

17. B. H. Gähwiler, P. Marbach, and A. J. Baertschi, *in* "Neuronal Communications" (B. J. Meyer and S. Kramer, eds.), p. 145. A. A. Balkema, Rotterdam, 1984.

18. J. E. Stern, T. Mitchell, V. L. Herzberg, and W. G. North, *Neuroendocrinology* **43,** 252 (1986).

19. S. Wray, B. H. Gähwiler, and H. Gainer, *Peptides* **9,** 1151 (1988).

20. M. V. Sofroniew, J. J. Dreifuss, and B. H. Gähwiler, *Brain Res. Bull.* **20,** 669 (1988).

21. S. Wray, R. T. Zoeller, and H. Gainer, *Mol. Endocrinol.* **3,** 1197 (1989).

22. S. Wray, K. Kusano, and H. Gainer, *Neuroendocrinology* **54,** 327 (1991).

23. S. Wray and H. Gainer, *in* "Progress in Brain Research" (J. Joose, R. M. Buijs, and F. J. H. Tilders, eds.), Vol. 92, p. 59. Elsevier Science, Amsterdam/New York, 1992.

24. H. Gainer and S. Wray, *Ann. N.Y. Acad. Sci.* **652,** 14 (1992).

25. L. Bertini, C. Kursner, R. C. Gaillard, R. Corder, and J. Z. Kiss, *Neuroendocrinology* **57,** 716 (1993).

26. B. H. Gähwiler, P. Sandoz, and J. J. Dreifuss, *Brain Res.* **151,** 245 (1978).

27. H. M. Geller and D. J. Woodward, *Exp. Neurol.* **64,** 535 (1979).

28. B. H. Gähwiler, *J. Neurobiol.* **12,** 187 (1981).

29. H. Geller, *in* "Advances in Physiological Sciences" (E. Stark, G. B. Makara,

B. Haluze, and G. Y. Rappay, eds.), Vol. 14, p. 107. Akademiai Kiado, Budapest, 1981.

30. F. Baldino, Jr., and B. Wolfson, *Brain Res.* **325,** 161 (1985).
31. H. Gainer, K. Kusano, and S. Wray, *Regul. Pept.* **45,** 25 (1993).
32. A. van den Pol, J-P. Wuarin, and F. E. Dudek, *Science* **250,** 1276 (1990).
33. F. Baldino, Jr., G. A. Higgins, M. T. Moke, and B. Wolfson, *Peptides* **6,** 249 (1985).
34. B. Wolfson, R. W. Manning, L. G. Davis, and F. Baldino, Jr., *Dev. Brain Res.* **18,** 241 (1985).
35. S. Wray, M. Castel, and H. Gainer, *Microsc. Res. Tech.* **24,** 46 (1993).
36. E. B. Masurovsky, H. H. Benitez, and M. R. Murray, *J. Comp. Neurol.* **143,** 263 (1971).
37. H. J. Romijn, B. M. de Jong, and J. M. Ruijter, *J. Neurosci. Methods* **23,** 75 (1988).
38. J. Paul, "Cell and Tissue Culture." Churchill–Livingstone, New York, 1975.
39. C. D. Toran-Allerand, *in* "Methods in Neuroscience." Vol. 2. "Cell Cultures" (P. M. Conn, ed.) p. 275. Academic Press, New York, 1990.
40. H. R. Maurer, *in* "Animal Cell Culture: A Practical Approach" (R. I. Freshney, ed.), p. 13. IRL Press, Oxford, 1986.
41. I. Llano, A. Marty, J. W. Johnson, P. Ascher, and B. H. Gähwiler, *Proc. Natl. Acad. Sci. U.S.A.* **85,** 3221 (1988).
42. M. G. Honig and R. I. Hume, *J. Cell Biol.* **103,** 171 (1986).
43. L. C. Katz, A. Burkhalter, and W. J. Dreyer, *Nature (London)* **310,** 498 (1984).
44. H. Geller, *Dev. Brain Res.* **1,** 89 (1981).
45. S. Wray, and G. Hoffman, *J. Comp. Neurol.* **252,** 522 (1986).
46. S. Wray, S. Key, and H. Gainer, *Soc. Neurosci.* **17,** 175.6 (1991).
47. M. Morris, R. L. Eskay, and D. K. Sundberg, *in* "Methods in Enzymology" (P. M. Conn, ed.), Vol. 124, p. 359. Academic Press, San Diego, 1986.

Section II

Electrophysiological and Ionic Events in Pulsatility

[3] Electrophysiological Analysis of Neuroendocrine Neuronal Activity in Hypothalamic Slices

Martin J. Kelly and Oline K. Rønnekleiv

Introduction

Ultimately, the pulsatile release of peptide hormones depends on the excitability of hypothalamic neurosecretory neurons. Twenty years ago, the electrical activity of magnocellular vasopressin and oxytocin neurons was correlated with physiological perturbations (1, 2). Based on these observations, there has been a systematic study of magnocellular neurons both *in vivo* and *in vitro* correlating changes in neuronal excitability with altered secretion of vasopressin and oxytocin [see (3–5)]. Although this approach has met with success in the study of the magnocellular neurons of the supraoptic and the paraventricular nuclei, it has not been successful in making the same correlation between electrical activity and peptide release in hypothalamic parvocellular neurons. The problem has been that it is difficult to identify parvocellular neurons because the preoptic area and hypothalamus contain a heterogenous mixture of different phenotypes some of which are neurosecretory and others are not. Therefore, it has been necessary to label the neurons with a dye and then perform immunocytochemistry to identify the phenotype. Intracellular recordings made with electrodes filled with Lucifer Yellow or Procion Yellow have allowed some characterization of vasopressin (6, 7) and luteinizing the hormone-releasing hormone-containing neurons (8, 9). Moreover, we have established the utility of the hypothalamic slice preparation in the study of the electrophysiology associated with pulsatile hormone release (8). However, characterization of conductances has been limited because of the limited current-passing capacity of these dye-filled electrodes. Utilizing the biotinylated compound biocytin in the recording pipette (10), we have been able to record and identify parvocellular neurosecretory neurons and characterize the conductances underlying their spontaneous and synaptically induced activity utilizing voltage-clamp analysis. This chapter describes the techniques that we have developed that have allowed single-electrode voltage-clamp recordings followed by immunocytochemical identification of parvocellular neurosecretory neurons in hypothalamic slices.

Methodology

Preparation and Maintenance of Hypothalamic Slices

Female guinea pigs (Topeka; 350–600 g), born and raised in our colony, are ovariectomized under ketamine (33 mg/kg)/xylazine (6 mg/kg) anesthetic 6–10 days prior to subcutaneous injection with estradiol benzoate (EB; 25 μg in 100 μl oil) or oil and are decapitated 24 hr after the injection. The brain is removed, the hypothalamus is dissected, and coronal slices of 450-μm thickness are cut on a vibratome. Ten slices are cut extending from caudal hypothalamus ($\approx$ slice 10) to the organum vasculosum of the lamina terminalis ($\approx$ slice 1) (Fig. 1). The slices are maintained in a Plexiglas chamber submerged in oxygenated medium (see below) at room temperature until being transferred to an interface recording chamber. In the recording chamber (Fig. 2) the slice is maintained in an oxygenated (95% O_2, 5% CO_2) environment at 35 ± 1°C and is perfused at 200–500 μl/min with a modified Krebs–Ringer buffer (in mM: NaCl, 124; KCl, 5; NaH_2PO_4, 1.25; $MgSO_4$, 2; $CaCl_2$, 2; $NaHCO_3$, 26; dextrose, 10; HEPES ($C_8H_{18}N_2O_4S$), 10; Boehringer-Mannheim, Indianapolis, IN). A 3 × stock solution, which includes NaCl, 372 mM; KCl, 15 mM, NaH_2PO_4, 7.8 mM; HEPES, 30 mM, is made up weekly and stored at 4°C. The day before the experiment 3 liters of stock is diluted 1 : 3 and 10 mM dextrose is added. On the day of the experiment 26 mM $NaHCO_3$ is added to the slice medium, and the mixture is saturated with 95% O_2/5% CO_2 ($\approx$15 min aeration). Finally, 2 mM $MgSO_4$ and 2 mM $CaCl_2$ are added to the solution. The pH (measured at room temperature) is 7.30–7.40 and the osmolarity is 305–308 mOsm. The solution is continually aerated during the experiment. Alternatively, a slice is submerged in the same medium which flows through the chamber at 1.5 ml/min. In order to accommodate the submerged slice, a platform with nylon netting is inserted into the inner Plexiglas chamber approximately 500 μm below the surface (Fig. 2). The submerged slice facilitates pharmacological studies on the cells (see below).

In addition, we have used rats for *in vitro* electrophysiological studies. Young female Sprague–Dawley rats are obtained from Charles River (Wilmington, MA). Rats weighing 140–250 g and exhibiting 4- or 5-day estrous cycles are used on the day of proestrus, or ovariectomized under tribromethanol (2.5% w/v; 1 ml/kg; Aldrich Chemical Co., Milwaukee, WI) anesthesia and 1 week later given a subcutaneous injection of EB (25 μg in 100 μl oil). The procedure for the preparation and maintenance of rat hypothalamic slices is the same as that described above for the guinea pig.

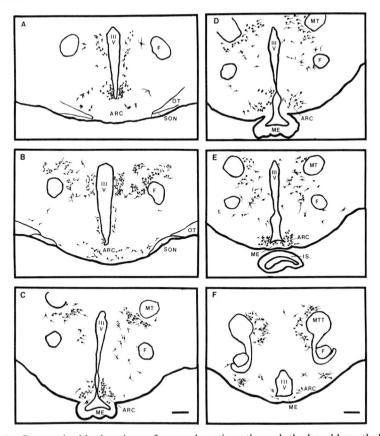

FIG. 1   Camera lucida drawings of coronal sections through the basal hypothalamus of the female guinea pig illustrating the distribution of neurons containing immunoreactive TH. (A–F) Slices 6–10. (A) The level of slice 6 which is the most rostral part of the ARC. At this level the TH neurons are found primarily in the periventricular area. (B) Slice 7, in which scattered TH neurons are found in the ARC. (C and D) Slices 8 and 9, respectively, both of which contain a high concentration of ARC TH neurons. (E and F) The rostral and caudal parts of slice 10, respectively. A relative high concentration of TH neurons are present in the rostral part of slice 10, whereas the caudal part of slice 10 contains a few scattered neurons. The distribution of neurons containing β-endorphin in the guinea pig hypothalamus has been illustrated elsewhere (43a). ARC, arucate nucleus; F, fornix; ME, median eminence; MT, mamillothalamic tract; MTT, mamillothalamotegmental tract; OT, optic tract; SON, supraoptic nucleus; IIIV, third ventricle. Bar = 500 μm.

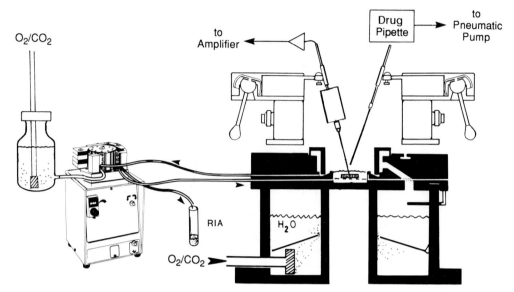

FIG. 2   Schematic of Plexiglas chamber used for recording from hypothalamic slices. A slice is submerged inside of a 1-ml chamber. A balanced salt solution which is preheated and saturated with 95% O_2/5% CO_2 flows at 1.5 ml/min (controlled by Gilson pump) into the chamber containing the slice (incoming arrowheads). The effluent flows from the slice into a "moat" where it is pumped out into a test tube for radioimmunoassay or disposal. The air above the reservoir is kept saturated with O_2/CO_2. Temperatures are controlled by a bridge circuit which maintains the chamber and the water reservoir beneath the slice at 35°C. A Leitz joystick is used to advance the recording electrode, which is attached to the Axoclamp headstage, into the slice, and another micromanipulator is used to position the drug pipette(s) immediately above the slice. Drugs are delivered by controlled pressure ejection. The slice is placed on a nylon screen and secured with an EM grid (3HgC 50; Pella, Redding, CA). There is ~500 μl of fluid above the slice.

Intracellular Recording

Microelectrodes are made from borosilicate glass micropipettes [1 mm outer diameter [OD] and 0.59 inner diameter [ID], A-M Systems, Seattle, WA; or 1.20 O.D., 0.60 I.D., DAGAN, Minneapolis, MN] which are pulled on a Brown-Flaming P-87 Puller (Sutter Instruments, Novato, CA). Tip sizes range from 0.25 to 0.50 μm in diameter (measured via Sutter Instruments' scanning electron microscope) and when filled with a 2% biocytin (Sigma, St. Louis, MO) solution in 1.75 M KCl and 0.025 M Tris(hydroxymethyl)aminomethane (Tris; Gibco BRL, Gaithersburg, MD) have resistances of 80–150

MΩ. The biocytin solution is used in the electrode so that recorded neurons contain biocytin following intracellular recording and subsequently can be identified following reaction with a streptavidin–fluorophore conjugate [see (10, 11)]. An electrode is placed in an electrode holder (HL-2) in the Axoclamp 2A headstage ($H = 0.01\times$; Axon Instruments, Burlingame, CA) which is secured to a Leitz joystick (Rockleigh, NJ; Fig. 2). Penetration of neurons is achieved by mechanically advancing into the tissue at ≈ 2 μm and then applying a short, high-voltage pulse ("+ clear" on the Axoclamp 2A amplifier). "Ringing" into parvocellular neurons via the "buzz" button on the Axoclamp 2A has not been as successful for penetrating small parvocellular neurons. The initial injury discharge is reduced by applying a hyperpolarizing current of up to 100 pA. This current is maintained for as long as 5 min in order to allow the membrane potential to stabilize. The "holding" current is gradually reduced to 0; or the electrode is withdrawn from the cell if the membrane does not stabilize. Sometimes a small current (<50 pA) is continued to maintain the membrane potential below threshold for firing. Intracellular potentials are amplified and current is passed through the electrode using an Axoclamp 2A amplifier (Axon Instruments) in the bridge mode of operation. Current and voltage traces are recorded on a chart recorder (Gould 2200), digitized, recorded to Axo-Tape (Axon Instruments) and periodically stored on an FM tape recorder (Vetter Instruments, Rebersburg, PA).

Electrophysiological analyses are performed on cells that are recorded for at least 20 min and exhibit overshooting action potentials and membrane potentials of -50 mV or more negative, at which time the amplifier may be switched to single-electrode, voltage clamp (SEVC). SEVC recordings are made using a 1- to 3-kHz switching frequency, a 30% duty cycle, and a gain of 0.10 to 0.15 nA/V in accordance with the procedures of Finkel and Redman (12). Current–voltage (I/V) relationships are obtained either by hyperpolarizing the neuron to potentials more negative than -100 mV and then depolarizing at a rate of 1–2 mV/s with the output fed directly to an X–Y plotter ("steady-state" I/V; Recorder Series 200, San Marcos, TX) or by passing a series of depolarizing and hyperpolarizing rectangular step commands of at least 150 msec (step I/V). In current clamp (bridge mode of operation), voltage–current relationships are obtained by applying a series of depolarizing and hyperpolarizing current pulses (150 msec duration) and measuring the voltage at the end of each step. The apparent input resistance of the cell membrane is calculated from the slope of the voltage–current (V/I) plots in the region between -60 and -80 mV. An approximation of the membrane time constant (τ) is obtained by measuring the time required for a small current-induced voltage deflection to reach 63% of its final level. The determination of the τ is done on a Tektronics 2232 Digital Scope (Beaverton, OR), and we have found that there is less than a 10% error utilizing this method versus determining τ from exponential plots (13). Numerical data are expressed as means $\pm$ SEM. Comparisons between groups are evaluated using the χ^2 statistic and the level required for significance is set at $p < 0.05$ (14).

Pharmacology

Cells must exhibit a stable membrane potential for 30–40 min, during which membrane properties are examined, before any pharmacological studies are performed. Drug testing is done in both current clamp and SEVC. Tetrodotoxin (TTX 1–2 μM; Sigma, St. Louis, MO), a sodium-channel blocker, is superfused for 10 min before the beginning of drug testing. Likewise, potassium-channel blockers (15) are added to the salt solution superfusing the slices: tetraethylammonium chloride (TEA, 10 mM; Sigma) for blocking I_K and $I_{K,Ca}$; CsCl (1–2 mM; Sigma) for blocking I_h; and 4-aminopyridine (4AP, 2 mM, Sigma) for blocking I_A. Medium with a high concentration of Mg^{2+} (10 mM) and a low Ca^{2+} concentration (0.1 mM) is also superfused for blocking synaptic transmission to evaluate direct postsynaptic effects.

Tyr-D-Ala-Gly-MePhe-Gly-ol enkephalin (DAMGO; Peninsula Labs, Belmont, CA), an opioid agonist selective for μ-receptors (16, 17) has been used extensively by our lab for pharmacological studies (18–22). Therefore, we use the characterization of the μ-opioid response as an example of the studies which can be undertaken using the *in vitro* slice preparation. Since DAMGO takes up to 20 min to completely wash out, a cumulative dose–response curve to DAMGO is generated by measuring the membrane hyperpolarization caused by increasing concentrations of DAMGO (20 nM, 50 nM, 100 nM, 300 nM, 600 nM, 1 μM). The membrane hyperpolarization to DAMGO (versus outward current) is used because of the high R_{in} of many of the ARC neurons (>400 MΩ), i.e., small currents are needed to produce large hyperpolarizations. Solutions containing each concentration are applied for 6 min, which is sufficient time for the membrane potential to reach a new steady level ($\approx$4 min). The dose–response relationship is fitted by logistic equation:

$$V = V_{max} * \frac{[DAMGO]^n}{EC_{50}^n + [DAMGO]^n} \tag{1}$$

We have found that Eq. (1) fits the dose–response curves for the majority of the cells and allows the determination of the Hill coefficient (n), the predicted maximal hyperpolarization (V_{max}), and the concentration at which 50% of V_{max} is observed (EC_{50}). (Lagrange and Kelly, unpublished observations; Fig. 6).

After complete washout of 1 μM DAMGO and return to the original membrane potential, which takes about 20 min, a second series of DAMGO concentrations (100 nM to 50 μM) is applied in the presence of the nonselective, opioid antagonist naloxone (30 nM to 1 μM) in order to do a "Schild" analysis. In 1947, Schild introduced the term pA_2 as a measure of the strength of a competitive antagonist (23). Specifically, pA_2 is the negative logarithm of the molar concentration of the antagonist which produces an agonist dose ratio (EC_{50} of agonist in the presence of antagonist divided by the EC_{50} of agonist) of 2. Based on Gaddum's formulation of competitive theory (24), pA_2 is related to the dissociation constant of antagonist–receptor interaction. Therefore, if two agonists act on the same receptors, they can be expected to be antagonized by the same competitive antagonist and to lead to the same value of pA_2 for the antagonist. Moreover, pA_2 values can be compared between groups to determine if the affinity of the μ-opioid receptor for naloxone is different between experimental groups.

A more expedient method for applying drugs is via ejection of a concentrated solution of a drug (e.g., 10–20 μM DAMGO) via increasing pressure from a large-bore ($\approx$50 μm) micropipette positioned above the slice (Fig. 2). Responses to DAMGO are reproducible using an identical number of pressure pulses (2 to 8 psi) of 500 msec (Medical Systems Neurophore, Great Neck, NY). The onset of the response occurs within 2 min of application and the maximum response is observed 1–3 min following response onset. There is a 20- to 40-fold dilution of a drug applied with this "microdrop" technique by the time it reaches the cell membrane (25), but one is unable to determine exact concentrations using this method. We have used this technique most often with the interface slice system.

Pharmacological "occlusion" experiments are performed to ascertain the different receptor subtypes that are coupled to the same physiological response (cascade). We have looked at agonists which activate the inwardly rectifying potassium conductance (a G protein-coupled response). We have studied the effects of the $GABA_B$ agonist baclofen alone and in combination with DAMGO on ARC neurons (21, 22). For these experiments, a concentration of DAMGO is applied which gives a maximum hyperpolarization (>300 nM). The membrane potential is returned to its original resting level by passing depolarizing current ("voltage match"), and then a maximum concentration of baclofen (>40 μM) is applied. The nonadditivity (occlusion) of the baclofen and DAMGO responses indicates that the binding of the ligands to their respective receptors activates the same cascade. This strategy has been used effectively to assess where estrogen is acting in the receptor/G protein/K^+-channel cascade to affect μ-opioid-mediated hyperpolarization (see below) (22).

Histochemistry

Reagents

Paraformaldehyde stock solution (8% w/v): Paraformaldehyde is dissolved in distilled water at 60°C, and the solution is titrated with NaOH to clear it and then filtered through a 0.20-μm membrane filter.

Sörensen's buffer: Make two stock solutions, 67 mM $KH_2PO_4 \cdot H_2O$ and 67 mM Na_2HPO_4 in Milli-Q water; to make a buffer solution of pH 7.2, mix 19.6 ml of 67 mM KH_2PO_4 and 80.4 ml of 67 mM Na_2HPO_4.

Phosphate buffer (0.1 M): Make two stock solutions, 0.2 M $NaH_2PO_4 \cdot H_2O$ and 0.2 M Na_2HPO_4; for 1 liter of pH 7.2, mix 95 ml of 0.2 M $NaH_2PO_4 \cdot H_2O$, 405 ml of 0.2 M Na_2HPO_4, and 500 ml Milli-Q water.

Tris buffer: 8.5 mM Na_2HPO_4, 3.5 mM KH_2PO_4, 120 mM NaCl, 41 mM tris(hydroxmethyl)aminomethane; adjust the pH to 7.6.

Streptavidin diluent: 0.7% λ-carrageenan (Sigma, Type IV), 0.4% Triton X-100 in Tris buffer.

Antibody diluent: 0.7% λ-carrageenan (Type IV), 0.4% Triton X-100, and 3% bovine serum albumin in Tris buffer.

Poly-L-lysine (0.1%) for coating slides: 0.1% poly-L-lysine (MW > 300,000; Sigma) in Milli-Q water; aliquot in 1-ml vials; can be stored at −20°C for 3–4 months.

Streptavidin–Fluorescein Isothiocyanate (FITC) Staining

Following intracellular recordings made with biocytin-filled electrodes, the 450- to 500-μm slices are fixed in 4% paraformaldehyde in 0.03 M Sörensen's phosphate buffer (PB) (pH 7.4; 80% potassium phosphate, 20% sodium phosphate, each mixed at 0.067 M) for 90–180 min and then soaked overnight in PB (0.1 M, pH 7.2) containing 30% sucrose. Each slice is then rapidly frozen and sectioned at 16 μm thickness on a cryostat; the sections are mounted on poly-L-lysine-coated slides and stored frozen at −20°C. All of the slides from a given slice are then washed with buffer, and streptavidin–FITC (1 : 600, Jackson Laboratories) is applied for 2 hr. The reaction is terminated by washing the slides with 0.1 M PB. The slides with the sections are dried at room temperature and then stored in the freezer at −20°C. The slides are scanned for the injected neuron with a Leitz Dialux 20 microscope (Rockleigh, NJ) outfitted with incident-light epifluorescence generated by a 100-W mercury vapor lamp through an I_2 filter cube (excitation filter bandpass 450–490 nm). The wider band H_2 filter (390–490 nM) is also used for scanning the sections but is not as suitable for photography. The FITC staining of the injected cells is photographed through Leitz PlanApo objectives ($\times 25$, $\times 40$ oil, $\times 63$ oil). Tri-X-Pan (ASA 400; Eastman Kodak, Rochester, NY) is used for black/white photography and Scotch Chrome 640T (ASA 640; 3M, St. Paul, MN) is used for color photography. Exposure times range from 50 to 70 sec for the black/white and from 10 to 25 sec for color photography.

Immunocytochemistry for Tyrosine Hydroxylase (TH)

After localization of the biocytin-filled neurons, the slides containing the appropriate sections are processed for the presence of TH using fluorescence immunohistochemistry. We utilize several electrophysiological criteria together with the anatomical location (slices 7, 8, 9 and rostral part of slice 10; Fig. 1) for assigning a cell for TH immunostaining. These include the presence of an I_h, a low-threshold spike (LTS), and the response to DAMGO (26). If we anticipate that a recorded cell contains TH, we incubate the slice in medium containing $1 \mu M$ forskolin for 30 to 60 min. Also, the slice is fixed for a longer period in 4% paraformaldehyde (120–180 min). Forskolin treatment *in vivo* has been shown to increase tyrosine hydroxylase activity (27), and we found *in vitro* treatment will increase TH immunoreactivity. Moreover, the antibody against TH is considered to label only DA-containing cells as there are no noradrenergic or adrenergic neurons in the arcuate nucleus (ARC) (28, 29). The section with the biocytin-identified neuron is washed and incubated 48 hr with an affinity-purified tyrosine hydroxylase antiserum (Pel-Freeze; 1:1000) followed by 30 min PB wash and a 2-hr incubation with a donkey anti-rabbit gamma globulin conjugated to CY3 (Jackson Laboratories; 1:100). CY3 is a very brilliant fluorophore which works well to detect the faint immunostaining of ARC TH neurons (Fig. 3). The sections are washed for 60 min with sodium phosphate buffer under continuous agitation, and coverslips are applied using a glycerol phosphate buffer (2:1 v/v; pH 7.6) containing 5% N-propyl gallate. A cell is considered immunoreactive for TH if the staining of the soma is unequivocally above background fluorescence and follows the outline of the soma as revealed by streptavidin–FITC staining (Fig. 3). The immunostained cells are photographed through a Leitz M_2 filter (539–553 nM) with Tri-X-Pan (10–25 sec exposure) or Scotch Chrome 640T (exposure 3–15 sec) as described above. The FITC staining can be seen using the I_2 or H_2 filter cubes, but the FITC staining is not observed with the M_2 filter (little or no "bleed through"). In contrast, the CY3 or the Texas Red fluorophores will bleed through when observed with the I_2 filter cube. Therefore, we always use FITC to identify the biocytin-injected neuron.

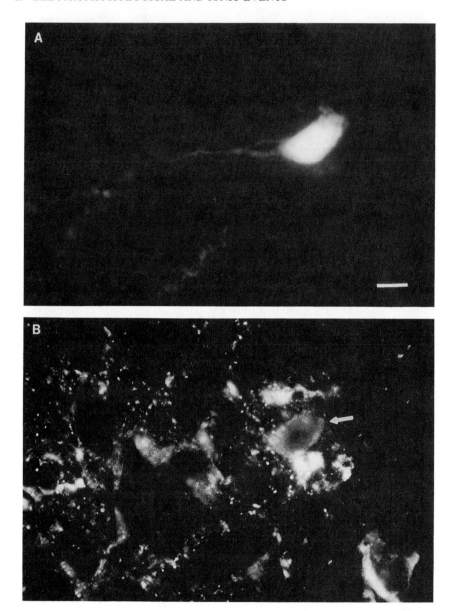

FIG. 3   Double labeling of arcuate (A12) dopamine neurons. (A) Biocytin–streptavidin–FITC labeling of a neuron in the ventromedial ARC in slice 7. Several fibers are visible exiting from the fusiform soma and projecting laterally. (B) TH staining of neuron is evenly distributed throughout the soma (arrow). This cell is intermingled in an area of the ARC nucleus in which there are a cluster of dopamine neurons. Scale bar, 10 μm.

Immunocytochemistry for β-Endorphin

After localization and documentation of the biocytin-filled neuron, the slide containing the appropriate section is processed for immunocytochemical staining of β-endorphin. We utilize several electrophysiological criteria together with the anatomical location (slices 6, 7, 8, 9 or 10; Fig. 1) for assigning a cell for β-endorphin immunostaining. β-Endorphin neurons show an irregular firing pattern and exhibit both an instantaneous ($I_{K,ir}$) and time-dependent inward rectification (I_h) and respond to DAMGO (20). Slices that we anticipate contain β-endorphin neurons are normally fixed for 90–120 min and then are processed as outlined above. The section with the biocytin-identified neuron is washed and incubated 48 hr with an antiserum to α-endorphin (R13) (30), an antiserum to β-endorphin (BE-2) (31), or a combination of both at a 1 : 1000 dilution followed by a 30-min PB wash and 2-hr incubation with donkey anti-rabbit immunoglobulin G conjugated to Texas Red (IGG-Texas Red, Jackson Labs; 1 : 100). The sections are washed five times for 30 min each with phosphate buffer under continuous agitation, then a coverslip is applied with glycerol phosphate buffer (2 : 1; pH 7.6) containing 5% n-propyl gallate. The long washing procedure is needed to reduce background levels of Texas Red in the tissue sections. The specific binding to β-endorphin neurons is very resistent to the washing. A cell is considered immunoreactive for β-endorphin if the staining of the soma is unequivocally above background fluorescence. The various POMC cleavage products are colocalized in hypothalamic neurons (32). Therefore, in order to optimize our chances of identifying endorphin neurons, we often mix two different endorphin antibodies (R13 and BE2) directed against different parts of POMC. The immunostained cells are photographed through a Leitz M_2 filter cube as described above.

Results and Discussion

Streptavidin–FITC Labeling of ARC Neurons

Ninety percent of the neurons that are recorded in the ARC have been identified morphologically following intracellular recording with biocytin-filled electrodes (mean recording time of 97 ± 8 min, $N = 130$) and the streptavidin–FITC reaction. These cells are located in the ARC as well as the cell-poor zone immediately lateral to the ventrolateral ARC (Fig. 1). Based on a subjective scale for judging the fluorescence intensity of cell somata staining ranging from "1+" for low intensity to "4+" for high intensity, all of the neurons which have been recorded for 20 min or longer, with one exception, have been judged to be 2+ or greater in intensity.

Moreover, the intensity of the FITC staining of cells correlates with the time of recording (11).

Morphology of TH-Containing Neurons: Prototypical Parvocellular Neurosecretory Neurons

Approximately 12% of the streptavidin–FITC-identified neurons are identified as containing TH following immunocytochemistry. Frequently, the proximal dendrites as well as the somata are stained. TH-identified neurons are located under the third ventricle in the rostral ARC and in the medial, ventrolateral, and ventromedial aspects of the medial and caudal ARC (Fig. 1). The size of the somata varies from small (8×11 μm) to large (20×20 μm) for "parvocellular" hypothalamic neurons (33, 34) with a mean length by width profile of $14.9 \pm 4.4 \times 11.5 \pm 3.1$ μm (mean $\pm$ SD). Two to four fibers typically radiate from the cell body (Fig. 3). Camera lucida drawings (Leitz drawing tube) are used to trace distal processes which extend over 100 μm in both the rostrocaudal and the dorsoventral direction. Numerous varicosities, which are documented by drawings and photography, are observed along the distal processes of the TH-containing neurons.

Electrophysiological Characterization of TH-Containing Neurons

A12 dopamine (TH-positive neurons) has a membrane potential of -60 ± 2 mV, an apparent input resistance of 348 ± 44 MΩ, and a membrane time constant of 20 ± 3 msec. Most of the cells are silent or fire at 2.5 Hz or less (mean firing rate 2.5 ± 0.9 Hz) in the slice. However, these neurons can be induced to fire continuously in a bursting pattern at rates greater than 20 Hz (unpublished observations). Threshold for the onset of the fastest rising phase of the action potential (-49 ± 1 mV), the amplitude of the fast action potential (67 ± 3 mV), and the duration of the action potential (0.8 ± 0.1 msec measured at $\frac{1}{3}$ amplitude) is measured on a digital oscilloscope. Arcuate dopamine neurons do not exhibit a "shoulder" on the falling phase of the action potential, which is indicative of a high-threshold Ca^{2+} spike (Fig. 4A), and they exhibit a long-lasting after-hyperpolarization following repetitive action potentials ("burst," Fig. 4B). This after-hyperpolarization decays to $\frac{1}{2}$ its magnitude in approximately 1.5 sec. The after-hyperpolarization that can be induced by a current pulse that is 0.2 nA above the threshold for induction of an action potential varies in amplitude from 6 to 9 mV (7.5 ± 0.5 mV).

A low-threshold and small-amplitude depolarizing potential is observed in

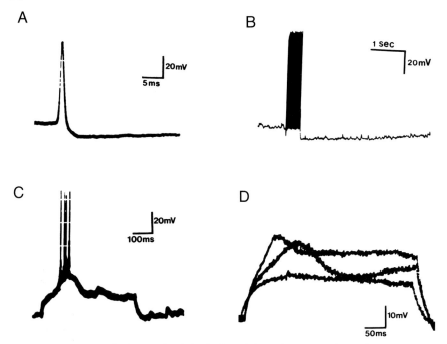

Fig. 4   Example of electrophysiological activity of arcuate dopamine neuron recorded in the slice. (A) An oscilloscope trace of a typical action potential during
spontaneous firing. Start of the fast rising phase occurred at −50 mV, and no shoulder
was present on the descending phase of the spike. (B) A 400-msec depolarizing
current pulse (220 pA) induced rapid sustained firing. The cell exhibited an after-
hyperpolarization of 9 mV at the end of the pulse and slowly recovered to the resting
membrane potential (−66 mV). (C) An oscilloscope trace showing a LTS that induced
four action potentials. This cell was held at −90 mV with negative current (110 pA),
then a depolarizing pulse was administered. The LTS was approximately 20 mV in
amplitude and 100 msec in duration. (D) Three superimposed traces showing the
membrane voltage defections induced by depolarizing current pulses of 30, 40, and
50 pA. The 30-pA current pulse did not elicit a LTS. The cell was held at −85 mV
with 60 pA to deinactivate the LTS, which could not be induced from the resting
membrane potential of −62 mV. The LTS is observed in isolation due to the presence
of 1 μM TTX in the medium, which eliminated fast action potentials. [Reproduced
with permission from Loose *et al.* (26).]

TH-positive neurons. The LTS that is induced by step depolarization to
between −65 and −60 mV from a membrane potential of −70 mV or more
negative causes a regenerative depolarizing potential that usually evokes one
to four, higher threshold, Na$^+$ action potentials (Fig. 4C). Perfusion with
TTX (1–2 μM) eliminates the fast Na$^+$ action potentials, but not the LTS.

In TTX, low-threshold spikes of 10–20 mV in amplitude and 40 to 100 msec in total duration are induced by depolarizing current pulses when the cell is held at −90 mV (Fig. 4D). When the membrane potential is held at −70 to −80 mV, the LTS is of smaller amplitude but similar duration. Hyperpolarizing current pulses of 20–80 msec are insufficient to deinactivate the conductance underlying the LTS even when the membrane potential is driven from −60 mV to very negative potentials (−110 mV). However, a 400-msec hyperpolarizing pulse to −90 mV allows sufficient deinactivation to occur so that an LTS is induced at the end of the pulse. The LTS is eliminated by perfusion of the slice with medium containing 10 mM Mg^{2+} and 0.1 mM Ca^{2+}, but is unaffected by K^+ channel blockers, e.g., Cs^+ (1–2 mM) or 4-aminopyridine (2 mM) or 4-aminopyridine (2 mM). In voltage-clamp recordings, a transient inward Ca^{2+} current ($I_{Ca,T}$) which peaks in 30–50 msec and returns to baseline within 200–250 msec is associated with the LTS (35). Moreover, the $I_{Ca,T}$ is insensitive to TTX and is blocked by 100–500 μM NiCl (35). Therefore, the LTS that we have identified in hypothalamic (A12 dopamine) neurons is similar to the low-threshold spike that was first described in thalamic neurons (36, 37) as it exhibits similar pharmacologic and voltage-dependent characteristics. ARC dopamine neurons are significantly more likely to exhibit an LTS than are other ARC neurons.

In current-clamp recordings, a hyperpolarizing current pulse of 400 msec elicits a time-dependent rectifying conductance in the majority of A12 dopamine neurons. This rectification appears as a delayed depolarization of the voltage deflection. The "sag" observed under current-clamp conditions is found to be associated with an inward current (I_h) under voltage-clamp conditions (26). The inward current becomes apparent when the membrane potential is hyperpolarized beyond approximately −70 mV and becomes larger and reaches maximal activation more quickly with greater hyperpolarization. Perfusion with Cs^+ (1–2 mM) eliminates both the sag in current clamp and the underlying current (I_h) in voltage clamp. TTX has no effect on the I_h nor do the potassium channel antagonists 4-aminopyridine (2 mM) and TEA (10 mM). In addition to the slower time-dependent rectifier, a rapidly activating, inwardly rectifying current is observed on hyperpolarization of the membrane ($I_{K,ir}$). This instantaneous inward rectifier is blocked by Cs^+ (1–2 μM). Both the instantaneous and the time-dependent rectifications in A12 dopamine neurons are similar, physiologically and pharmacologically, to conductances that have been described previously in other central nervous system neurons (38–41).

The presence of several endogenous currents, I_h, $I_{Ca,T}$, and $I_{K,Ca}$, in the parvocellular neurosecretory (e.g., A12 dopamine) neurons is essential for the oscillatory behavior in the firing pattern (bursting). Indeed, these same currents have been identified in bursting thalamic neurons (42, 43).

Morphology of β-Endorphin Neurons: Local Circuit and Long-Projection Neurons

Approximately 10% of the recorded neurons are identified as containing β-endorphin. β-Endorphin cells are small (mean diameters: 10.8×15.2 μm) oval or fusiform neurons or slightly larger (mean diameters: 14.0×19.3 μm) pyramidal neurons. β-Endorphin cells are distributed in the medial ARC and in the lateral arcuate extending over the pars tuberalis. Both of these areas have been shown to be densely populated with immunoreactive β-endorphin neurons (43a). The concentration of the granules in the perimeter of the cell soma is a characteristic of the staining of β-endorphin neurons in which colchicine pretreatment is not used (20). Two morphological characteristics of the identified β-endorphin neurons are the presence of thick proximal dendrites and of varicosities in the peripheral dendrites. About 10% of the β-endorphin neurons appear to be "dye-coupled" (where small molecular weight compounds will diffuse via a gap junction from the recorded cell to an adjacent cell) to another neuron which is not immunoreactive for β-endorphin (20).

Electrophysiological Characterization of β-Endorphin Neurons

β-Endorphin neurons have a RMP of -56 ± 2 mV, R_{in} of 439 ± 66 MΩ, and a τ of 17.5 ± 2.4 msec; all of these passive membrane properties do not differ from ARC dopamine neurons. However, β-endorphin neurons usually exhibit an irregular firing pattern (5.9 ± 2.2 Hz) or are silent. β-Endorphin neurons typically show a high incidence of synaptic activity (IPSPs) which is blocked by the GABA$_A$ antagonist bicuculline (10 μM; Sigma). Action potentials are 63 ± 4 mV in amplitude, measured from the initiation of the fast rising phase which activates at approximately -50 mV, and are 0.8 ± 0.1 msec in duration (measured at $\frac{1}{3}$ amplitude). The V/I relationship between -60 and -120 mV appears to be nonlinear, and the curvature in the V/I plots occurs in a voltage range around E_{K+}. The apparent R_{in} in the potential range of -60 to -80 mV is greater than the R_{in} in the potential range of -100 to -120 mV (calculated inward rectification ratio: 1.5 ± 0.1). β-Endorphin cells exhibit both I_h and $I_{K,ir}$ that activate below ≈ -80 mV. As with dopamine neurons, this current is blocked with 2 mM Cs$^+$. The lack of an LTS gives these neurons a very different firing pattern than that of the dopamine neurons and probably reflects their greater role as modulatory rather than neurosecretory neurons.

Pharmacology: Effects of DAMGO and Baclofen on ARC Dopamine and β-Endorphin Neurons

DAMGO hyperpolarizes the membrane and/or induces and outward current in voltage clamp in all ARC dopamine and β-endorphin neurons. The DAMGO-induced hyperpolarization (14 ± 3 mV for dopamine and 12 ± 2 mV for β-endorphin) is accompanied in every case by a decrease in R_{in} ($44 \pm 7\%$ for dopamine cells and 38 ± 4 for β-endorphin cells). The DAMGO-induced hyperpolarization is reversed by naloxone, an opioid receptor antagonist. The induced outward current when neurons are held at -60 mV in voltage clamp varies from 40 to 180 pA (93 ± 44 pA for dopamine neurons and 55 ± 14 pA for β-endorphin neurons). Steady-state I/V plots are generated in order to identify the ionic conductance responsible for the outward current (Fig. 5). The intersection of these I/V plots under control conditions and in the presence of the opioid agonist is -94 ± 2 mV, which is at E_{K+} (Fig. 5). A further verification that a K^+ conductance is activated is obtained by varying the extracellular concentration of K^+ from 2.5 to 10 mM. A plot of the reversal potential, again determined by the intersection of the I/V plots, versus the K^+ concentrations is a straight line with a slope of 58.0 mV per log unit as predicted by the Nernst equation (19). The DAMGO-induced hyperpolarization is a direct, postsynaptic action since TTX (1–2 μM) does not block the effect. The DAMGO-induced conductance increase is voltage sensitive such that the conductance increase is larger at more hyperpolarized membrane potentials. The conductance increase due to DAMGO is obtained

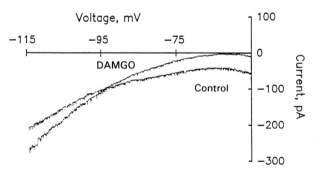

FIG. 5 Steady-state current–voltage plots of a voltage-clamped cell which shows that DAMGO increases the slope conductance of the current–voltage relationship, and the reversal potential of the DAMGO-induced current in the cell was -95 mV. Traces are obtained online during a slow (1 mV/sec) ramp depolarization from a -115-mV holding potential. The postsynaptic current fluctuations have been truncated. [Reproduced with permission from Loose *et al.* (26).]

by subtracting the total membrane current before DAMGO administration from that present after DAMGO application. The magnitude of the inward rectification of the DAMGO-induced current is quantified by comparing the conductance increase caused by DAMGO near -70 and near -100 mV (3.1 ± 0.7 nS versus 6.4 ± 1.2 nS). Therefore, DAMGO's effects occur via opening inwardly rectifying K^+ channels.

Although DAMGO is highly selective for μ-opioid receptors, we have tested several other agonists and antagonists on ARC neurons. The effects of DAMGO are totally blocked by 1 μM naloxone. The κ-selective agonist U50,488H (Upjohn, Kalamazoo, MI) is without any effects. The δ-selective agonist Try-D-Pen-Gly-Phe-D-Pen (Peninsula) causes a small hyperpolarization (4 mV) in a few unidentified ARC neurons, but has no effect on β-endorphin neurons. Therefore, the μ-receptor appears to be an autoreceptor for β-endorphin neurons (20).

Modulation of G Protein Cascade by Estrogen: Combined in Vivo and in Vitro Experiments

The modulation of the μ-opioid response has been studied using the slice preparation. To discriminate between long-term (genomic) and short-term (nongenomic) actions of estrogen two different protocols are followed. For the long-term studies, female guinea pigs are pretreated in vivo with estradiol benzoate or oil, and 24 hr later the animals are sacrificed and slices are prepared. Serum estrogen levels are measured in the trunk blood by radioimmunoassay to ascertain that the pretreatment regime has mimicked preovulatory conditions (100 to 150 pg/ml of estrogen) (22). The potency of DAMGO to hyperpolarize ARC neurons is compared in EB-treated and oil-treated animals by generating dose–response relationships (membrane hyperpolarization versus concentration of DAMGO). Estrogen treatment significantly decreases the potency of DAMGO (Fig. 6). However, the maximum membrane hyperpolarization or accompanying decrease in R_{in} is equivalent, which indicates that the number of ligand-gated K^+ channels and the conductance state of the channels are unaltered. The EC_{50} increased over three-fold by estrogen pretreatment. [The concentrations of DAMGO (20 nM to 1 μM) are below those at which desensitization is shown to occur (44), which is an important consideration when doing these type of pharmacological studies.] This would indicate that estrogen treatment decreases the number of μ-opioid receptors or alters the G protein coupling of the μ-receptor to the K^+ channel.

Following a washout of DAMGO and a return to the original resting membrane potential, a Schild analysis is done. A second cumulative dose–

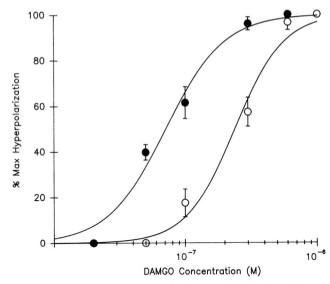

FIG. 6   Composite dose–response curves for the μ-opioid-induced hyperpolarization of ARC neurons recorded from ovariectomized, oil-treated females (filled circles, $N = 7$ cells) and from ovariectomized, EB-treated females (open circles, $N = 8$ cells). A logistic equation (1) was used to fit the curve to the points. The EC_{50} for the EB-treated group (240 nM) was significantly ($p < 0.001$) greater than that for the oil-treated group (70 nM). [Adapted with permission from Kelly $et\ al.$ (22).]

response curve (100 nM to 50 μM) is generated in the presence of the opioid antagonist naloxone (30 nM, 100 nM, or 1 μM) (Fig. 7). Since the pA_2 value for naloxone antagonism is not different between the two groups (8.13 $\pm$ 0.11 for the oil-treated group; 8.22 $\pm$ 0.17 for the estrogen-treated group), the antagonism (antagonist affinity) of the μ-opioid response by naloxone does not change with estrogen treatment.

For studies on short-term actions of estrogen, slices are prepared from ovariectomized, oil-treated animals. Basic membrane properties are measured and a complete dose–response curve to DAMGO is generated. Then 100 nM estrogen is superfused into the chamber for 20–30 min and, immediately afterward, a second dose–response relationship to DAMGO is generated. With this protocol we have measured a significant shift in the EC_{50} similar to what has been measured with 24 hr exposure to estrogen (45). These actions are directly on the cell in which we are recording because treatment has been done in the presence of TTX.

The μ-opioid and the GABA$_B$ receptors are coupled to the same inwardly rectifying potassium conductance based on occlusion experiments (21). We have utilized this fact to ascertain where in the receptor/G protein/K$^+$-

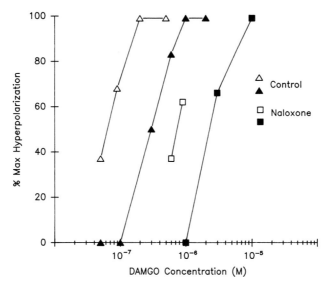

FIG. 7   Dose–response curve from arcuate neurons from an ovariectomized, oil-treated female guinea pig (open symbols) and from an ovariectomized, EB-treated guinea pig (closed symbols). In the presence of 100 nM naloxone, the dose–response curve was shifted to the right by approximately 1 log unit in both groups (squares). The K_e for naloxone was equivalent in both cases. Calculated pA_2 values are not significantly different between both groups of animals (oil-treated: 8.13 ± 0.17; EB-treated: 8.22 ± 0.17). [Adapted with permission from Kelly *et al.* (22).]

channel cascade estrogen is acting to "desensitize" the μ-opioid response; we have investigated the potency of baclofen, a GABA$_B$ agonist, to hyperpolarize ARC neurons. The dose–response relationship for the GABA$_B$ agonist baclofen also is shifted 3.3-fold rightward following estrogen treatment without an alteration in the maximal response or a decrease in R_{in}. We conclude from these experiments that estrogen is acting downstream from the binding of DAMGO and baclofen to their respective receptors since the steroid affects both the potency of the DAMGO and baclofen response, and a possible site of action is at the G protein such that coupling of the receptors to the inwardly rectifying K$^+$ channel is less effective.

Summary

We have described the use of the hypothalamic slice preparation in studying the membrane properties of the parvocellular neurosecretory neurons *in situ* as it relates to cell firing and hormone release. Stable intracellular recordings for up to 6 hr offer the possibility of doing extensive pharmacological testing to determine specific receptor subtypes and second messenger cascades that are associated with activation of these receptors. Moreover, slices from adult animals are utilized such that synaptic plasticity in afferent pathways can be studied. Most importantly, following the electrophysiological and pharmacological analysis of individual neurons, it is possible to identify the cell phenotype with intracellular biocytin followed by immunocytochemistry. We are currently developing an *in situ* hybridization technique in order to identify a greater number of different phenotypes within the heterogenous population of arcuate neurons.

Acknowledgments

The work presented in this chapter was supported by PHS Grants HD 16793 and DA 05158. M.J.K. was a recipient of a Research Career Development Award (HD 00718). The authors thank Mrs. Martha Bosch and Mr. Barry Naylor for their technical assistance.

References

1. J. B. Wakerley and D. W. Lincoln, *J. Endocrinol.* **57,** 477 (1973).
2. J. B. Wakerley, D. A. Poulain, and D. A. Brown, *Brain Res.* **148,** 425 (1978).
3. D. A. Poulain and J. B. Wakerley, *Neuroscience* **7,** 773 (1982).
4. C. W. Bourque and L. P. Renaud, *Front. Neuroendocrinol.* **11,** 183 (1990).
5. L. P. Renaud and C. W. Bourque, *Prog. Neurobiol.* **36,** 131 (1991).
6. P. Cobbett, K. G. Smithson, and G. I. Hatton, *Neuroscience* **16,** 885 (1985).
7. P. Cobbett, K. G. Smithson, and G. I. Hatton, *Brain Res.* **362,** 7 (1986).
8. M. J. Kelly, T. P. Condon, J. E. Levine, and O. K. Ronnekleiv, *Brain Res.* **345,** 264 (1985).
9. T. P. Condon, O. K. Ronnekleiv, and M. J. Kelly, *Neuroendocrinology* **50,** (1989).
10. K. Horikawa and W. E. Armstrong, *J. Neurosci. Methods* **25,** 1 (1988).
11. O. K. Ronnekleiv, M. D. Loose, K. R. Erickson, and M. J. Kelly, *BioTechniques* **9,** 432 (1990).
12. A. S. Finkel and S. J. Redman, *in* ''Voltage and Patch Clamping with Microelectrodes'' (T. G. Smith, Jr., H. Lecar, S. J. Redman, and P. W. Gage, eds.), p. 95. American Physiological Society, Bethesda, MD, 1985.
13. J. J. B. Jack, D. Noble, and R. W. Tsien, ''Electric Current Flow in Excitable Cells.'' Clarendon Press, Oxford, 1983.
14. S. Siegel, ''Nonparametric Statistics for the Behavioral Sciences.'' McGraw–Hill, New York, 1956.
15. B. Hille, ''Ionic Channels of Excitable Membranes,'' p. 115. Sinauer, MA, 1992.

16. B. K. Handa, A. C. Lane, A. H. Lord, B. A. Morgan, M. J. Rance, *et al. Eur. J. Pharmacol.* **70,** 531 (1981).

17. J. T. Williams and R. A. North, *Mol. Pharmacol.* **26,** 489 (1984).

18. M. D. Loose and M. J. Kelly, *Brain Res. Bull.* **22,** 819 (1989).

19. M. D. Loose and M. J. Kelly, *Brain Res.* **513,** 15 (1990).

20. M. J. Kelly, M. D. Loose, and O. K. Ronnekleiv, *Neuroendocrinology* **52,** 268 (1990).

21. M. D. Loose, O. K. Ronnekleiv, and M. J. Kelly, *Neuroendocrinology* **54,** 537 (1991).

22. M. J. Kelly, M. D. Loose, and O. K. Ronnekleiv, *J. Neurosci.* **12,** 2745 (1992).

23. H. O. Schild, *Br. J. Pharmacol.* **2,** 189 (1947).

24. J. H. Gaddum, *Pharmacol. Rev.* **9,** 211 (1957).

25. M. D. Loose, O. K. Ronnekleiv, and M. J. Kelly, *Soc. Neurosci. Abstr.* **15,** 1087 (1989).

26. M. D. Loose, O. K. Ronnekleiv, and M. J. Kelly, *J. Neurosci.* **10,** 3627 (1990).

27. V. Leviel, B. Guibert, J. Mallet, and N. Faucon-Biguet, *J. Neurosci. Res.* **30,** 427 (1991).

28. R. Y. Moore and F. E. Bloom, *Annu. Rev. Neurosci.* **2,** 113 (1979).

29. T. Hökfelt, R. Mårtensson, A. Björklund, S. Kleinau, and M. Goldstein, *in* "Handbook of Chemical Neuroanatomy" (A. Björklund and T. Hökfelt, eds.), p. 277. Elsevier Science, Amsterdam/New York, 1984.

30. E. Weber, C. J. Evans, J. K. Chang, and J. D. Barchas, *J. Neurochem.* **38,** 436 (1982).

31. J. R. Dave, N. Rubinstein, and R. L. Eskay, *Endocrinology (Baltimore)* **117,** 1389 (1985).

32. B. A. Eipper and R. E. Mains, *Endocrinol. Rev.* **1,** 1 (1980).

33. M. Bodoky and M. Réthelyi, *Exp. Brain Res.* **28,** 543 (1977).

34. A. N. Van den Pol, R. S. Herbst, and J. F. Powell, *Neurosci.* **13,** 1117 (1984).

35. K. R. Erickson, O. K. Ronnekleiv, and M. J. Kelly, *Neuroendocrinology* **57,** 789 (1993).

36. H. Jahnsen and R. R. Llinás, *J. Physiol. (London)* **349,** 205 (1984).

37. H. Jahnsen and R. R. Llinás, *J. Physiol. (London)* **349,** 227 (1984).

38. J. V. Halliwell and P. R. Adams, *Brain Res.* **250,** 71 (1982).

39. A. Constanti and M. Galvan, *J. Physiol. (London)* **385,** 153 (1983).

40. F. Crepel and J. Penit-Soria, *J. Physiol. (London)* **372,** 1 (1986).

41. J. T. Williams, W. F. Colmers, and Z. Z. Pan, *J. Neurosci.* **8,** 3499 (1988).

42. D. A. McCormick and H.-C. Pape, *J. Physiol. (London)* **431,** 291 (1990).

43. J. R. Huguenard and D. A. Prince, *J. Neurosci.* **12,** 3804 (1992).

43a. J. E. Thornton, M. D. Loose, M. J. Kelly, and O. K. Rönnekleiv, *J. Comp. Neurol.,* in press.

44. G. C. Harris and J. T. Williams, *J. Neurosci.* **11,** 2574 (1991).

45. A. H. Lagrange, O. K. Ronnekleiv, and M. J. Kelly, *Soc. Neurosci. Abstr.* **18,** 1373 (1992).

[4] Calcium Signaling and Episodic Secretory Responses of GnRH Neurons

Stanko S. Stojilkovic, Lazar Z. Krsmanovic,
Daniel J. Spergel, Melanija Tomic, and Kevin J. Catt

Introduction

Mammalian gonadotropin-releasing hormone (GnRH)-producing cells are located within the preoptic area or the mediobasal hypothalamus, depending on the species (1, 2). In contrast to other hypothalamic neurons, GnRH cells do not form a clearly defined nucleus within which the cells are closely adjacent and tightly connected. Despite their scattered locations, GnRH neurons are interconnected to form a network termed the "GnRH pulse generator" (3) that is responsible for the synchronized pattern of pulsatile GnRH release into the portal vessels *in vivo* (4) as well as from hypothalamic tissue *in vitro* (5, 6). Recently, dissociated GnRH neurons have been shown to retain the ability to form functional interconnections *in vitro* when cultured in a mixed population of hypothalamic cells and to generate a pattern of neuropeptide secretion similar to that observed *in vivo* and *in situ* (6). The finding that immortalized GT1-1 and GT1-7 (GT1) neuronal cells also show an oscillatory pattern of GnRH release further indicates that rhythmic activity is an intrinsic property of the GnRH neurons and is manifested in culture even in the absence of other cell types (6–8).

An increase in intracellular calcium concentration ($[Ca^{2+}]_i$) is required for the release of neurotransmitters from presynaptic terminals in many neurons (9). Thus, it is reasonable to postulate that the pulsatile nature of basal GnRH release as well as agonist-mediated modulation of basal GnRH release is associated with changes in $[Ca^{2+}]_i$. Unfortunately, the complexity of the structural organization of the hypothalamus and the difficulty of purifying GnRH-producing neurons have limited the analysis of Ca^{2+} signaling and the consequences of such signaling on GnRH release. However, the development of the GT1 immortalized GnRH neuronal cell line has provided a valuable model system in which to study Ca^{2+} signaling and neuropeptide secretion (10).

In this chapter, we describe studies on $[Ca^{2+}]_i$ in unstimulated GT1 neurons, as well as in response to high K^+, dihydropyridines, and endothelins, utilizing three different procedures for the measurement of $[Ca^{2+}]_i$: (a) in cells in suspension; (b) in individual single cells cultured on coverslips;

Methods in Neurosciences, Volume 20

and (c) in interconnected cells cultured on coverslips to form a monolayer network. Pituitary cells in suspension and single gonadotropes were employed as standards for the validation of $[Ca^{2+}]_i$ measurements in GT1 cells. The data indicate that the cell suspension method provides only a modicum of information, while the other methods are appropriate for the detailed analysis of Ca^{2+} signaling in GT1 cells. In addition, the comparison of $[Ca^{2+}]_i$ responses in single cells and in a cell network has potential value in studies on the dependence of Ca^{2+} signals on intercellular communication. The latter procedure also permits the comparison of Ca^{2+} signaling in GnRH neurons with that of the pulsatile secretory response of perifused GnRH neurons cultured on beads, which also form a neuronal network (8).

Experimental Procedures

Primary Culture of Hypothalamic Cells

Hypothalamic tissue is removed from fetuses of 17-day pregnant Sprague–Dawley rats. The borders of the excised hypothalami are delineated by the anterior margin of the optic chiasm, by the posterior margin of the mammilary bodies, and laterally by the hypothalamic sulci. After dissection, hypothalami are placed into ice-cold dissociation buffer consisting of 137 mM NaCl, 5 mM KCl, 0.7 mM Na_2HPO_4, 25 mM HEPES, 100 mg/liter gentamicin, pH 7.4. The preparation of hypothalamic cells is performed by minor modifications of the method described by Peterfreund and Vale (11). The tissues are washed and then incubated in a sterile flask with dissociation buffer supplemented with 0.2% collagenase (activity 149 U/mg; Worthington, Freehold, NJ), 0.4% bovine serum albumin, 0.2% glucose, and a pinch of DNase I (Sigma, St. Louis, MO). After 60 min of incubation in a 37°C water bath with shaking at 60 cycles min^{-1}, the tissue is gently triturated by repeated aspiration into a smooth-tipped Pasteur pipette. Incubation is continued for another 30 min, after which the tissue is finally dispersed. The dispersed cells are passed through sterile mesh (200 μm) into a 50-ml tube, pelleted by centrifugation for 10 min at 200 g, and then washed once in dissociation buffer and once in culture medium consisting of 500 ml Dulbecco's modified Eagle's medium (DMEM) containing 0.584 g/liter L-glutamine and 4.5 g/liter glucose (Sigma), mixed with 500 ml F-12 medium containing 0.146 g/liter L-glutamine, 1.802 g/liter glucose (Sigma), 100 μg/ml gentamicin, 2.438 g/liter sodium bicarbonate, and 10% heat-inactivated fetal calf serum (Gibco). Each fetal hypothalamus yields about 1.5×10^6 cells.

Primary Culture of Pituitary Cells

Experiments are performed on anterior pituitary cells from adult female Sprague–Dawley rats (200–250 g), either intact or 2 weeks postovariectomy, obtained from Charles River, Inc. (Wilmington, MA). Groups of 50 anterior pituitary glands are rinsed several times with 10 ml Ca^{2+}/Mg^{2+}-free Dulbecco's phosphate buffer solution (Biofluids, Rockville, MD) supplemented with 0.1% bovine serum albumin plus 100 units/ml penicillin and 10 μg/ml streptomycin (dispersion medium). The tissue is minced into 0.7-mm cubes using a tissue chopper (Brinkmann Instruments, Inc., Westbury, NY). The minced tissue is washed in dispersion medium several times and incubated for 1 hr in a water bath at 37°C with shaking (70–75 min^{-1}) in 50 ml prewarmed dispersion medium containing 75 mg trypsin (Gibco) and a pinch of DNase inhibitor (Sigma). After incubation, the medium is replaced by 50 ml of prewarmed dispersion medium containing 75 mg trypsin inhibitor (Sigma). After 10 min incubation with trypsin inhibitor at 37°C without shaking, the tissue is transferred into a 15-ml plastic tube.

The pituitary fragments are mechanically dispersed by repeated pipetting several times during a 20- to 30-min period. Each time, after the tissue settles to the bottom of the tube, the supernatant is transferred into a sterile 50-ml tube on ice. The pooled cells are then filtered through nylon mesh, pelleted by centrifugation, and then washed once in dispersion buffer and once in culture medium consisting of medium 199 with 10% horse serum, 100 u/ml penicillin, and 10 μg/ml streptomycin. Cells prepared from pituitaries of ovariectomized female rats contain about 25% gonadotropes, which respond to stimulation by agonists and high K^+ in a manner similar to the 10% of gonadotropes obtained from glands of intact females (12, 13).

GnRH Neuronal and Gonadotrope Cell Lines

The GnRH cell lines (GT1-1 and GT1-7) and gonadotrope cell line (αT3) (generously provided by Drs. Richard Weiner and Pamela Mellon, University of California, San Francisco, and University of California, San Diego) are grown in 75-ml culture flasks (Corning) in DMEM with L-glutamine (0.584 g/liter), glucose (4.5 g/liter), gentamicin (100 μg/ml), sodium bicarbonate (3.7 g/liter), and 10% heat-inactivated fetal calf serum. When cells reach confluence they are dispersed by 10 min trypsinization in phosphate-buffered saline containing 0.05% trypsin, 0.02% EDTA, 0.05% $NaHCO_3$, 0.2% DNase I, 0.1% glucose, and 0.01% gentamicin. The cells are pelleted by centrifugation for 10 min at 400 g, washed twice in culture medium, and cultured on Cytodex beads for perifusion studies, on coverslips for [Ca^{2+}]$_i$ measurements, or in culture plates for further growth. Culture medium is changed at 48-hr intervals.

Assay of Cytoplasmic Calcium in Single Cells

For [Ca^{2+}]$_i$ measurements, GT1 cells are plated (5 × 10^4/dish) in 35-mm petri dishes (Falcon, Oxnard, CA) containing 25-mm-diameter glass coverslips (Erie Scientific Co., Porstmouth, NH) coated with 0.01% poly-L-lysine (Sigma). After culture for 2 to 3 days, the medium is replaced with 2 ml of phenol red-free medium 199–Hanks' incubation medium (1.2 mM CaCl$_2$, 0.1% bovine serum albumin (BSA), 25 mM HEPES, 16.7 mM NaHCO$_3$, and 1% penicillin/streptomycin) containing 2 μM Indo-1 acetylmethyl (AM) (Molecular Probes; Eugene, OR). After incubation for 60 min at 37°C, the coverslips are washed twice with fresh incubation medium and maintained in the same medium in the dark at 22°C before fluorescence measurements.

After being washed, individual coverslips are transferred to a Leiden coverslip dish (Medical Systems Co., Greenvale, NY) with 1 ml phenol red-free medium 199, mounted on the stage of an inverted Diaphot microscope attached to a dual-emission microscopic fluorometer (Nikon, Garden City, NY), and examined at 22°C under a 40X or 100X oil immersion fluorescence objective. For excitation of Indo-1, the light beam from a 100-watt mercury arc lamp is reduced by a $\frac{1}{16}$th neutral density filter, passed through a 360-nm interference filter, and then reflected from a DM 400 dichroic mirror through a pinhole diaphragm, which is slightly smaller than the selected cell. The emergent beam is split by a DM 455 dichroic mirror and directed through 405 and 485-nm interference filters with a 20-nm bandpass. Each beam is monitored by an individual photomultiplier tube, and the ratio of intensities is calculated by a computer at 360-msec intervals throughout the experiments, using the FASTINCA program (University of Cincinnati Medical Center, Cincinnati, OH).

All [Ca^{2+}]$_i$ values are derived from a standard curve that is constructed by addition of increasing concentrations of Ca^{2+} (10–1500 nM) to 15 μM free Indo-1 (Molecular Probes). For background collection, the dual emission of an open area of the culture dish with medium 199 is recorded, since the intensity of the resulting fluorescence is almost identical to that of unloaded cells. After subtraction of the background from the emission of the specimen, the ratios of the net values are applied to the standard curve stored in the computer.

Assay of Cytoplasmic Calcium in Cell Suspensions

For $[Ca^{2+}]_i$ measurements, GT1 and αT3 cells are plated in six-well culture plates (Costar, Cambridge, MA) and allowed to reach 60–90% confluence in DMEM supplemented with 10% fetal bovine serum. After detachment by pretreatment in Ca^{2+}-free medium + 0.02% EDTA and 0.05% trypsin and preincubation for 30 min at 37°C in culture medium, the cells are centrifuged at 400 g for 5 min; washed twice; resuspended (2×10^6 cells/ml, 10 ml) in medium 199 containing Hanks' salts, 25 mM HEPES, and 1 μM Fura-2 AM (Calbiochem, San Diego, CA); and incubated for 30 min at 37°C. They are then diluted and centrifuged for 5 min at 100 g, washed twice in assay buffer (M199 with 1.2 mM $CaCl_2$, or in Ca^{2+}-deficient medium buffered with EGTA to around 180 nM $[Ca^{2+}]_e$), and kept in the dark at 22°C before use. Spectrofluorometric analyses of $[Ca^{2+}]_i$ are conducted at 32°C in a Delta Scan spectrofluorometer (Photon Technology International, South Brunswick, NJ) with excitation at 340 and 380 nm. The $[Ca^{2+}]_i$ values calculated from emission data at 500 nm are corrected for dye leakage and autofluorescence as described by Grynkiewicz et al. (14). Autofluorescence of cells not loaded with Fura-2 AM is negligible. $[Ca^{2+}]_i$ measurements in hypothalamic cells and pituitary cells in primary culture are performed by the same procedure, except that the freshly dispersed cells are used after preincubation for 2 hr in medium 199 on ice.

Assay of Cytoplasmic Calcium in Monolayer Networks

Studies have shown that GT1 cells cultured on slides (15) and beads (8) form numerous interconnections within 36 hr. To analyze the Ca^{2+} signaling in such GnRH cell networks, cells are cultured (5×10^5 cells/cm^2) on rectangular coverslips (No. 1 thickness) coated with poly-L-lysine, thoroughly rinsed with distilled water, and sterilized by overnight exposure to UV light. The coverslips are maintained in a sterile petri dish, and the culture medium is changed every 2 days. After 2–3 days, when connections between the neurons are evident, the coverslips are washed in phenol red-free medium 199 containing 10 mM HEPES and 0.1% bovine serum albumin and incubated with 2 μM Fura-2 AM (Calbiochem or Molecular Probes) for 60 min at 37 or 22°C. For the measurement of $[Ca^{2+}]_i$ in the cell monolayer, the coverslip is inserted into an adjustable holder (Micron Systems, Sykesville, MD) that is fitted to a 4-ml quartz cuvette containing medium 199 or modified Krebs–Ringer buffer (140 mM NaCl, 4.7 mM KCl, 2.6 mM $CaCl_2$, 0.6 mM $MgCl_2$, 10 mM HEPES, 10 mM glucose, pH adjusted to 7.4 with NaOH,

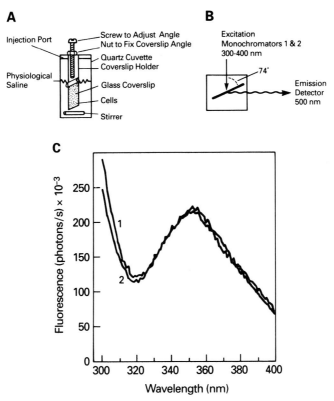

FIG. 1   Schematic representation of the experimental conditions for measurement of $[Ca^{2+}]_i$ in a monolayer network. (A and B) Arrangement for measuring $[Ca^{2+}]_i$ in a monolayer network of cells attached to a coverslip. (A) Front view; (B) top view. (C) Fluorescence spectra, after background correction, of a monolayer network of GT1 cells (ca. 10^6 cells/cm²) loaded with 2 μM Fura-2 AM for 1 hr at 22°C and then washed for 30 min. The spectra were obtained by exposing the cells to light from 300 to 400 nm and measuring the emitted light at 500 nm. Experiments were done in the timebase mode with 340 and 380 nm excitation after it was verified that the fluorescence spectra peaked at 340 nm and resembled each other as closely as possible.

osmolality adjusted to 300 mOsm) (Fig. 1A). The angle of the coverslip is adjusted such that two criteria are met:

1. The fluorescence spectra measured at 500 nm by the emission detector (Fig. 1B) during simultaneous scanning with both excitation monochromators from 300 to 400 nm should peak at 340 ± 10 nm with large fluorescence signals (200×10^3 photons/sec in Fig. 1C) after subtraction of the fluorescence

of a coverslip of cells not loaded with Fura-2 AM (20×10^3 photons/sec; not shown). The presence of such fluorescence spectra indicates that Fura-2 loading is adequate.

2. The fluorescence spectra from the two excitation monochromators match each other as closely as possible, i.e., the channels (1 and 2 in Fig. 1C) are balanced. Channel balance guards against possible artifacts by ensuring that in the timebase mode a change in $[Ca^{2+}]_i$ is reported by Fura-2 only when a change in the fluorescence due to 340 nM excitation, indicating a change in the concentration of Fura-2 bound to $[Ca^{2+}]_i$, is equal and opposite to a change in the fluorescence due to 380 nm excitation, due to the concomitant change in the concentration of unbound Fura-2. The coverslip angle that satisfies these two criteria is one of 16° between the coverslip and detector (Fig. 1B) when the cells are located on the side of the coverslip facing away from the excitation monochromators.

Values for $[Ca^{2+}]_i$ are determined according to the formula of Grynkiewicz *et al.* (14): $[Ca^{2+}]_i = K_d (R - R_{min})/(R_{max} - R) (F_{max_{380}}/F_{min_{380}})$, where $R = F_{340}/F_{380}$ and $K_d = 224$ nM, the dissociation constant for the Ca^{2+} Fura-2 complex in the presence of 1 mM Mg^{2+}. R_{min} is obtained by exposing the cells to a mixture of EGTA (10 mM), Tris (30 mM), and ionomycin (10 μM; Ref. 15). R_{max} is obtained by adding 100 mM $CaCl_2$ to the mixture. Ionomycin (Calbiochem) rather than Triton X-100 is used to permeabilize the cells to Ca^{2+} since the detergent detaches the cells from the coverslip.

Perifusion Procedure

Attachment of the cells to Cytodex beads (Pharmacia, Piscataway, NJ) is performed in 50-ml tubes containing 1.5×10^7 cells, 0.3 ml preswollen Cytodex-2, and 30 ml DMEM, with L-glutamine (0.584 g/liter), glucose (4.5 g/liter), and 100 μg/ml gentamicin supplemented with 10% fetal calf serum, incubated for 24 hr in 5% CO_2/air. The next day, cells are transferred into 60-mm dishes (total incubation volume of 7.5 ml culture medium) and cultured for 7 to 10 days. The culture medium is changed every 3 days. Before each perifusion, the cell–bead mixture is collected by sedimentation; resuspended in Krebs–Ringer buffer containing 1 mg/ml BSA, 1 mg/ml glucose, 20 μM bacitracin, pH 7.4; gassed with 95% O_2/5% CO_2 for 1 hr; and loaded into a temperature-controlled 0.5 ml chamber (Endotronics; Minneapolis, MN). The multiple microchamber module is used with a chamber volume of 500 μl. Cells are perifused with media at a flow rate of 10 ml/hr at 37°C for at least 1 hr, before being tested, to establish a stable baseline. Drugs are made up in the appropriate test medium, with normal Ca^{2+} (1.25 mM), or in Ca^{2+}-deficient medium (200 nM). Fractions are collected every 5 min and stored at $-20°C$ prior to radioimmunoassays. GnRH assay is performed as previously described (17), using ^{125}I-GnRH (from Amersham, Arlington Heights, IL), unlabeled GnRH (from Peninsula, Belmont, CA), and primary antibody (donated by Dr. V. D. Ramirez, University of Illinois, Urbana, IL). The intra- and interassay coefficients of variation at 80% binding in standard samples (15 pg/ml) were 12 and 14%, respectively.

Calcium Signaling in GnRH Neurons

General Observations

In many cell types, Ca^{2+} signaling in response to agonist stimulation and activation of voltage-sensitive calcium channels (VSCC) can be examined in cell suspensions (18). For example, Fig. 2A shows the spike amplitude of $[Ca^{2+}]_i$ in rat pituitary cells in response to activation of endothelin receptors, as well as in response to stimulation of Ca^{2+} entry through VSCC by K^+-induced depolarization and by the calcium-channel agonist, Bay K 8644. In contrast, the $[Ca^{2+}]_i$ responses of dispersed hypothalamic cells to the same stimuli were only slightly above the baseline (Fig. 2B).

The GT1 neuronal cells also showed very small Ca^{2+} responses to endothelin, high K^+, and Bay K 8644 (Fig. 3B), while the αT3 gonadotroph cell

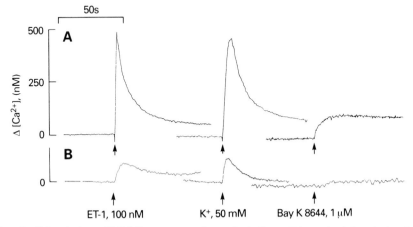

FIG. 2   Stimulation of $[Ca^{2+}]_i$ responses by endothelin-1, K^+-evoked depolarization, and Bay K 8644 in suspensions of pituitary (A) and hypothalamic (B) cells.

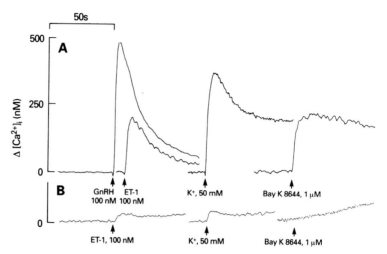

FIG. 3   Effects of endothelin, GnRH, and depolarization of cells by high K^+ and Bay K 8644 on $[Ca^{2+}]_i$ in suspensions of αT3 pituitary cells (A) and GT1 neuronal cells (B).

line [derived by a procedure similar to that of the GT1 cell line (10, 18)] responded with amplitudes comparable to those of other endocrine cells (Fig. 3A). At present, the reason for this difference between these neuroendocrine and endocrine cells, both expressing VSCC, is unclear. The experimental conditions for the data shown in Figs. 2 and 3 were identical. Since loss of axons and dendrites is evident after dispersion of both primary cultures and GT1 cells, it is probable that the VSCC are not distributed uniformly over the perikarya, axons, and dendrites. Alternatively, these data could indicate that the small amplitudes of Ca^{2+} signaling in GnRH neurons are characteristic of these cells.

To address these questions, we utilized an alternative system for $[Ca^{2+}]_i$ measurement in which the cells were attached to coverslips (16). Depending on the initial density of cells and duration of culture, the cells were either isolated or had developed interneuronal connections. Analyses of the Ca^{2+}-signaling responses both in single cells and in the monolayer neuronal network are shown in Fig. 4. It is clear that the Ca^{2+} responses in attached single GT1 cells (Fig. 4B) and in the neuronal network (Fig. 4C) are significantly higher than those in suspension. The responses are comparable to those observed in pituitary cells in suspension (Figs. 2 and 3) and in single pituitary gonadotropes attached to coverslips (Fig. 4A). Thus, these data suggest that the integrity of GnRH neurons or attachment to a substrate is required for normal Ca^{2+} signaling within the cells in response to activation

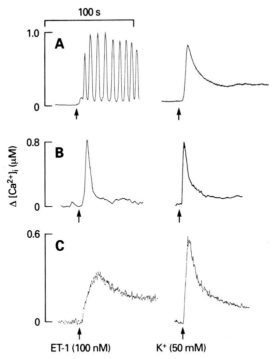

FIG. 4   Comparison of the amplitudes of Ca^{2+} responses in single pituitary gonado-tropes (A), single GT1 cells (B), and GT1 cells in a monolayer network (C).

of Ca^{2+}-mobilizing receptors, as well as in response to activation of Ca^{2+} entry through VSCC.

Basal [Ca^{2+}]$_i$ in GT1 Cells

In general, two types of resting [Ca^{2+}]$_i$ signals were recorded from single GT1-7 cells. About one-third of the cells were quiescent, with a stable resting [Ca^{2+}]$_i$ level around 200 nM. However, the majority of the GT1-7 cells showed episodes of prominent spontaneous fluctuations, with random frequency and amplitude, and a variable basal [Ca^{2+}]$_i$ level (from 150 to 600 nM). Several examples of such spontaneous [Ca^{2+}]$_i$ fluctuations are shown in Figs. 5A–5F. Spontaneous [Ca^{2+}]$_i$ fluctuations were dependent on Ca^{2+} entry, since they were abolished when cells were exposed to Ca^{2+}-deficient medium (Fig. 5G). Spontaneous fluctuations were also abolished by addition of the Ca^{2+}-channel

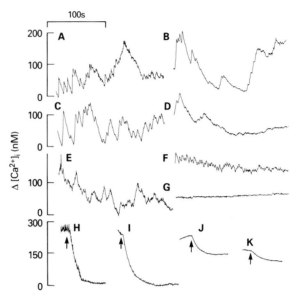

FIG. 5   Spontaneous fluctuations of $[Ca^{2+}]_i$ in single GT1 cells. Basal $[Ca^{2+}]_i$ in the presence of 1.25 mM (A–F) and 20 nM (G) extracellular Ca^{2+}. Inhibitory effects of the Ca^{2+}-channel blocker, nifedipine, on basal $[Ca^{2+}]_i$ (H–K).

antagonist, nifedipine (Figs. 5H–5K), suggesting that Ca^{2+} entry through VSCC participates in their generation or maintenance.

Baseline $[Ca^{2+}]_i$ in the monolayer network was slightly below that observed in single cells (about 200 nM) and did not fluctuate. However, as in single cells, basal $[Ca^{2+}]_i$ was also reduced by nifedipine in a dose-dependent manner with an IC_{50} of 0.9 $\pm$ 0.2 μM (mean $\pm$ SEM) (Fig. 6A). Basal $[Ca^{2+}]_i$ levels in both single cells (not shown) and in the GnRH neuronal network (Fig. 6B) were increased by application of the calcium-channel agonist, Bay K 8644, in a dose-dependent manner (IC_{50} of 1.0 $\pm$ 0.04 μM).

Depolarization-Induced Ca^{2+} Signaling in GT1 Cells

Elevation of K^+ also induced a rapid increase in $[Ca^{2+}]_i$ in single cells and in GT1 cell networks, followed by an exponential decrease to a steady-state level (Fig. 6C). Such a profile of Ca^{2+} response to depolarization by high K^+ is consistent with the presence of L-type VSCC and with changes in their activation–inactivation kinetics to produce a biphasic response (12). In agreement with this mechanism, addition of nifedipine terminated the steady-

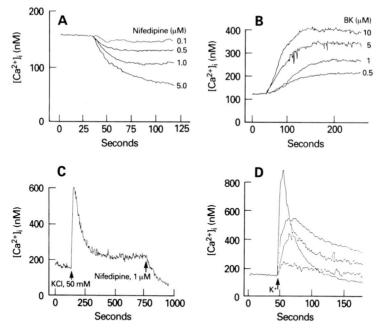

FIG. 6   Effects of depolarization of cells by high K^+ and dihydropyridines on $[Ca^{2+}]_i$ in GT1 cells in a monolayer network. (A) The dose-dependent inhibitory effect of nifedipine on $[Ca^{2+}]_i$. (B) The dose-dependent effects of Ca^{2+}-channel agonist, Bay K 8644, on $[Ca^{2+}]_i$. (C) Nifedipine sensitivity of K^+-induced $[Ca^{2+}]_i$ response in GT1-1 cells. (D) Dose-dependent effects of high K^+ on $[Ca^{2+}]_i$; from top to bottom: 75, 50, 35, and 25 mM KCl. [Derived with permission from Krsmanovic *et al.* (6).]

state $[Ca^{2+}]_i$ response (Fig. 6C). The effects of high K^+ on the $[Ca^{2+}]_i$ response were evident over a wide range of K^+ concentrations (Fig. 6D).

Agonist-Induced Ca²⁺ Signaling in Hypothalamic and GT1 Cells

Primary cultures of hypothalamic cells were found to secrete the potent calcium-mobilizing peptide, endothelin (17). Endothelin receptors were also identified in GT1 cells, as well as in primary cultures of hypothalamic cells, and exhibited higher affinity for endothelin-1 and endothelin-2 than for endothelin-3 (17). In accord with these findings, single GT1 cells and the monolayer network showed a biphasic $[Ca^{2+}]_i$ response to endothelins, with an early spike phase followed by a sustained plateau phase. At the same concentra-

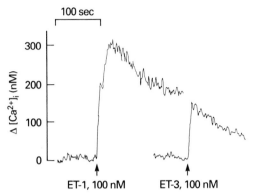

FIG. 7   Comparison of $[Ca^{2+}]_i$ responses to endothelin-1 and endothelin-3 in GT1 cells in a monolayer network.

tions, endothelin-1 induced a larger $[Ca^{2+}]_i$ response than endothelin-3 (Fig. 7).

An obvious difference in the amplitudes of Ca^{2+} responses in endothelin-1 (100 nM)-stimulated single GT1 cells and monolayer networks was observed [Fig. 4; spike amplitude of $\Delta[Ca^{2+}]_i$ in nM: single cells, 806 ± 17 ($n = 7$) vs monolayer network 397 ± 31 ($n = 3$)]. Under similar experimental conditions, K^+ (60 mM)-mediated depolarization of GT1 cells led to comparable profiles of Ca^{2+} responses in the two cell types [spike amplitude of $\Delta[Ca^{2+}]_i$ in nM: single cells, 695 ± 28 ($n = 5$) vs neuronal networks, 637 ± 49 ($n = 8$)]. These data suggest that the ability of endothelins to induce a $[Ca^{2+}]_i$ response in GnRH cells decreases with the integration of single cells into a neuronal network.

Correlation between $[Ca^{2+}]_i$ and Secretory Responses of GnRH Neurons

Perifused cultured hypothalamic cells and GnRH neuronal cell lines were found to spontaneously secrete GnRH in a pulsatile manner (6–8). In general, the secretory responses of hypothalamic cultures and GT1 cells paralleled the $[Ca^{2+}]_i$ signaling in those cells: (a) The pulsatile release of GnRH from perifused primary cultures and GT1 cells depended on extracellular Ca^{2+}; lowering $[Ca^{2+}]_e$ to 100 nM by addition of EGTA completely abolished pulsatile GnRH secretion; and recovery of the GnRH secretory pattern was observed after returning Ca^{2+} to the perifusion medium (6). (b) Activation of

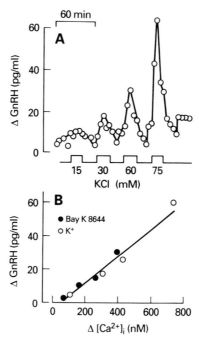

FIG. 8   Correlation between $[Ca^{2+}]_i$ and secretory response to GnRH neurons. (A) Dose-dependent effects of high K^+ on GnRH release in perifused GT1 cells. (B) Linear relationship between the spike amplitudes of $[Ca^{2+}]_i$ and secretory responses in GT1 cells; $r = 0.97$. [Derived with permission from Krsmanovic *et al.* (6).]

VSCC by high K^+-induced depolarization in cultured hypothalamic neurons, GT1-1 neuronal cells (6, 7), and perifused hypothalamic explants (20, 21) increased GnRH release. (c) The amplitude of K^+-induced and spontaneous pulsatile GnRH release from hypothalamic explants, as well as from cultured hypothalamic neurons and GT1 neuronal cells, was sensitive to blockade by the dihydropyridine calcium-channel antagonist, nifedipine (6). (d) The dihydropyridine calcium-channel agonist, Bay K 8644, increased basal GnRH release and further amplified the K^+-induced secretory response (6). These findings indicate that hypothalamic neurons exhibit spontaneous activity via voltage-sensitive Ca^{2+} channels, which leads to elevation of $[Ca^{2+}]_i$ and GnRH release.

The present data provide additional evidence to support the conclusion that the $[Ca^{2+}]_i$ and secretory responses are interrelated, although it has yet to be shown that they occur with similar time courses. Figure 8A illustrates the dose-dependent effects of high K^+ on GnRH release in perifused GT1 cells cultured on beads. Such changes in the secretory responses were not related to changes in the medium osmolality, which was kept constant by adjustment of the NaCl concentration. The amplitudes of such GnRH secretory responses correlate with the amplitudes of $[Ca^{2+}]_i$ responses to the same K^+ concentrations. The Bay K 8644-induced rises in $[Ca^{2+}]_i$ also correlate with the amplitudes of GnRH responses to the same drug.

Conclusions

1. Ca^{2+} signaling in GnRH neurons can be analyzed when the integrity of the cells is preserved; dispersion of cells and presumably the concurrent cell detachment and damage of axons and dendrites attenuate the amplitudes of Ca^{2+} responses to Ca^{2+}-mobilizing as well as depolarizing agents.

2. Studies can be performed on single cells or cells incorporated in a neuronal network, depending on the initial density of cells and the age of culture. Both systems are appropriate for the analysis of Ca^{2+} signaling. The latter procedure is more useful for comparison with the secretory response in perifused cells, since in both cases the cells are integrated into a complex neuronal network (8).

3. A comparison of Ca^{2+} signaling in single cells vs cells in a network should permit the analysis of the differences that occur as consequences of the integration of cells into a more complex morphological and physiological system.

4. Single cells exhibit prominent spontaneous fluctuations in $[Ca^{2+}]_i$, with random frequencies and amplitudes that depend on entry of Ca^{2+} through VSCC. Cells in a network also show functional VSCC channels that display sensitivities to nifedipine and Bay K 8644 similar to those in single cells.

5. The extracellular $[Ca^{2+}]$ dependence of GnRH release from perifused hypothalamic cells parallels that of Ca^{2+} signaling and is consistent with the hypothesis that the electrical activity of GnRH neurons is a driving force in promoting Ca^{2+} entry and activation of Ca^{2+}-dependent GnRH exocytosis. In accord with this, a temporal correlation between the electrical activity of the arcuate nucleus and peripheral luteinizing hormone concentrations has been observed in rhesus monkeys (22).

6. The spontaneous fluctuations in $[Ca^{2+}]_i$ in GnRH-producing neurons can be modulated by activation of endothelin receptors, which predominantly activate a Ca^{2+} mobilization pathway (23). Since primary cultures of hypothalamic neurons also secrete endothelin (17), it is possible that this vasoactive peptide has the capacity to regulate neurosecretion and could participate in the hypothalamic control of anterior pituitary function and gonadotropin secretion. The larger amplitude of the endothelin-induced Ca^{2+}

responses in single cells vs cells in a network indicates that the sensitivity of the system to agonist stimulation is determined by the degree of connectivity between the cells.

7. The rises in $[Ca^{2+}]_i$ caused by activation of Ca^{2+} entry through VSCC and by agonist-induced mobilization of Ca^{2+}, both measured in the monolayer network, correlate with the increased secretion of GnRH in perifused GT1 cells. These findings indicate that in GnRH neurons, as in other neuronal cells, secretion is determined by rises in $[Ca^{2+}]_i$ that result from electrical and/or agonist stimulation.

Acknowledgments

L.Z.K. is on leave from the Institute of Biology, University of Novi Sad, Yugoslavia, and is supported by a grant from Sigma-Tau, Rome, Italy. D.J.S. is the recipient of a National Research Council—ADAMHA/NIH Research Associateship in Neuroscience. M.T. is on leave from the Faculty of Science, University of Zagreb, Croatia.

References

1. G. Chieffi, R. Pierantoni, and S. Fasano, *Intern. Rev. Cytol.* **127,** 1 (1991).
2. J. C. King and E. L. P. Anthony, *Peptides* **5** (Suppl. 1), 195 (1984).
3. E. Knobil, *Recent Prog. Hormone Res.* **36,** 53 (1980).
4. I. J. Clarke and J. T. Cummins, *Endocrinology (Baltimore)* **111,** 1737 (1982).
5. J. P. Bourguignon and P. Franchimont, *Endocrinology (Baltimore)* **114,** 1941 (1984).
6. L. Z. Krsmanovic, S. S. Stojilkovic, F. Merelli, S. M. Dufour, M. A. Virmani, and K. J. Catt, *Proc. Natl. Acad. Sci. U.S.A.* **89,** 8462 (1992).
7. G. M. Escalera, A. L. H. Choi, and R. I. Weiner, *Proc. Natl. Acad. Sci. U.S.A.* **89,** 1852 (1992).
8. W. C. Wetsel, M. M. Valenca, I. Merchenthaler, Z. Liposits, F. J. Lopez, R. I. Weiner, P. L. Mellon, and A. Negro-Vilar, *Proc. Natl. Acad. Sci. U.S.A.* **89,** 4149, 1992.
9. R. Llinas, M. Sugimori, and R. B. Silver, *Science* **256,** 677 (1992).
10. P. L. Mellon, J. J. Windle, P. C. Goldsmith, C. A. Padula, J. L. Roberts, and R. I. Weiner, *Neuron* **5,** 1 (1990).
11. R. A. Peterfreund and W. Vale, *Brain Res.* **239,** 463 (1982).
12. S. S. Stojilkovic, T. Iida, M. A. Virmani, S.-I. Izumi, E. Rojas, and K. J. Catt, *Proc. Natl. Acad. Sci. U.S.A.* **87,** 8855 (1990).
13. T. Iida, S. S. Stojilkovic, S.-I. Izumi, and K. J. Catt, *Mol. Endocrinol.* **5,** 949 (1991).
14. G. Grynkiewicz, M. Poenie, and R. W. Tsien, *J. Biol. Chem.* **260,** 3440 (1985).
15. Z. Liposits, I. Merchenthaler, W. C. Wetsel, J. J. Reid, P. L. Mellon, R. I. Weiner, and A. Negro-Vilar, *Endocrinology (Baltimore)* **129,** 1575 (1991).

16. M. I. Kotlikoff, R. K. Murray, and E. E. Reynolds, *Am. J. Physiol.* **253,** C561 (1987).

17. L. Z. Krsmanovic, S. S. Stojilkovic, T. Balla, S. A. Damluji, R. I. Weiner, and K. J. Catt, *Proc. Natl. Acad. Sci. U.S.A.* **88,** 11,124 (1991).

18. S. S. Stojilkovic and K. J. Catt, *Endocr. Rev.* **13,** 256 (1992).

19. J. J. Windle, R. I. Weiner, and P. L. Mellon, *Mol. Endocrinol.* **4,** 597 (1990).

20. S. V. Drouva, J. Epelbaum, M. Hery, L. T. Arancibia, E. Laplante, and C. Kordon, *Neuroendocrinology* **32,** 155 (1981).

21. H. Bigdeli and P. J. Snyder, *Endocrinology (Baltimore)* **103,** 281 (1978).

22. C. L. Williams, J. C. Thalabard, K. T. O'Byrne, P. M. Grosser, M. Nishihara, J. Hotchkiss, and E. Knobil, *Proc. Natl. Acad. Sci. U.S.A.* **87,** 8580 (1990).

23. S. S. Stojilkovic and K. J. Catt, *Trends Pharmacol. Sci.* **13,** 385 (1992).

[5] Patch-Clamp Studies on Identified Pituitary Gonadotropes *in Vitro*

Amy Tse and Bertil Hille

Introduction

Secretion of hormones from endocrine cells in the anterior pituitary regulates a variety of physiological functions including reproduction, lactation, growth, and metabolism. However, until recently cellular mechanisms underlying the stimulus–secretion coupling in these cells have been hard to study for two reasons: (i) It was difficult to isolate specific cell types from the heterogenous population of anterior pituitary cells; and (ii) the intracellular environment could not be manipulated or monitored accurately.

The gigaseal and patch-clamp recording methods of Hamill *et al.* (1) open up new approaches to cellular signaling questions. In the whole-cell configuration of this technique, a large-tipped pipette is in direct contact with the cytoplasmic compartment. The intracellular environment can then be altered by diffusing various activators or inhibitors of second messenger pathways, caged molecules, and ion-selective fluorescent indicator dyes into the cell. Hence roles of specific second messengers in cellular responses can be readily assessed at the single-cell level. At the same time it is possible to use the recording pipette to monitor exocytosis and endocytosis of secretory granules at high temporal resolution by an electrical method, membrane capacitance measurement. This method measures vesicular secretion from single cells by monitoring the resulting increases in cell membrane surface area. These techniques allow us to examine the molecular mechanisms underlying the stimulus–secretion coupling in endocrine cells.

To study anterior pituitary cells, it would be ideal to have a homogenous population of a specific cell type. For the more abundant cell types such as lactotropes or somatotropes which typically constitute nearly 50 and 35% of the entire anterior pituitary cell population, a highly enriched preparation can be obtained with Percoll-gradient centrifugation (2). However, similar enrichment of less-abundant cell types such as gonadotropes (typically 5–10% of the anterior pituitary cells) is less successful. The yield of gonadotropes can be increased by ovariectomy or by taking advantage of special anatomical features of certain animals, such as the pars tuberalis of sheep which bears mostly gonadotropes. For single-cell gigaseal work it is possible to work with an identified cell in a mixed cell population. In principle, the cell might be identified by binding of a fluorescent ligand (3), by calcium or electrophysiological responses to specific hormones, or because it secretes a certain hormone. The reverse hemolytic plaque assay (4) identifies specific cell types by the hormone(s) they secrete. In this assay, each pituitary cell is surrounded by a monolayer of erythrocytes preconjugated with a specific antihormone antibody. When stimulated by the appropriate secretagogue, the pituitary cells of interest will secrete the hormone into the medium. Binding of hormone to the antibodies on adjacent erythrocytes sensitizes the erythrocytes to lysis by complement, and, as a consequence, pituitary cells that secrete the right hormone will be surrounded by a zone of lysed erythrocytes (a plaque).

Here, we describe a plaque procedure to identify individual rat gonadotropes, which secrete luteinizing hormone and follicle-stimulating hormone in response to gonadotropin-releasing hormone (GnRH). We also illustrate how the stimulus–secretion coupling in gonadotropes is examined by adapting the whole-cell method for measuring intracellular Ca^{2+} and membrane capacitance.

Cell Preparation

Dissociation of Anterior Pituitary Cells

The anterior lobe of the pituitary gland is removed from the adult (35–45 days) rat (Sprague–Dawley) euthanized with CO_2. Since the ability of gonadotropes to secrete luteinizing hormone (LH) varies at different stages of the estrous cycle (5), we use only male rats. Anterior pituitary cells are enzymatically isolated using a procedure modified from that described for melanotropes (6). The dissected anterior pituitary gland is bathed in 2 ml of solution A, which contains the following (in mM): 137 NaCl; 5 KCl; 0.7 Na_2HPO_4; 10 glucose; 25 HEPES; 50 units/ml penicillin G and 150 μg/ml of streptomycin (Gibco), pH 7.4, with NaOH. Using a sterile scalpel blade, we cut the gland into small pieces. The pieces are harvested as a pellet by low-speed centrifugation (150 g for 5 min) and then resuspended in 1 ml of solution A supplemented with 2 mg/ml of collagenase type V (Sigma), 4 mg/ml bovine serum albumin fraction V (BSA; Sigma), and 20 μg/ml of deoxyribonuclease I (Sigma). After being incubated at 37°C for 30 min, the tissue is triturated 20–30 times with a Pasteur pipette fire-polished to narrow its tip. The suspension is mixed with 1 ml of solution A supplemented with 0.5 mg trypsin type XIII (Sigma) and 4 mg/ml of BSA and then incubated at 37°C for 15 min. Single cells are obtained by triturating the tissue suspension 40–50 times with a fire-polished Pasteur pipette. Cells are centrifuged

(150 g for 5 min) into a pellet and then resuspended in 200 μl of solution B which contains 0.1% BSA, 50 units/ml of penicillin G, and 50 μg/ml of streptomycin in Dulbecco's modified Eagle's medium (DMEM; Gibco).

Identification of Gonadotropes

Individual gonadotropes are identified by a reverse hemolytic plaque assay. Sheep erythrocytes (Colorado Serum Co; used within 21 days of collection) are first conjugated with *Staphylococcus aureus*-derived protein A (Sigma) using chromium chloride (0.2 mg/ml; Sigma) as the catalytic agent as described by Smith *et al.* (4). The pituitary cell suspension is mixed with an equal volume (200 μl) of 18% (v/v) erythrocytes in solution B at room temperature and infused via capillary action into a modified Cunningham chamber (7).

In our experiments, the bottom half of the Cunningham chamber is also used as a recording chamber. For recording current, membrane potential, or capacitance, any 35-mm plastic culture dish is suitable. However, for experiments in which an inverted microscope and fluorometry are employed to monitor intracellular calcium concentration ($[Ca^{2+}]_i$), it is essential that the bottom of the recording chamber be composed of thin glass instead of plastic because (i) the UV light used for excitation of fluorescent dye is largely absorbed by plastic; (ii) the large-numerical aperture oil objective typically employed for calcium measurement has a short working distance; and (iii) plastic can be dissolved by immersion oil. A thin glass-bottomed Cunningham chamber is constructed as follows. A circular hole of approximately 20 mm diameter is drilled in the bottom of a 35-mm plastic culture dish (Falcon). A 25-mm circular glass coverslip (VWR: No. 2) is cemented onto the bottom of the culture dish with Sylgard 184 elastomer (Dow Corning). The chamber is rinsed with 100% methanol and then several times with distilled water to remove any grease. To facilitate cell attachment, the bottom of the chamber is coated by adding 1 ml of 1% gelatin solution (Sigma). After 5 min, the solution is removed and the chamber is allowed to dry under UV light. The coating procedure is repeated with a 0.8 mg/ml concanavalin A solution (Sigma). We have less success with conventional polylysine coating. The roof of the Cunningham chamber is constructed by attaching a 12-mm circular coverslip onto two pieces of 3M double-sided Scotch tape (Cat. No. 136) placed approximately 10 mm apart on the bottom of the chamber. The volume of such a Cunningham chamber is approximately 8 μl.

The cell mixture (10–15 μl) is infused from one side of the chamber and slowly pulled across the chamber via capillary action with piece of Kimwipe. The chamber is incubated at 37°C for 1 hr in a 5% CO_2 incubator. Solution

B (20 μl) is then infused into the chamber to wash away any unattached cells, leaving a monolayer of cells stuck to the bottom of the chamber. Each pituitary cell should be surrounded by erythrocytes. Plaque formation is then initiated by infusing the chamber with 20 μl of solution B supplemented with 50 nM GnRH (Peninsula), rabbit polyclonal antibodies to rat LH (American Biochem), or bovine LH (courtesy of Dr. D. Leong, University of Virginia) at 1 : 50 dilution. After a 2-hr incubation at 37°C, the chamber is infused with 20 μl of solution B, followed by 20 μl guinea-pig complement at 1 : 50 dilution (Gibco) in solution B. Plaques can be observed after 30 min of incubation at 37°C. The complement reaction is terminated by infusing the chamber twice with 20 μl of solution B. To facilitate the removal of the double-sided Scotch tape, about 1 ml of solution C which contains 10% horse serum (Gibco), 50 units/ml of penicillin G, and 50 μg/ml of streptomycin in DMEM is added to the chamber, and the chamber is incubated for another 15 min at 37°C. Then the Scotch tape and the coverslip that forms the roof of the chamber are removed with a pair of fine-tipped forceps. Finally another 2 ml of solution C is added to the recording chamber. Plaques remain identifiable for up to 5 days under standard culture conditions.

Electrophysiological Recording

We employ standard whole-cell gigaseal techniques (8, 9). Gigaseals are relatively difficult to form on cells identified with the reverse hemolytic plaque assay, probably because the cell surface is cluttered with lysed erythrocytes and serum proteins. The probility of gigaseal formation is significantly improved by perfusing the cells with standard physiological saline for 5–10 min before attempting a seal.

For studying the effect of GnRH on gonadotropes, we routinely employ a rich internal (pipette) solution with 120 mM potassium aspartate, 20 mM KCl, 0.1 mM Na_4GTP, 2 mM $MgCl_2$, 2 mM Na_2ATP, and 20 mM HEPES (pH 7.4 with KOH). Figure 1 shows a typical electrophysiological response to GnRH application in an identified gonadotrope under voltage-clamp conditions. GnRH (1–10 nM) reliably initiates an oscillatory Ca^{2+}-activated K^+ current which is sensitive to the bee venom apamin (10). This current oscillation is a consequence of a G protein-initiated, rhythmic release of intracellular Ca^{2+} from the inositol triphosphate (IP_3)-sensitive stores. Because, during the response, GTP will be hydrolyzed by activated G proteins and ATP will be hydrolyzed by Ca^{2+} pumping, it is essential to include both GTP and ATP in the pipette solution to ensure a continuous supply of these nucleotides to the cytoplasm. Otherwise, endogenous GTP and ATP would gradually dialyze from the cell into the pipette during whole-cell recording. With our

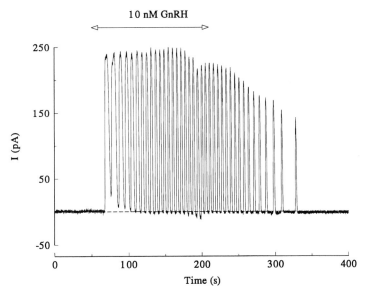

FIG. 1   Oscillations of membrane current induced by GnRH. The cell was voltage clamped at −50 mV in physiological saline. GnRH solution was perfused into the bath during the period marked with arrows. In cells challenged with GnRH continuously, the current oscillations persist without decrement.

internal solution, GnRH responses can persist for more than 30 min of whole-cell recording.

We omit Ca^{2+} chelators from the pipette solution to avoid blunting the Ca^{2+} rise that mediates the GnRH response. However, the absence of a Ca^{2+} chelator increases the tendency of the ruptured membrane to reform under the pipette tip, thus interrupting whole-cell recording, particularly at elevated $[Ca^{2+}]_i$. It is helpful, therefore, to use pipettes with fairly large tips. Ours are made from hematocrit glass (VWR Scientific), and the tip is coated with Sylgard 184 silicone elastomer (Dow Corning) and then fire-polished. Pipette resistances are typically 1.5–3 MΩ after being filled with internal solution, and, during whole-cell recording, the series resistance is typically between 5 and 10 MΩ.

An alternative to the whole-cell method is the perforated-patch technique (11), where the patch membrane is not broken open but rather is lightly permeabilized with an antibiotic like nystatin. This has the advantage of disturbing the cytoplasmic environment less and minimizing the loss of metabolites and cytoplasmic proteins. We have employed the perforated-patch technique on gonadotropes and observed GnRH responses similar to those recorded with the whole-cell method, suggesting fortunately that cytoplasmic elements essential for the GnRH response are mostly conserved during whole-cell recording under our experimental conditions.

An advantage of whole-cell over perforated-patch recording is that intracellular activators or inhibitors of second messenger systems can be dialyzed into the cell via the recording pipette. For example, one line of evidence for the involvement of G proteins in the GnRH-induced Ca^{2+} oscillations in gonadotropes is the suppression of the response by intracellular dialysis of GDPβS, an inhibitor of G protein function. For small spherical cells such as gonadotropes (cell diameter 12–18 μm), molecules from the pipette can diffuse rapidly into the cell. The rate at which substances diffuse from the pipette into the cell has been measured in various systems and can be described by empirical equations with measurable quantities. We use the equation of Pusch and Neher (12),

$$\tau = (0.60 \pm 0.17) \, R_A M^{1/3} \, (r/7.68)^3 \tag{1}$$

where τ is the diffusion time constant in seconds, R_A is the pipette series resistance in MΩ, M is the molecular weight of the substance, and r is the cell radius in micrometers. According to this equation, for a gonadotrope with cell radius of 8 μm and a pipette series resistance of 5 MΩ, the diffusion of GDPβS (MW 477) into the cell will have a predicted time constant of ~27 sec.

Measurement of $[Ca^{2+}]_i$

Several fluorescent dyes have been optimized for optical measurements of $[Ca^{2+}]_i$ by the ratio method (13). They can be either dialyzed into the cell in the free-acid form via the patch pipette or loaded into cells using the membrane-permeant acetoxymethyl (AM) ester form, which is hydrolyzed inside the cell to yield the free acid. The AM-loading method is simpler, but may present problems such as compartmentalization of dye or incomplete ester cleavage. Use of AM loading is described by Stojilkovic et al. in Chapter 4, this volume. We describe here loading of the dye Indo-1 via the patch pipette, which we have used since we were already doing electrophysiology.

Our measurements are made with an inverted Nikon Diaphot epifluorescence microscope as shown schematically in Fig. 2. Light from an HBO 100-W mercury lamp (Nikon) is passed through an electronic shutter (Uniblitz, VS25E2WO), two neutral-density filters (0.7 and 1.0; Rolyn optics), an adjustable diaphragm (Nikon), and then a bandpass filter (365 ± 15 nm; Omega). The resultant light is reflected into the epiillumination light path of the micro-

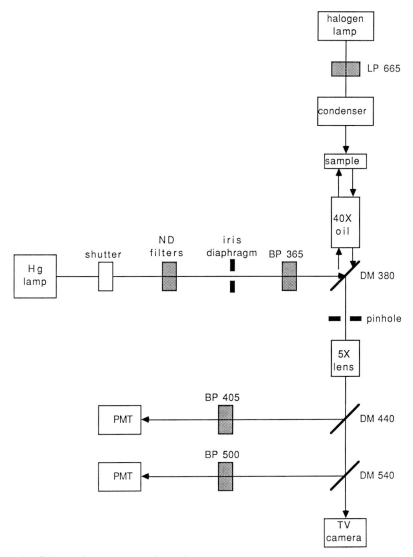

FIG. 2   Schematic representation of the optical setup for Indo fluorometry. For conventional brightfield and video viewing of the cells, light from the halogen lamp of the microscope was longpass filtered at 665 nm. Optics for Indo fluorometry are as described in text. LP, longpass filter; ND, neutral density; DM, dichroic mirror; BP, bandpass filter; and PMT, photomultiplier tubes.

scope via a dichroic mirror (380 nm) and then delivered via a 40X, 1.3 NA UV fluor oil objective (Nikon) to excite Indo-1 in the cell. The fluorescence (<390 nm) from the cell passes through the dichroic mirror to a 1-mm pinhole which is inserted before a 5X projection lens in the video port of the microscope. The adjustable diaphragm of the illuminator is set to illuminate a 25-μm circular spot on the stage and the 1-mm pinhole restricts the light collection to the same spot (25 μm = 1 mm/40). This "confocal" arrangement helps to reduce background fluorescence from Indo-1 in the pipette. Fluorescence is then collected by two photon-counting photomultiplier tubes (Hamamatsu, H3460-04) at 405 and 500 nm. The discriminator logic levels of the photomultiplier tubes are translated to TTL signals and counted by a CYCTM-10 counter card (Cyber Research) plugged into a PC computer. The computer controls the frequency of measurements, the duration of the shutter opening, and the duration of the photon counting. The shutter is normally closed to avoid photodynamic damage and bleaching of dye. It is commanded to open 7–9 msec before counting begins, allowing enough time to reach full opening. Fluorescence at the two wavelengths is counted simultaneously for 5–20 msec and stored on the computer, along with the time at which the measurement is made. The background counts measured after forming a cell-attached seal, but before breakthrough, are subtracted. Fluorescence is typically measured at 100- to 500-msec intervals. It is essential to use a nonfluorescent immersion oil.

An advantage of the pipette-loading method for dyes is that one can reproducibly achieve and maintain the same intracellular dye concentration each time. In order to avoid damping the Ca signal, the intracellular concentration of Indo-1 should be low; however, sufficient dye must be present to give a fluorescence intensity well above background. We typically use 0.1 mM Indo-1 and see a fluorescence 30–50 times above background. An example of the time course of dialysis of Indo-1 (MW 838) is shown in Fig. 3. The time-dependent increase of the two fluorescence signals is well described by single exponentials with time constants near 65 sec, values about twice that predicted by Eq. (1). Thus, Indo-1 dialysis is essentially complete within 200 sec after the establishment of whole-cell mode. Because calcium measurements are based on fluorescence ratios, measurements can begin before the diffusional steady state is reached.

In some experiments, membrane current or capacitance is monitored simultaneously with $[Ca^{2+}]_i$. To synchronize these signals, the ratio (R) of the fluorescence (405 nm/500 nm) is calculated on-line and output via a digital-to-analog converter to one of the four channels in an FM tape recorder (Racal). Current or capacitance signals are recorded on the other channels simultaneously. The data are digitized later.

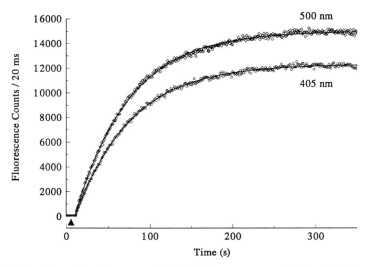

FIG. 3   Time-dependent increase of Indo-1 fluorescence at 405 and 500 nm. The triangle marks the time at which whole-cell recording was established. Background at both wavelengths is subtracted (typically 200–400 counts/20 msec). The solid lines are exponential fits with time constants of 65.6 sec at 405 nm and 64.5 sec at 500 nm. The cell membrane capacitance was 5 pF and the pipette series resistance was 6 MΩ.

$[Ca^{2+}]_i$ is calculated from the ratio (R) of fluorescence (405 nm/500 nm), using the equation (15),

$$[Ca^{2+}]_i = K^* (R - R_{min})/(R_{max} - R) \qquad (2)$$

where R_{min} is the fluorescence ratio of Ca^{2+}-free Indo-1 and R_{max} is the ratio of Ca^{2+}-bound Indo-1. $K^* = K_d (S_{f2}/S_{b2})$ where K_d is the dissociation constant of the Ca^{2+}-bound Indo-1 complex, and S_{f2} and S_{b2} are the fluorescence of the Ca^{2+}-free and Ca^{2+}-bound form of Indo-1 at 500 nm.

Calibrations are performed by measuring Indo fluorescence from groups of gonadotropes dialyzed with three pipette solutions. R_{min} is measured in cells loaded with (in mM) 62 potassium aspartate, 50 HEPES, 50 EGTA, 0.1 Indo-1, pH 7.40 (with KOH); R_{max} is measured in cells loaded with (in mM) 136 potassium aspartate, 50 HEPES, 15 $CaCl_2$, 0.1 Indo-1, pH 7.40 (with KOH). K^* is calculated from Eq. (2) using the ratio obtained from cells loaded with (in mM) 60 potassium aspartate, 50 HEPES, 20 EGTA, 15 $CaCl_2$, 0.1 Indo-1, pH 7.40, which has a calculated free Ca^{2+} concentration of 146 nM at 24°C (16). The calibration constants tend to vary as the output characteristics of the lamp change slowly during its 200-hr lifetime. Therefore, we normally recalibrate every 60–70 lamp hours. Since these calibrations, particularly R_{max}, also change significantly with slight changes in alignment of the optics, we always recalibrate if any of the filters or the position of the lamp is altered.

An alternative method of calibration is to determine the calibration constants from miniature cuvettes filled with pipette solutions. However, we found that this procedure yeilds calibration constants that would overestimate the free [Ca^{2+}] inside cells. It is generally agreed that the fluorescence properties of these dyes are affected by the local viscosity and by protein binding.

Photolysis of Caged Compounds

Caged compounds, which can be converted to biologically active molecules by photolysis, are valuable tools in studies of intracellular messenger pathways. Short pulses of UV light (360 nm) from a flash lamp or laser are typically used for photolysis (17), and the result is a rapid increase in the concentration of active molecules. As Indo-1 is excited by light of similar wavelengths, caged compounds can be photolyzed during Indo fluorometry. Although the intensity of illumination during fluorometry is much lower than that of a flash lamp, under our experimental conditions, caged compounds can be included in the pipette solution and will be slowly photolyzed when the open time of the light-controlling shutter is lengthened during Indo measurements. Figure 4 shows an example of photolysis of caged IP$_3$ (10 μM) in a gonadotrope. Because the UV illumination was focused via the objective (see Fig. 2), only the caged IP$_3$ in the cell and in the tip of the pipette photolyzes. Under this condition, sufficient IP$_3$ was liberated to induce a couple of [Ca^{2+}]$_i$ oscillations (Fig. 4). The caged IP$_3$ in the unilluminated part of the pipette will dialyze into the cell continuously. Therefore, such photolysis of IP$_3$ can be repeated many times, as long as sufficient time is allowed between attempts so that more caged IP$_3$ can dialyze into the cell.

Measurement of Secretion

Most studies of pituitary secretion assay the hormone released from a large population of cells and are limited to sampling intervals longer than 1 sec. The capacitance method, on the other hand, measures changes of plasma membrane surface area in a single cell with a sensitivity approaching one

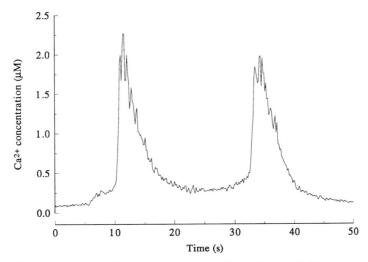

FIG. 4 Slow photolysis of intracellular caged IP$_3$ induces [Ca^{2+}]$_i$ oscillations in gonadotropes. The pipette contained 10 μM caged IP$_3$. To increase UV light illumination on the cell, the shutter was opened for 85 msec every 100 msec, throughout the 50-sec period of the experiment. Sufficient IP$_3$ was generated in the cell to elicit a couple of Ca^{2+} oscillations. The fluorescence at 405 and 500 nm was integrated for 5 msec.

vesicle and on a time scale of milliseconds. Furthermore, since it is based on the whole-cell gigaseal method, one can simultaneously do electrophysiology and dialyze in test molecules. Because biological membranes have a rather constant specific capacitance of 10 fF/μm^2, any increase in membrane area is associated with a proportional increase of the membrane capacitance. For example, in gonadotropes, the secretory vesicle has a diameter of about 200 nm and thus should contribute a 1.3 fF increase in membrane capacitance during exocytosis.

Several methods exist to determine capacitance. Some of the latest patch-clamp amplifiers can monitor capacitance automatically and continuously without further apparatus. Most workers, however, use a sinewave excitation and analyze the resulting currents either by a computer program (18) or by a lock-in amplifier (19). We use a two-phase lock-in amplifier in our experiments because it can monitor small capacitance changes with low background noise. The theory of this technique has been extensively reviewed (19, 20) and variants of this technique have also been described (21).

For accurate measurement of small changes in membrane capacitance, the tip of the pipette must be coated (e.g., with Slygard 184 elastomer) to reduce the pipette capacitance. Using the fast transient cancellation circuit of the patch-clamp amplifier, we carefully cancel any remaining stray capacitance from the pipette and the headstage of the amplifier after forming of a cell-attached seal. Following the establishment of the whole-cell configuration, the series resistance of the pipette and the membrane capacitance of the cell are also neutralized by the patch-clamp amplifier and the cell is voltage clamped at a holding potential of -70 mV. An 800-Hz sinusoidal wave of 30-mV peak-to-peak amplitude (generated by the lock-in amplifier) is then superimposed on the holding potential. Since the output of the lock-in amplifier is proportional to the amplitude of the sinusoidal wave, a large-amplitude sinusoidal wave will increase the resolution of the output signals. However, the capacitance measurement is based on the assumption that the membrane conductance of the cell is unchanging in the range of voltages covered by the sinusoidal wave. Therefore, when superimposed on the holding potential, the amplitude of the sinusoidal wave should remain in a range where most voltage-gated ion channels are closed. The choice for the frequency of sinusoidal wave is governed by several factors including the cell membrane capacitance, the series resistance of the pipette electrode, and the leakage conductance of the cell. The lock-in amplifier can measure changes in capacitance only when $\omega < G_a/C_m$ (ω is the angular frequency, G_a is the series conductance of the pipette, and C_m is the cell membrane capacitance). For example, when recording from a 5-pF gonadotrope with a pipette series resistance of 10 MΩ ($G_a = 0.1$ μS), the upper limit of the angular frequency ω is 2×10^4 radian/sec or 3.2 kHz. Up to the limit set by G_a/C_m, the signal-to-noise ratio of the lock-in amplifier's output increases with the frequency of the sinusoidal wave. However, a higher frequency sinusoidal wave will contribute larger error in the capacitance measurement if the pipette series resistance is unstable during the time course of the experiment. For gonadotropes, we determined empirically that a frequency of 800 Hz is appropriate.

The two-phase lock-in amplifier has two outputs, a real component signal (Y_1) and an imaginary component (Y_2). When the phase angle of the amplifier is set correctly, Y_1 will be proportional to $\Delta G_m - \Delta G_a \omega^2 C_m^2/G_a^2$ (G_m = membrane conductance) and Y_2 will be proportional to changes in membrane capacitance (ΔC_m). There are two methods to set the phase angle in the lock-in amplifier. In the first method, the phase is found by slightly deflecting the setting of the whole-cell capacitance compensation circuit in the patch-clamp amplifier (to simulate small changes in membrane capacitance) while adjusting the phase-angle setting on the lock-in amplifier until the change is maximal in Y_2 and minimal in Y_1. In the second method, the phase is set by simulating changes in series resistance. This is done by installing a 1-MΩ resistor between the bath electrode and the electrical ground. This resistor is switched momentarily in and out, and the phase-angle setting in the lock-

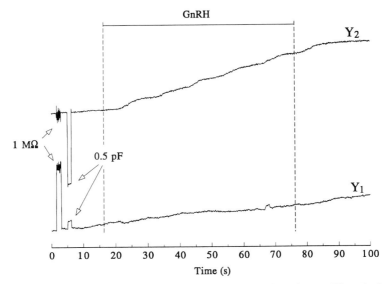

FIG. 5   Calibrating the real and imaginary outputs of a lock-in amplifier. Switching
in the 1-MΩ resistor resulted in a large deflection in Y_1 but little change in Y_2,
indicating that the phase angle in the lock-in amplifier was set correctly. The setting
of the whole-cell capacitance neutralization in the patch-clamp amplifier was then
decreased momentarily by 0.5 pF which resulted in the downward deflection of Y_2.
The amplitude of this deflection in Y_2 was later used as a calibration (0.5 pF) for
calculating changes in membrane capacitance. GnRH (50 nM) was pressure applied
from a puffer pipette (which also contained 1 μM apamin) during the period indicated
by the bars and the C_m signal (Y_2) increased in waves of exocytosis. The small change
in Y_1 probably reflects a slight increase in pipette series resistance.

in amplifier is adjusted until the change is maximal in Y_1 and minimal in Y_2.
These methods give similar results; however, the second approach is more
effective in reducing the errors in the measurement of capacitance change
(Y_2) due to changes of pipette series resistance. Figure 5 shows the two
outputs of the lock-in amplifier when the phase was set by this method. After
the correct phase-angle setting in the lock-in amplifier is found, the setting
of the whole-cell capacitance neutralization in the patch-clamp amplifier is
deflected by 0.5 pF, and the corresponding change in Y_2 is used for calibrating
the membrane capacitance changes.

The major source of error in capacitance measurements is that the phase
angle can change significantly due to large variations in the parameters C_m,
G_a, and G_m during the experiments. For gonadotropes, the variations in C_m
are usually small and thus contribute little error. However, GnRH application

results in oscillation of Ca^{2+}-activated potassium current, which in turn gives rise to periodic variations in G_m. Therefore, in the experiment shown in Fig. 5, apamin was included in the bath solution to block the Ca^{2+}-activated potassium conductance. To minimize changes in G_a, we use low-resistance pipettes. Since the output signal Y_1 is dependent on both G_m and G_a, the stable Y_1 signal in Fig. 5 indicates that variations in G_a and G_m are minimal under our experimental conditions. Another source of error is fluctuations in bathing solution levels during agonist application. An unstable solution level leads to changes in both Y_1 and Y_2 signals. Therefore, we prefer to apply GnRH by pressure from a puffer pipette while the cell is continuously perfused. Figure 5 shows an example of the GnRH effect on the membrane capacitance of a gonadotrope. The membrane capacitance of this cell increases approximately 0.5 pF, reflecting an exocytosis of roughly 400 secretory vesicles.

Summary

This chapter describes techniques used to examine the mechanisms underlying the GnRH response in gonadotropes. Similar procedures should be applicable for studying the stimulus–secretion coupling in other pituitary cells.

Acknowledgments

We thank Drs. W. Almers and F. W. Tse for assistance on experiments with calcium and capacitance measurements and Drs. F. W. Tse, J. Herrington, A. Iwata, and J. Kirillova for reading the manuscript. This work was supported by NIH Grants NS-08174 and HD-12629 and awards from the McKnight Foundation, the W. M. Keck Foundation, and the Mellon Foundation.

References

1. O. P. Hamill, A. Marty, E. Neher, B. Sakmann, and F. J. Sigworth, *Pfluegers Arch.* **391,** 85 (1981).
2. W. T. Mason and C. D. Ingram, *in* "Methods in Enzymology" (P. M. Conn, ed.), Vol. 124, p. 207. Academic Press, San Diego, 1986.)
3. C. Marchetti, G. V. Childs, and A. M. Brown, *Am. J. Physiol.* **252,** E340 (1987).
4. P. F. Smith, E. H. Luque, and J. D. Neill, *in* "Methods in Enzymology" (P. M. Conn, ed.), Vol. 124, p. 443. Academic Press, San Diego, 1986.

5. P. F. Smith, L. S. Frawley, and J. D. Neill, *Endocrinology* (*Baltimore*) **115,** 2484 (1984).

6. P. Thomas, A. Surprenant, and W. Almers, *Neuron* **5,** 723 (1990).

7. A. J. Cunningham and A. Szenberg, *Immunology* **14,** 599 (1968).

8. B. Sakmann and E. Neher, "Single Channel Recording." Plenum, New York, 1983.

9. B. Rudy and L. E. Iverson, *in* "Methods in Enzymology," (B. Rudy and L. E. Iverson, eds.), Vol. 207. Academic Press, San Diego, 1992.

10. A. Tse and B. Hille, *Science* **255,** 462 (1992).

11. R. Horn and A. Marty, *J. Gen. Physiol.* **92,** 145 (1988).

12. M. Pusch and E. Neher, *Pfluegers Arch.* **411,** 204 (1988).

13. R. Y. Tsien, *Trends Neurosci.* **11,** 419 (1988).

14. S. S. Stojilkovic, L. Z. Kramenovic, D. J. Spergel, M. Tomic, and K. J. Catt, Chapter 4, this volume.

15. G. Grynkiewicz, M. Poenie, and R. Y. Tsien, *J. Biol. Chem.* **260,** 3440 (1985).

16. J. R. Blinks, W. G. Wier, P. Hess, and F. G. Prendergast, *Prog. Biophys. Mol. Biol.* **40,** 1 (1982).

17. J. W. Walker, A. V. Somlyo, Y. E. Goldman, A. P. Somlyo, and D. R. Trentham, *Nature* (*London*) **327,** 249 (1987).

18. C. Joshi and J. M. Fernandez, *Biophys. J.* **53,** 885 (1988).

19. M. Lindau and E. Neher, *Pfluegers Arch.* **411,** 137 (1988).

20. M. Lindau, *Q. Rev. Biophys.* **24,** 75 (1991).

21. R. Zorec, F. Henigman, W. T. Mason, and M. Kordas, "Methods in Neuroscience," Vol. 4, p. 194. Academic Press, San Diego, 1990.

[6] Electrophysiological Analysis of GnRH Pulse Generator Activity in the Rhesus Monkey

Kevin T. O'Byrne and Ernst Knobil

Introduction

The rhythmic pulsatile pattern of luteinizing hormone (LH) secretion, first noted in primates (1, 2) and subsequently in all mammals studied (3), is consequent to the episodic discharge of gonadotropin-releasing hormone (GnRH) into the hypophysial portal blood (4–7). This finding gave rise to the concept of a neural "oscillator" or "pulse generator" in the central nervous system that is responsible for the rhythmic activation of GnRH cells and the release of the neurohormone from their terminals. In the rhesus monkey, using the classic neuroendocrine techniques of radiofrequency lesions (8) and surgical disconnection (9), the GnRH pulse generator has been localized to the arcuate nuclear region of the mediobasal hypothalamus.

Many strategies have been used to monitor GnRH pulse generator activity, in addition to the detection of LH pulses in the peripheral blood. These have included the measurement of GnRH pulses in pituitary portal blood (4–7; Caraty *et al.*, chapter 9, this volume), in cerebrospinal fluid (10), and in hypothalamic extracellular fluid sampled by microperfusion (11, 12; Terasawa, chapter 10, this volume) and microdialysis (13; Levine *et al.*, chapter 8, this volume). Efforts in our own laboratory have centered on monitoring the electrophysiological correlates of GnRH pulse generator activity* in the rhesus monkey. This approach was based on the supposition that each bolus of GnRH released into the hypophyseal portal blood must be the consequence of the synchronous discharge of a large number of GnRH neurons. Knowing its location and having an unambiguous marker of its activity (LH pulses in the peripheral circulation), our strategy was to place recording electrodes in the mediobasal hypothalamus in the hope of finding evidence for the changes in electrical activity associated with the rhythmic activation of GnRH cells.

* The GnRH pulse generator is defined as the neuronal construct that eventuates in the pulsatile discharge of LH into the peripheral circulation. The activity of the GnRH pulse generator can be assessed by the monitoring of pulsatile LH secretion and/or any antecedent or associated event such as GnRH release, the electrophysiological manifestations of an associated neurosecretory process, as used here, or other cognate phenomena.

Methods in Neurosciences, Volume 20

The multiunit recording technique, described earlier for the study of the hypothalamic magnocellular system in the rhesus monkey by Hayward was initially employed (14). Early experiments utilizing single, acutely placed tungsten electrodes to record hypothalamic multiunit activity (MUA) in monkeys, while largely unsuccessful, occasionally yielded evidence of striking MUA increases (MUA volleys) correlated with pulses of LH as measured in the peripheral circulation (15, 16). The paucity of successful electrode placements in the monkey was atttributed to the sparsity of active sites in the hypothalamus and led us to change our strategy to the stereotaxic bilateral implantation of chronic multiple electrode arrays that essentially blanketed the entire mediobasal hypothalamus. This approach yielded unambiguous and reproducible electrophysiologic evidence of GnRH pulse generator activity in the rhesus monkey (17).

Preparation and Implantation of Recording Electrodes

Construction of Electrodes

Multiple electrode arrays are implanted bilaterally in the mediobasal hypothalamus in each monkey. Each electrode assembly, modified from a previously described design (18), consists of nine 50-μm insulated Nichrome wires (California Fine Wire Company, Grover City, CA) encased in a 22-gauge stainless steel tube and square cut with a pair of sharp scissors to extend 3–5 mm beyond its tip (Fig. 1). Each recording wire is secured with epoxy solder (E-Solder No. 3021, Acme, New Haven, CT) to a separate contact pin on a mini connector (Augat 8058-IG34, Augat, Inc., Attleboro, MA) attached to the head of the tube and the contacts encased in dental acrylic cement (Modern Materials, Miles, Inc., South Bend, IN). The impedance of each electrode is measured in normal saline *in vitro* (electrode impedance tester, Model IMP-1, BAK Electronics, Inc., Clarksburg, MD). An upper limit of 300 kΩ is acceptable for use. The electrodes are gently teased into an evenly spaced splay measuring 4–5 mm in the anterior–posterior axis and about 1 mm in the mediolateral axis. The flexible electrodes are retracted into an outer 18-gauge guide tube for protection during implantation. Extension of the retracted electrodes is prevented during implantation by locating a plastic spacer, exactly 5 mm in depth, between the head of the outer guide tube and the Augat connector (Fig. 1) and the guide tube is held fast to the remainder of the assembly with three small strips of adhesive tape. The outer 18-gauge guide tube cut to a length of 32–36 mm, the inner 22-gauge tube, and its attachment to the Augat connector are constructed

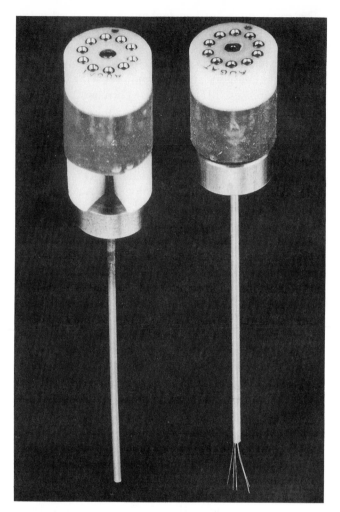

FIG. 1   The recording electrode assembly. A removable spacer between the electrode connector block and the head of the outer guide tube permits retraction of the recording wires within the guide tube (left). On the right, the spacer has been removed and the electrodes extruded (17).

in our machine shop. The electrodes have impedances of 100–300 kΩ measured *in vivo*.

Stereotaxic Procedures

The electrode assemblies are prealigned by placing them in electrode manipulators (David Kopf Instruments, Tujunga, CA) mounted on a stereotaxic frame (David Kopf Instruments). The manipulators are set to an angle of 8° from the vertical in the mediolateral axis and the tip of the electrodes is aligned with the center of the ear bar tips to obtain "ear bar zero" coordinates. The electrode assemblies and manipulators are gas-sterilized using ethylene oxide (Anprolene, H. W. Andersen Products, Inc., Chapel Hill, NC).

A radiographic technique is used to monitor the placement of the electrodes in the mediobasal hypothalamus. The animals are anesthetized with sodium pentobarbital (Nembutal, 25 mg/kg) and mounted in the stereotaxic frame which is accurately aligned with the X-ray beam for a lateral exposure, using specially constructed "alignment rods" demarcating ear bar zero in the vertical and horizontal planes. The left and right vertical alignment rods are held in Kopf electrode manipulators mounted on the stereotaxic frame and the horizontal alignment rods are inserted into special sockets machined in the side of the ear bars. Using the light beam from the X-ray head the stereotaxic frame is adjusted until the shadows cast by the two sets of alignment rods are superimposed. Alignment is verified roentgenographically.

Asepsis is maintained throughout the implantation procedure. The scalp is scrubbed with an antiseptic solution (Cliniscrub, Clinipad Co., Guilford, CT), an 8-cm midline incision made, the skin retracted, and the periosteum removed from the exposed calvaria. A radioopaque dye (Amipaque, 200 mg iodine/ml, Winthrop Pharmaceuticals, NY) is injected into a lateral ventricle using a 22-gauge, 63.5-mm-long, spinal needle (Becton–Dickinson Co., Franklin Lakes, NJ) initially filled with normal saline inserted, through a hole trephined in the skull, 19 mm anterior to ear bar zero and 2 mm laterally from the midline to a depth of 20 mm below the dura. Following entry of the needle into the ventricle, identified by a sudden drop in the saline meniscus in the hub of the spinal needle, 0.3 ml of the radioopaque solution is infused and a lateral X-ray exposure made 30 sec later with a 108-msec exposure at 74 kV using a mobile X-ray unit (Model KCD-IOM-6C = B, Toshiba Corp., Shibaura Electric Co., Ltd., Tokyo). The X-ray film (Kodak type XRP) is developed by a Kodak RP X-OMAT processor (Model M7B, Eastman–Kodak Co., Rochester, NY). The stereotaxic coordinates of the target chosen to be 1–1.5 mm posterior and 1 mm dorsal to the infundibular recess of the third ventricle and 0.4 mm lateral to the midline are calculated from the ventriculogram after appropriate magnification corrections are made using a Hewlett–Packard calculator (Model HP-41CV, Hewlett–Packard, Corvallis, OR) programmed with the appropriate trigonometric equations. After two holes are drilled in the skull and the underlying dura is punctured the two electrode assemblies are lowered simultaneously to within 5 mm of the target. The spacer between the outer guide and the Augat connector is then removed and the electrode wires are extruded from the guide tube to splay out within the arcuate area. The electrode assemblies are then secured to the calvaria by four stainless steel screws and dental acrylic cement impregnated with Vancomycin (Eli Lilly & Co., Indianapolis, IN). Placement of the electrode tips is verified at the end of the procedure by a final X-ray (Fig. 2).

Recording of Neuronal Activity

Restrained Animals

The rhesus monkeys (*Macaca mulatta;* 5–10 kg) used in these studies are obtained from the University of Pittsburgh Primate Research Laboratory. They are fed once daily with Purina monkey chow, supplemented with fresh fruit three times weekly. Water is available *ad libitum*. The monkeys are placed in primate chairs (BAK MC-D; BAK Electronics, Inc.) located in a shielded recording room. Using a "hard-wired" system (Fig. 3) the electrodes are connected to a high-impedance probe (Model CFP-1020, $> 10^3$ MΩ, BAK Electronics, Inc.) using an Augat connector plugged into the socket on the animal's head. The signals are then passed through Grass high-input impedance modules (Model H1P511E, 10^{10} Ω; Grass Instruments, Quincy, MA) to a bank of Grass P511 amplifiers (Grass Instruments) to provide amplification (50,000×) and filtering (300 Hz–1 KHz bandwidth). The probe is mounted within a protective cylindrical plastic container (hat) which is then affixed by four screws to a Plexiglas adapter ring attached to the animal's acrylic head platform (Fig. 3). The noise level of this recording system is less than 10 μV. Peak amplitude of the MUA signal ranged from 15 to 40 μV. MUA discharge frequencies following amplitude discrimination (19) using a window discriminator (WPI Model 121, WP Instruments, Inc., New Haven, CT) are processed as activity rates, in 1-min bins, using a data acquisition system (Dataquest III, Data Sciences, St. Paul, MN) on an IBM-XT computer. The discrimination level on the window discriminator is usually set to give 1000–2000 counts/min. Before connecting the probe to the monkey the system is tested with a signal generator (Model Omnical 2001, WP Instruments, Inc.). During each experiment MUA signals from nine electrodes are recorded and analyzed simultaneously.

Throughout the recording sessions, blood samples (1 ml) are collected at 10-min intervals from chronic indwelling cardiac catheters. The distal end of the catheter is tunneled subcutaneously to the back of the head and attached to a vascular access port consisting of a blunt needle hub covered with a rubber injection cap. This assembly is encased in silicone adhesive (Dow Corning Co., Midland, MI), coated in Vancomycin (Eli Lilly & Co.), placed subcutaneously, and accessed by transcutaneous penetration with a 21-gauge butterfly needle (Abbott Hospitals, Inc., North Chicago, IL) (17).

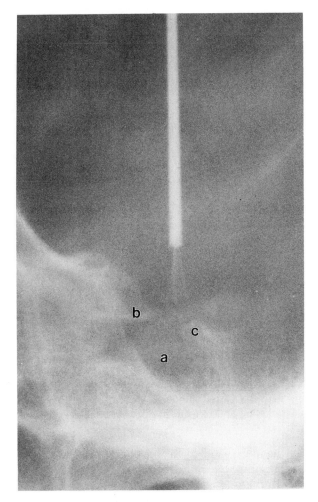

F IG. 2   Example of a lateral X-ray showing the electrode wires extruded from the guide tube splayed in the arcuate region of the mediobasal hypothalamus. a, Sella turcica; b, anterior clinoid process; c, posterior clinoid process.

Before the butterfly needle is introduced into the subcutaneous port the overlying skin is shaved and scrubbed thoroughly with an antiseptic solution (Cliniscrub, Clinipad Co.). The LH concentrations in serum of ovariectomized animals are determined by radioimmunoassay (RIA) (17) and, in intact monkeys, by bioassay (20). In our initial studies it was noted that pulses of LH could be observed in restrained ovariectomized monkeys but not in

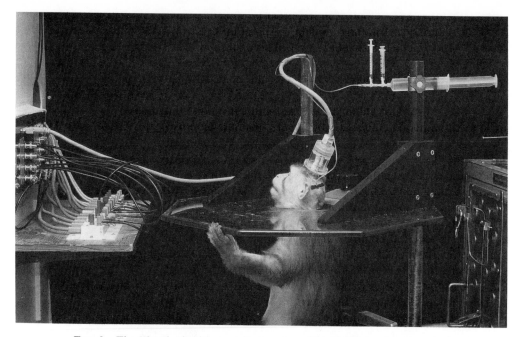

Fig. 3 The "hard-wired" recording system. The high-impedance probe is mounted in a plastic housing affixed to the acrylic electrode platform of the rhesus monkey placed in a primate chair. The probe leads to a panel of terminals which connect to a bank of Grass high-input impedance modules mounted on the shelf that in turn connect to the Grass amplifiers located outside the shielded recording room. For blood sampling a butterfly needle is inserted in the subcutaneous vascular access port.

intact animals handled in the same manner (1). After habituation to chair restraint, however, pulsatile LH secretion was reestablished suggesting that the perturbations associated with catching and restraint in primate chairs resulted in the arrest of GnRH pulse generator activity. For this reason, all ovary-intact animals are now habituated to primate chairs on a schedule of 6-hr restraint once or twice per month (21).

All the electrodes are "screened" for the characteristic MUA volleys associated with the initiation of each LH pulse in the peripheral circulation (Fig. 4) and the active ones identified for use in subsequent studies.

Unrestrained Monkeys

A radiotelemetric recording system has been developed to exploit the possibility of the continuous monitoring of GnRH pulse generator activity in unrestrained monkeys in physiological settings for unlimited periods of time.

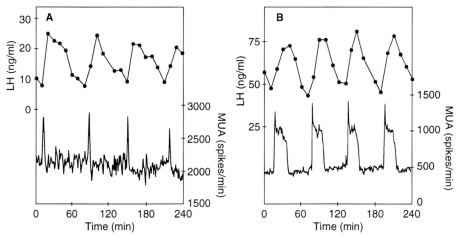

FIG. 4   Multiunit electrical activity (MUA) recorded from the mediobasal hypothalamus and LH pulses measured in the peripheral circulation in an ovary-intact animal on Day 5 of the follicular phase of the menstrual cycle (A) and in a long-term (8 months) ovariectomized monkey (B). The duration of the MUA volleys in the intact animal approximates the duration of the "overshoot" in the ovariectomized monkey (30).

For this purpose, single-channel wide-band FM transmitters (Petron Industries, Houston, TX) are constructed using low-power complementary metal-oxide silicon integrated circuitry, a nondifferential input amplifier with an input noise of 10–12 μV peak-to-peak and impedance of 10^{10} Ω, a voltage regulator, and a voltage-controlled Hartley oscillator. The normal operating band is 95–108 MHz. The signal deviation is $\pm$50 KHz with a 50 μV peak input signal. Powered by 3.0-V lithium batteries (Type CR 2477.IB, Renata SA. CH-4452 Itingen, Switzerland), the transmitters operate continuously for more than 30 days. The transmitter is mounted within a protective cylindrical plastic container which is then affixed by four screws to a plastic adapter ring attached to the animal's acrylic head platform (Fig. 5), and the connection between the transmitter and the selected electrode is established. However, before mounting the transmitter on the monkey the system is tested with a signal generator.

For recording of telemetered signals the monkeys are housed singly in Lucite-sided fiberglass or metal cages placed in shielded recording rooms with controlled illumination. The MUA signal is transmitted to a conventional FM receiver system (IC-R7000, ICOM Incorporated, Osaka, Japan or AR-2002, AOR Ltd., Tokyo, Japan) from a whip receiving antenna positioned above the cage. The signal is amplified 2400- to 5000-fold by the receiver and activity rates are computed and displayed using the Dataquest III system

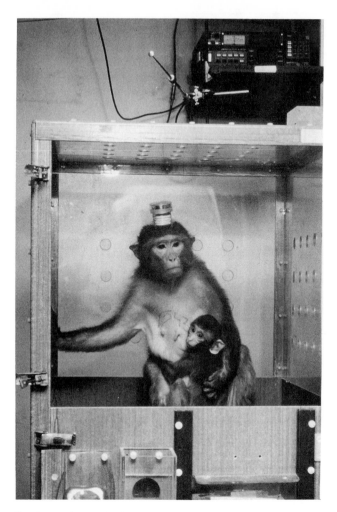

Fig. 5   Radiotelemetric monitoring of hypothalamic GnRH pulse generator activity in a postpartum lactating rhesus monkey. The neuronal signal has been continuously recorded from this particular monkey for 2 years. The transmitter is mounted within a plastic screw-top cylindrical container (top hat) affixed to the animal's acrylic electrode platform. The battery is located directly beneath the screw cap and is changed once a month. The transmitting antenna is coiled and taped to the bottom half of the inner surface of the plastic hat. The MUA signal is transmitted to a conventional FM receiver from a whip receiving antenna positioned above the Lucite-sided fiberglass cage.

as described for the hard-wired recording system. The addition of a remote blood sampling system (Alice King Chatham, Hawthorne, CA) permits frequent withdrawal of blood for measurement of pituitary and ovarian hormones from the unrestrained monkeys.

Electrophysiological Correlates of GnRH Pulse Generator Activity in the Rhesus Monkey

An invariable synchrony between abrupt increases in frequency of hypothalamic multiunit electrical activity (MUA volleys) and the initiation of LH pulses measured in the peripheral circulation (Fig. 4) is observed in a variety of experimental circumstances (17, 20–30) with the conclusion that these volleys represent the electrophysiological manifestations of GnRH pulse generator activity. At present, it is not clear whether the electrical activity underlying the operation of the pulse generator is recorded from GnRH cells, from GnRH fibers, or from other neuronal elements which eventually impinge on GnRH cells. This is because the diameter of the electrode tips is much larger than the structures near which they are found (31). The active sites, however, seem to correspond to the distribution of the GnRH neurons and their axons within the mediobasal hypothalamus (31, 32).

While the duration of the MUA volley in intact monkeys is but 2 to 3 min, it is some 10 times longer in chronically ovariectomized animals (Fig. 4). In the latter the volley is characterized by an initial "overshoot" followed by a plateau of increased frequency and a return to baseline as precipitous as the initiation of the signal (17). In the presence of the ovary the entire signal seems to be limited to this overshoot, but this is of a lesser maximum discharge rate (30). In other words, the acceleration of firing is greater in the ovariectomized than in the intact monkey. The administration of estrogen to ovariectomized animals reduces the duration of their MUA volleys to that of intact monkeys within 6 hr (25). Curiously, however, it takes some 6 weeks following ovariectomy for the MUA volley duration characteristic of castrates to be achieved (30).

Spike Analysis of the Hypothalamic Multiunit Activity

The use of MUA recording techniques cannot distinguish between an increase in the firing frequency of individual neurons and the recruitment of a population of neurons that is otherwise silent. Because unit recording from hypothalamic neurons *in vivo*, which can be expected to increase their firing rates but once an hour, has not been possible an alternative approach is used to gain insight into the behavior of the components of the MUA volleys: a spike analysis program (Discovery Software, Brainwave System Corporation, Bloomfield, CO) which can extract single-unit activity from the multiunit signal. To perform this analysis, the multiunit signal is digitized and the component spikes in the MUA are classified according to several spike waveform parameters, such as spike height, duration, and slope, and appropriately displayed. Their firing rates can then be compared with one another and with that of the MUA volley (33). Of 40 single units identified in this manner from 28 multiunit recordings 24 increased while 4 decreased their firing rate synchronously with the MUA volley. The remainder did not change their frequency of firing. No evidence of recruitment of new units during the MUA volley was found. The synchrony between the cells that began to "burst" at the same time as the initiation of the MUA volley was not very precise, a lag of seconds not being uncommon. This, however, was very difficult to quantitate because the time that a burst actually begins cannot be precisely identified. It would appear from these findings that the MUA volleys that reflect the activity of the GnRH pulse generator represent the synchronized increase in the firing rate of single units in the mediobasal hypothalamus and the simultaneous decrease in the firing rate of a smaller population of others (33).

Operational Characteristics

The success rate of recording MUA volleys associated with GnRH pulse generator activity was 25% in the intact and 75% in the ovariectomized monkeys. The reason for this marked difference is not known, but it is tempting to speculate that the increase in the maximum increment in neuronal discharge rate during the MUA volleys following ovariectomy (30) facilitate their detection.

Those electrodes which show clear MUA volleys are identified for use in subsequent studies. Animals which have pulsatile LH secretion without accompanying unambiguous changes in electrical activity cannot be utilized and the electrodes are removed and a new set implanted. If MUA volleys and pulsatile LH secretion are both absent the reestablishment of LH pulses is awaited and the animals are rescreened. MUA volleys have been recorded from the third and fourth set of implanted electrodes. In individual animals the MUA volleys have been recorded from 1 to 9 of the 18 electrodes in the bilateral array for as long as 6 years; the longest interval studied to date.

To reduce infection at the base of the electrode platform Gentamicine (Schering Co., Bloomfield, NJ) is added to the acrylic cement (1 g Gentamicine to 17 g acrylic powder). This has been successfully used for about 6 years as effective prophylaxis. However, a number of platforms have become detached due to cranial erosion at the screw anchorage sites associated with the emergence of a Gentamicine-resistant *Staphylococcus aureus* (GRSA). The problem is overcome by switching to Vancomycin (Eli Lilly & Co.) to which GRSA are sensitive. Vancomycin (1 g) is thoroughly mixed with 20 g of powder component of the acrylic cement prior to the addition of the liquid monomer.

Summary of Principal Results Using Electrophysiological Techniques

This electrophysiological approach provides an unambiguous, on-line, marker of GnRH pulse generator activity in the rhesus monkey. More recently, similar observations have been made in the rat (34) and the goat (35; Nishihara *et al.*, chapter 7, this volume). The establishment of the radiotelemetry system permits continuous monitoring of pulse generator activity for extended periods and thereby the study of what transpires during the 28-day menstrual cycle (20), gestation, the long period of lactational amenorrhea, and the period preceding the advent of puberty. Computerized spike discrimination analysis, which reveals single action potentials in the hypothalamic multiunit signal, may provide an approach to the investigation of signal synchronization.

Acknowledgment

This work was supported by Grants HD 8610 and HD 17638 from the National Institutes of Health and by grants from the Clayton and Ellwood Foundations.

References

1. D. J. Dierschke, A. N. Bhattacharya, L. E. Atkinson, and E. Knobil, *Endocrinology (Baltimore)* **87,** 850 (1970).
2. J. Dolais, A-J. Valleron, A-M. Grapin, and G. Rosselin, *C. R. Acad. Sci. Paris* **270,** 3123 (1970).
3. C. R. Pohl and E. Knobil, *Annu. Rev. Physiol.* **44,** 583 (1982).
4. P. W. Carmel, S. Araki, and M. Ferin, *Endocrinology (Baltimore)* **99,** 243 (1976).
5. I. J. Clarke and J. T. Cummins, *Endocrinology (Baltimore)* **111,** 1737 (1982).
6. A. Caraty, A. Locatelli, and G. B. Martin, *J. Endocrinol.* **123,** 375 (1989).

7. S. M. Moenter, A. Caraty, A. Locatelli, and F. J. Karsch, *Endocrinology (Baltimore)* **129,** 1175 (1991).

8. T. M. Plant, L. C. Krey, J. Moossy, J. T. McCormack, D. L. Hess, and E. Knobil, *Endocrinology (Baltimore)* **102,** 52 (1978).

9. L. C. Krey, W. R. Butler, and E. Knobil, *Endocrinology (Baltimore)* **96,** 1073 (1975).

10. D. A. Van Vugt, W. D. Diefenbach, E. Alston, and M. Ferin, *Endocrinology (Baltimore)* **117,** 1550 (1985).

11. J. E. Levine, R. L. Norman, P. M. Gliessman, T. T. Oyama, D. R. Bangsberg, and H. G. Spies, *Endocrinology (Baltimore)* **117,** 711 (1985).

12. M. Gearing and E. Terasawa, *Brain Res. Bull.* **21,** 117 (1988).

13. J. E. Levine and K. D. Powell, *in* "Methods in Enzymology" (P. M. Conn, ed.), Vol. 168, p. 166. Academic Press, San Diego, 1989.

14. J. N. Hayward, *Physiol. Rev.* **57,** 574 (1977).

15. B. Dufy, L. Dufy-Barbe, J-D. Vincent, and E. Knobil, *J. Physiol. (Paris)* **75,** 105 (1979).

16. E. Knobil, *Biol. Reprod.* **24,** 44 (1981).

17. R. C. Wilson, J. S. Kesner, J-M. Kaufman, T. Uemura, T. Akema, and E. Knobil, *Neuroendocrinology* **39,** 256 (1984).

18. S. L. Chorover and A-M. DeLuca, *Physiol. Behav.* **9,** 671 (1972).

19. J. S. Buchwald, S. B. Holstein, and D. S. Weber, *in* "Bioelectric Recording Techniques" (R. F. Thompson and M. M. Patterson, eds.), Part A, p. 201. Academic Press, New York, 1973.

20. K. T. O'Byrne, J-C. Thalabard, P. M. Grosser, R. C. Wilson, C. L. Williams, M-D. Chen, D. Ladendorf, J. Hotchkiss, and E. Knobil, *Endocrinology (Baltimore)* **129,** 1207 (1991).

21. M-D. Chen, K. T. O'Byrne, S. E. Chiappini, J. Hotchkiss, and E. Knobil, *Neuroendocrinology* **56,** 666 (1992).

22. J-M. Kaufman, J. S. Kesner, R. C. Wilson, and E. Knobil, *Endocrinology (Baltimore)* **116,** 1327 (1985).

23. J. S. Kesner, J-M. Kaufman, R. C. Wilson, G. Kuroda, and E. Knobil, *Neuroendocrinology* **42,** 109 (1986).

24. J. S. Kesner, J-M. Kaufman, R. C. Wilson, G. Kuroda, and E. Knobil, *Neuroendocrinology* **43,** 686 (1986).

25. J. S. Kesner, R. C. Wilson, J-M Kaufman, J. Hotchkiss, Y. Chen, H. Yamamoto, R. R. Pardo, and E. Knobil, *Proc. Natl. Acad. Sci. U.S.A.* **84,** 8745 (1987).

26. C. L. Williams, M. Nishihara, J-C. Thalabard, P. M. Grosser, J. Hotchkiss, and E. Knobil, *Neuroendocrinology* **52,** 133 (1990).

27. C. L. Williams, M. Nishihara, J-C. Thalabard, K. T. O'Byrne, P. M. Grosser, J. Hotchkiss, and E. Knobil, *Neuroendocrinology* **52,** 225 (1990).

28. C. L. Williams, J-C. Thalabard, K. T. O'Byrne, P. M. Grosser, M. Nishihara, J. Hotchkiss, and E. Knobil, *Proc. Natl. Acad. Sci. U.S.A.* **87,** 8580 (1990).

29. P. M. Grosser, K. T. O'Byrne, C. L. Williams, J-C. Thalabard, J. Hotchkiss, and E. Knobil, *Neuroendocrinology,* **57,** 115 (1993).

30. K. T. O'Byrne, M-D. Chen, M. Nishihara, C. L. Williams, J-C. Thalabard, J. Hotchkiss, and E. Knobil, *Neuroendocrinology,* **57,** 588 (1993).

31. A-J. Silverman, R. Wilson, J. S. Kesner, and E. Knobil, *Neuroendocrinology* **44,** 168 (1986).

32. A. J. Silverman, J. L. Antunes, G. M. Abrams, G. Nilaver, R. Thau, J. A. Robinson, M. Ferin, and L. C. Krey, *J. Comp. Neurol.* **211,** 309 (1982).

33. H. Cardenas, K. T. O'Byrne, T. Ördög, and E. Knobil, *Proc. Natl. Acad. Sci. U.S.A.* **90,** 9630 (1993).

34. F. Kimura, M. Nishihara, H. Hiruma, and T. Funabashi, *Neuroendocrinology* **53,** 97 (1991).

35. Y. Mori, M. Nishihara, T. Tanaka, T. Shimizu, M. Yamaguchi, Y. Takeuchi, and K. Hoshino, *Neuroendocrinology* **53,** 392 (1991).

[7] In Vivo Electrophysiological Monitoring of the GnRH Pulse Generator in Rats and Goats

Masugi Nishihara, Yuji Mori, Mi-Jeong Yoo, and Michio Takahashi

Introduction

The hypothalamic pulse generator which regulates intermittent discharges of gonadotropin-releasing hormone (GnRH) into the pituitary portal circulation and thereby modulates the pulsatile secretion of gonadotropin has been recognized as a key determinant of reproductive function in mammals (1). Each species of animal has its own characteristics of the pulsatile pattern, e.g., the interval between pulses of luteinizing hormone (LH) in the ovariectomized monkey, goat, and rat is about 60, 40, and 20 min, respectively (2). Prolongation of the pulse interval is known to result in the regression of gonadal function and infertility. Thus, many internal and external environmental factors including sex steroids, stress, suckling, and photoperiod first modify the electrical activity of the GnRH pulse generator, which then affects the pulsatile pattern of gonadotropin secretion and, eventually, reproductive function.

For the study of neuroendocrine mechanisms controlling reproductive function, attempts have been made to determine the electrical events associated with the activity of the hypothalamic GnRH pulse generator. Characteristic increases in electrical activity coincident with the initiation of each LH pulse were first described by Knobil's group in the mediobasal hypothalamus (MBH) of the ovariectomized rhesus monkey (3). Similar electrical activity was then reported by Kawakami *et al.* (4) in the MBH, but not in the medial preoptic area (MPO), of the ovariectomized rat. In these early studies, single, acutely placed electrodes were utilized to record hypothalamic multiunit activity (MUA) in anesthetized animals. Recordings of greater clarity were subsequently obtained by Knobil's group (5) in both anesthetized and conscious rhesus monkeys using multiple recording electrodes permanently placed in the MBH. They have further developed a radiotelemetric system for continuous monitoring of the hypothalamic MUA throughout the menstrual cycle of unrestrained rhesus monkeys (6; O'Byrne and Knobil, Chapter 6, this volume).

Methods in Neurosciences, Volume 20

We have successfully recorded characteristic increases in the neuronal activity associated with pulsatile LH secretion in the MBH of freely moving rats (7–9) and goats (10–12) by means of an MUA recording technique, which is an adaptation of one that has been developed by Knobil's group for use in the rhesus monkey. One of the major modifications is that we are using a compact head-mounted buffer amplifier to stabilize the neuronal signals without interfering with the movement of animals. The unitary relationship between periodical increases in the electrical activity (MUA volleys) and LH pulses in the circulation is well maintained even under a variety of experimental conditions in all three species of animals examined, providing evidence that these MUA volleys are the consequence of GnRH pulse generator activity. In this chapter, a procedure that has permitted permanent recording of electrophysiological manifestation of GnRH pulse generator activity in awake, freely behaving rats and goats is described.

Procedures

Electrode Construction

The electrode assembly for the rat consists of four 75-μm Teflon-insulated platinum (90%)–iridium (10%) wires (A-M Systems, 7770, Everett, WA) encased in a stainless steel tube (guide tube) with an outer diameter of 0.65 mm and a shaft length of 15 mm. All Teflon, platinum, and iridium are both chemically and biologically inert and suitable for chronic implantation in the brain. In early studies, we also used stainless steel wire, but when used as an electrode it usually resulted in a gradual increase in noise level with time after implantation. Straight lengths of insulated platinum–iridium wires approximately 25 mm long are cut with a pair of scissors. One end of the wires is burned with a small flame to remove insulation, connected to an IC socket having 8 pins (10 × 10 mm) with solder, and covered with dental acrylic (Fig. 1). The other end is cut to extend about 1 mm beyond the tip of the guide tube and thus insulation is removed from the electrode only at the end of each electrode tip. The wires are slightly bent to splay out. The guide tube is also connected to one of the pins of the IC socket with a fine stainless steel wire and used as ground. The DC resistance between each electrode and ground (guide tube) measured in physiological saline is 50–100 kΩ.

The electrode assembly for the goat is a modification of that for the rat and resembles more the one for the monkey described by Knobil's group (5). Since the larger size of the goat brain permits us to implant the electrodes into the bilateral MBH simultaneously, two 23-gauge stainless steel guide

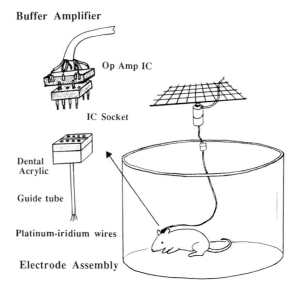

FIG. 1   A schematic of the electrode assembly and the buffer amplifier for recording MUA from the rat. The electrode assembly consists of four platinum–iridium wires encased in a stainless steel tube (guide tube) and is implanted unilaterally. The buffer amplifier is fabricated with an operational amplifier (op amp) IC and IC socket.

tubes with a length of 45–50 mm, each of which encases four 75-μm Teflon-insulated platinum–iridium wires, are installed in the assembly as shown in Fig. 2. The distance between the guide tubes is 4 mm. One end of the platinum–iridium wires is terminated at an IC socket having 14 pins (10 × 17.5 mm), and the other end is cut to extend 3 mm beyond the tip of the guide tube and bent to splay out. These recording wires are retracted into an outer 19-gauge guide tube and the spacer is inserted between the electrode connector block and the head of the outer guide tube. During the implantation, the spacer is removed and the flexible electrodes are extruded as described below.

Buffer Amplifier

At recording, a buffer amplifier is plugged directly into the electrode assembly keeping the connection minimum to reduce noise interference. The buffer amplifier is made using an operational amplifier IC (Texas Instruments, TL084, Dallas, TX) to form a voltage follower circuit. This circuit provides a high input impedance and low output impedance and thus enables the noise level along the signal path to be reduced. The head-mounted voltage follower

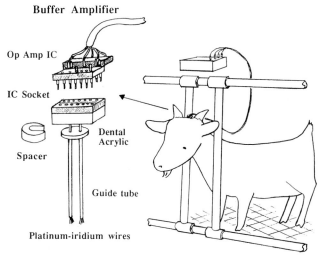

Buffer Amplifier

Op Amp IC

IC Socket

Spacer

Dental
Acrylic

Guide tube

Platinum-iridium wires

Electrode Assembly

FIG. 2   A schematic of the electrode assembly and the buffer amplifier for recording MUA from the goat. Two stainless steel guide tubes, each of which encases four platinum-iridium wires, are installed in the electrode assembly for bilateral implantation. The recording wires are retracted within the outer guide tubes and extruded during implantation by removing the spacer. The buffer amplifier is fabricated with an operational amplifier (op amp) IC and IC socket.

should be made as compact as possible in order not to interfere with the movement of the animals, especially in the case of the rat. For this reason, it is fabricated with only a few electronic components, i.e., an IC and IC socket as shown Figs. 1 and 2. Since four voltage follower circuits can be installed on TL084, signals from four electrodes can be fed into the IC. All pins of the IC except for those of noninverse input, which initiate the signal input from the electrodes, are gently turned over and connected directly to the cables. The pin of the inverse input and that of the output of the IC are combined and serve the signal output to the differential amplifier. It has been reported that a similar type of buffer amplifier has been successfully used to record increases in MUA associated with copulatory behavior from the MPO of the freely moving male rat (13).

Animals and Surgical Preparation

For MUA recording in the rat, we currently use ovariectomized female rats of the Wistar–Imamichi strain. Animals are maintained under controlled lighting conditions (light on from 05:00 to 19:00 hr) and receive food and water *ad libitum*. All animals are ovariectomized under ether anesthesia at the age of 8 weeks, and 4–9 weeks later they are fitted with permanently implanted electrode arrays under sodium pentobarbital anesthesia (30 mg/ kg). The implantation is performed with the rat placed in a stereotaxic apparatus (Narishige, SR-5, Tokyo, Japan). The electrode assembly is secured to a micromanipulator by a clamp and implanted into the target site of the medial basal hypothalamus unilaterally so that the tip of the electrode is aimed at the coordinates given in the Atlas of Albe-Fessard *et al.* (14). The interaural line is used as reference for the determination of anteroposterior and dorsoventral coordinates (5.8 and 0.1 mm, respectively). The lateral coordinate (0.3 mm) is determined by using the sagittal suture as zero. The electrode assembly is secured to the skull with stainless steel anchor screws and dental acrylic. After a recovery period of a few days, MUA signals are recorded from freely moving animals. At the end of the experiments, an anodal direct current (200 μA) is passed through the electrodes for 10 sec under sodium pentobarbital anesthesia to make small electrolytic lesions at the tip of the electrodes, and the animals are then sacrificed by cardiac perfusion with 10% formalin. Then the brains are removed and stored in the formalin solution. Frozen sections (60 μm thickness) are prepared for histological confirmation of the recording sites.

As for the goat, adult female Shiba goats from a closed colony of the University of Tokyo are used. They are indigenous Japanese goats with a relatively small body size, the adult female weighing about 20 kg, and are nonseasonal breeders under natural daylight (15). In the case of ovariectomized animals, the ovaries are removed bilaterally under halothane anesthesia at least a month before electrode implantation. The stereotaxic instrument for the Shiba goat is illustrated in Fig. 3. It is a modification of the apparatus, originally designed for cats and dogs (Narisige, SN-2), to fit for the goat head (16). The major modifications are that the distance between the anterior–posterior (AP) bars is widened to be 200 mm and that the ear bars and the head holder are newly designed so that the external auditory meati (horizontal zero) is positioned 30 mm above the upper ridge of the AP bars. The lower extremities of the eye bars are adjusted to be exactly 25 mm below the horizontal zero which passes through the meeting point of the ear bars and is equal to the lower margin of the orbit. This method allows the basis encephali to be held horizontally no matter how large the cranium is. Under halothane anesthesia, the head of the goat is mounted in the stereotaxic instrument, and a median incision is made into the scalp. After the calvarium is exposed, a small hole is drilled and a spinal needle attached to a micromanipulator is lowered until the tip reaches the lateral ventricle. Through this needle, 0.5 ml of radioopaque material, Iopamidol (Iopamiron 370, Schering, Berlin, Germany), is injected slowly and a lateral radiograph is taken 30 sec

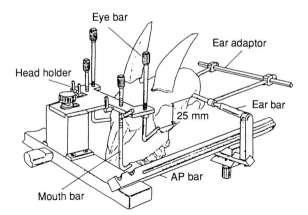

Eye bar

Ear adaptor

Head holder

Ear bar

25 mm

AP bar

Mouth bar

FIG. 3   A schematic of a goat skull positioned in the stereotaxic instrument. A set of ear adapters is inserted into the external auditory meati, and the front head is supported by a head holder consisting of two angled eye bars resting on the lower orbital margins and two mouth bars holding the maxilla.

later. Using the radiograph, in which the infundibular recess of the third ventricle is visualized, the stereotaxic coordinates are calculated so that the tip of the electrodes is placed in the arcuate nucleus–median eminence region of the hypothalamus. First, the electrode assembly is lowered until the tip of the outer guide tube reaches 3 mm above the target, and the tube is fixed to the calvaria with dental acrylic. Then the spacer is removed and the electrodes are extruded to splay out at the target region. Figure 4 is a radiograph showing the final position of the electrodes. The whole assembly is secured to the calvaria using anchor screws and dental acrylic. After a recovery period of 1 week or longer, MUA signals are recorded from conscious animals.

Blood Sampling and Hormone Assays

To assure synchrony between hypothalamic electrical activity and LH pulses, it is necessary to monitor LH levels in peripheral circulation. For blood sampling in rats, a silastic cannula is inserted under ether anesthesia through the jugular vein to reach the right atrium a day before sampling experiments. The distal end of the cannula is tunneled subcutaneously to the back of the neck. A blood sample (120 μl) is withdrawn through the indwelling cannula without anesthesia at 6-min intervals and an equal volume of heparinized saline (10 IU/ml) is replaced after each bleeding. This blood-

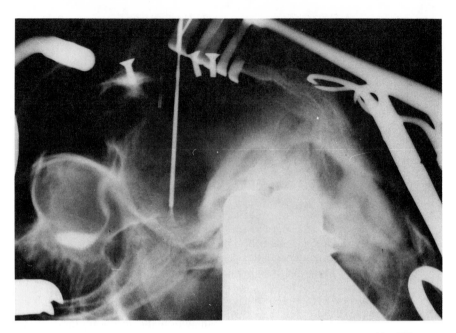

FIG. 4 A fluoroventriculogram of the goat. Radioopaque material injected into the lateral ventricle through the cannula is diffused into the third ventricle. The tips of the electrodes are extruded from the guide tube to splay out within the MBH.

sampling procedure does not affect the interval between the MUA volleys for as long as 4 hr. Serum LH is measured by radioimmunoassay with materials supplied by NIDDK and expressed in terms of NIH-LH-RP-3.

As for blood sampling in goats, a vinyl chloride catheter with an outer diameter of 1.32 mm and a length of 70 cm is placed in the jugular vein under sedation with ketamine HCl and xylazine HCl a day before sampling (17). Blood samples (500 μl) are collected every 6 min, and plasma LH is measured by radioimmunoassay (18) and expressed in terms of NIADDK-oLH-25.

Recording of MUA and Data Analysis

The whole-recording system is shown schematically in Fig. 5. During experimental sessions, the animals are kept in individual cages and allowed free access to food and water in a Faraday cage. The animals are habituated to the recording room several times before actual recordings are attempted. Signals are passed through a buffer amplifier directly connected to the elec-

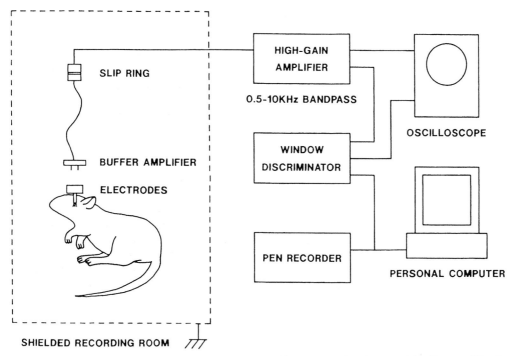

FIG. 5   A schematic of the MUA recording system for the rat. A buffer amplifier is plugged directly onto the electrode assembly permanently implanted in the MBH. Electrical signals are relayed by slip ring for further amplification, filtration, and processing.

trode assembly, amplified by means of a high-gain differential amplifier (Nihon Kohden, MEG 2100, Tokyo, Japan) with low and high cut-off frequencies of 500 Hz and 10 kHz, respectively, and monitored visually on an oscilloscope (Nihon Kohden, VC 10). Tether entanglement resulting from turning behavior of the animals is prevented by an intervening slip ring commutator (Airflyte Electronics, CAY-675-12, Bayonne, NJ) which is used to relay signals between buffer and differential amplifiers. Action potentials are differentiated by their amplitudes and the spike numbers beyond a certain amplitude are counted by using a spike counter (Nihon Kohden, MET 1100). In our recording system, the noise level is ordinarily less than ± 10 μV, and peak amplitudes of MUA signals range from ± 20 to ± 50 μV. MUA signals are recorded in terms of spikes per second on a chart recorder (Nihon Kohden, RTA 1200) as shown in Fig. 6 to analyze the exact firing pattern, and also simultaneously stored and displayed in terms of spikes per minute using a

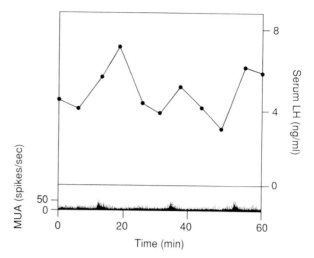

Fig. 6   A ratemeter record of MUA volleys on a chart recorder expressed in terms of spikes per second and serum LH profiles in an ovariectomized rat.

personal computer (NEC, PC-9801 RX, Tokyo, Japan), as shown in Fig. 7, for data storage and processing after the signals are fed into an interface (Dia Medical System, DPC-1310-PI, Tokyo, Japan). Signals are also stored on a magnetic tape by a digital tape recorder (Sony Magnescale, PC 204, Tokyo, Japan) for an off-line analysis.

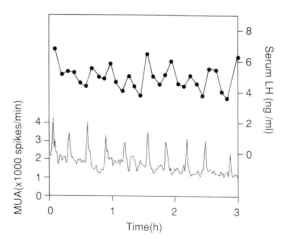

Fig. 7   Correlation between MUA volleys expressed in terms of spikes per minute and LH pulses in an ovariectomized rat.

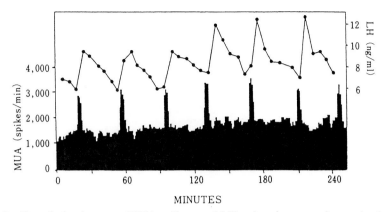

FIG. 8   Correlation between MUA volleys and LH pulses in an ovariectomized goat.

In the case of recording the unit activity from freely behaving animals, it is essential to suppress electrical artifacts originating from the movement of both the animals and cables. To minimize the artifacts due to the movement of the animals, such as mixing of the electromyogram, signals between two electrodes are amplified by a differential amplifier in which common input from the two electrodes is rejected. Since the electrode assembly consists of four or eight electrodes, we attempt to record neuronal activity by using different combinations of electrodes and determine the one from which the most stable signals can be obtained. Further, as mentioned above, a compact voltage follower circuit is plugged directly onto the electrode assembly permanently implanted in the MBH in order to reduce artifacts caused by the movement of the cable. Despite these efforts to reduce movement-induced electrical artifacts, at present about 10% of rats implanted with electrodes give off stable MUA signals associated with LH pulses. In the case of goats, however, the MUA volleys can be recorded from more than 70% of the animals implanted with electrodes. This difference in the success rate may be due partially to the difference in the size of the target area and/or in the intensity of the movement of animals.

A representative example of ratemeter records of MUA signals on a chart recorder obtained from the MBH of an ovariectomized rat is shown in Fig. 6. Explosive rises in MUA are coincident with or slightly precede the initiation of each LH pulse. Each MUA volley is characterized by an initial overshoot followed by a gradual decrease to the baseline activity. The mean duration and interval of MUA volleys are about 2 and 20 min, respectively (7). The correlation between MUA volleys and LH pulses in an ovariectomized goat is shown in Fig. 8. The duration of the episodes of increased

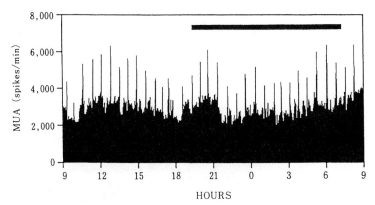

FIG. 9   The profile of MUA volleys recorded over 24 hr in an ovariectomized goat. The dark period is indicated by the shaded bar.

MUA and the interval between them in the goat are about 4 and 40 min, respectively (10). The firing pattern resembles that recorded in rats more than in monkeys (5) in terms of relatively short durations.

The MUA recording system permits permanent monitoring of GnRH pulse generator activity in awake, freely moving animals. Figure 9 shows the representative profile of MUA volleys recorded from an ovariectomized goat over 24 hr. While the frequency of MUA volleys during the dark phase has been reported to be markedly reduced in the monkey (6) and increased in the rat (9) as compared with that during the light phase, the volley frequency in the goat does not change throughout the day. This suggests that the circadian oscillation of the GnRH pulse generator activity varies from species to species.

Conclusions

By means of MUA recording techniques, the electrophysiological manifestation of the hypothalamic pulse generator governing the secretion of GnRH has been demonstrated not only in the primate, but also in the rodent and ruminant. The techniques, however, do not permit the electrical activity of single elements to be quantified, and the precise cellular nature of the electrical activity recorded has not yet been determined. The vast majority of GnRH-containing perikarya are immunohistochemically identified in the MPO in both the rodent (19) and ruminant (20, 21), while those in the primate are located in the MBH (22). Despite the apparent interspecies differences in the distribution of the cell bodies of GnRH neurons, the MUA volleys associated with LH pulses have always been recorded from the same region of the hypothalamus, i.e., the MBH, and never the MPO. This may indicate that MUA volleys are recorded from the axonal tract or terminal field of GnRH neurons. An alternative explanation is that the recorded action potentials are from a neuronal oscillator, if any, resident in the MBH which then activates GnRH neurons.

While there are several methodological limitations, the present procedure nevertheless offers many advantages, and using the MUA as an index, it is now possible to access directly the hypothalamic controlling system of pulsatile GnRH secretion. The MUA recording techniques permit the permanent monitoring of the electrical activity of GnRH pulse generator in real time from freely behaving animals. This is an advantage, especially for small animals such as rats from which frequent blood sampling over a long period is difficult. Further, experimental treatments can be applied at known intervals from the onset of MUA volley, i.e., the initiation of LH pulse. Although many drugs and hormones used for the neuroendocrinological study act on both the pituitary and the hypothalamic levels, monitoring of MUA makes it possible to evaluate their direct hypothalamic actions. Moreover, the MUA volleys can be used as a simple and direct index of the effect of stress, pheromones, cytokines, opioid peptides, etc., on reproductive function since these electrical activities are very sensitive to factors affecting gonadotropin secretion and are easy to evaluate (7, 12, 23, 24). The MUA studies in the different species of animals, i.e., the rat, goat, and monkey, will promote a better understanding of the organization of the pulse-generating system and of brain control of reproductive function in mammals.

Acknowledgments

We are grateful to Dr. E. Knobil (The University of Texas) for his contribution to the development of the MUA recording system for the rat and goat. This work was supported in part by Grants 01770110, 02454101, 03660308, 03304024, and 05454117 from the Ministry of Education, Science, and Culture, Japan.

References

1. E. Knobil, *Recent Prog. Horm. Res.* **36,** 53 (1980).
2. M. Nishihara, H. Hiruma, and F. Kimura, *in* "Brain Control of the Reproductive System" (A. Yokoyama, ed.), p. 69. CRC Press, Boca Raton, FL, 1992.
3. E. Knobil, *Biol. Reprod.* **24,** 44 (1981).

4. M. Kawakami, T. Uemura, and R. Hayashi, *Neuroendocrinology* **35,** 63 (1982).

5. R. C. Wilson, J. S. Kesner, J.-M. Kaufman, T. Uemura, T. Akema, and E. Knobil, *Neuroendocrinology* **39,** 256 (1984).

6. K. T. O'Byrne, J.-C. Thalabard, P. M. Grosser, R. C. Wilson, C. L. Williams, M.-D. Chen, D. Ladendorf, J. Hotchikiss, and E. Knobil, *Endocrinology (Baltimore)* **129,** 1207 (1991).

7. F. Kimura, M. Nishihara, H. Hiruma, and T. Funabashi, *Neuroendocrinology* **53,** 92 (1991).

8. M. Nishihara, H. Hiruma, and F. Kimura, *Neuroendocrinology* **54,** 321 (1991).

9. H. Hirmua, M. Nishihara, and F. Kimura, *Brain Res.* **582,** 119 (1992).

10. Y. Mori, M. Nishihara, T. Tanaka, T. Shimizu, M. Yamaguchi, Y. Takeuchi, and K. Hoshino, *Neuroendocrinology* **53,** 392 (1991).

11. T. Tanaka, Y. Mori, and K. Hoshino, *Neuroendocrinology* **56,** 641 (1992).

12. K. Ito, T. Tanaka, and Y. Mori, *Neuroendocrinology.* **57,** 634 (1993).

13. T. Horio, T. Shimura, M. Hanada, and M. Shimokochi, *Neurosci. Res.* **3,** 311 (1986).

14. D. Albe-Fessard, F. Stutinsky, and S. Libouban, "Atlas stereotaxique du diencephale du rat blanc." Centre National de la Recherche Scientifique, Paris, 1986.

15. Y. Mori, K. Maeda, T. Sawasaki, and Y. Kano, *Jpn. J. Anim. Reprod.* **4,** 239 (1984).

16. Y. Mori, Y. Takeuchi, M. Shimada, S. Hayashi, and K. Hoshino, *Jpn. J. Vet. Sci.* **52,** 339 (1990).

17. Y. Mori, Y. Kano, and T. Sawasaki, *Jpn. J. Vet. Sci.* **45,** 667 (1983).

18. Y. Mori and Y. Kano, *J. Reprod. Fertil.* **72,** 223 (1984).

19. H. Kawano and S. Daikoku, *Neuroendocrinology* **32,** 179 (1981).

20. M. N. Lheman, J. E. Robinson, F. J. Karsch, and A. J. Silverman, *J. Comp. Neurol.* **244,** 19 (1986).

21. T. Hamada, T. Shimizu, M. Ichikawa, and Y. Mori, *J. Reprod. Dev.* **38,** 143 (1992).

22. A. J. Silverman, J. L. Antunes, G. M. Abrams, G. Nilaver, R. Thau, J. A. Robinson, M. Ferin, and L. C. Krey, *J. Comp. Neurol.* **211,** 309 (1982).

23. C. L. Williams, M. Nishihara, J.-C. Thalabard, P. M. Grosser, J. Hotchikiss, and E. Knobil, *Neuroendocrinology* **52,** 113 (1990).

24. M. Nishihara, M.-J. Yoo, and M. Takahashi, "Ninth International Congress of Endocrinology, Nice," p. 412, 1992. [Abstract]

Central and Peripheral Sampling of Pulses *in Vivo*

[8] *In Vivo* Sampling and Administration of Hormone Pulses in Rodents

Jon E. Levine, Andrew M. Wolfe, Tarja Porkka-Heiskanen, John M. Meredith, Jeffrey R. Norgle, and Fred W. Turek

Introduction

Pulsatility is now recognized as a nearly ubiquitous functional feature of mammalian neuroendocrine systems. The existence of neuroendocrine "pulse generators" was first proposed on the basis of discoveries in rats (1) and monkeys (2) that pituitary hormone secretions, particularly those of luteinizing hormone (LH), occur in a regular, rhythmic fashion. It has since been documented by direct measurements that neurosecretions of neurohormones such as LH-releasing hormone (LHRH) are indeed pulsatile in most circumstances (3–6) and that this intermittent mode of release is both sufficient and necessary for the maintenance of pulsatile pituitary hormone secretion (7–9). Pulsatile neurohormone secretions, in turn, have been shown to be associated with rhythmic electrophysiological activity (10–12; see also Nishihara *et al.*, Chapter 7, and Knobil and O'Byrne, Chapter 6, this volume) of neurosecretory cells and/or neuronal groups providing afferents to these cells. The cellular basis of pulse generation and the mechanism(s) by which the activities of pulsing cells are synchronized remain to be characterized.

In general, two types of *in vivo* experimental methods have been employed in the analysis of pulsatility. One approach is to monitor *endogenous* pulses and assess changes in spontaneous or evoked pulsatility in differing physiological or experimental circumstances. The second strategy involves the administration of carefully controlled *exogenous* hormone pulses to subjects in which endogenous pulsatility is either minimal or absent and the observation of the physiological or cellular consequences of stimulation by a particular pulsatile pattern. In cases where the pulsatile stimulation is held constant in amplitude and frequency during an experimental manipulation, this model has been referred to as a "hypothalamic clamp" approach (8, 13–15). Both types of experimental strategies have been used with success in rodents, ruminants, and primates, and a wealth of information has been gained regarding the neural and endocrine control of pulsatility and neuropeptidergic regulation of pituitary function.

For most investigators, practical considerations dictate the use of rodents in studying neuroendocrine pulsatility. Rodents are robust, are relatively

Methods in Neurosciences, Volume 20

inexpensive to purchase and house, and require much less elaborate surgical and experimental equipment and facilities than do other mammalian experimental subjects. In studies of pulsatility, however, these advantages are often counterbalanced by the technical disadvantages of the diminutive tissues, organs, and vessels in rodents which make sampling and chronic pulse administration more problematic. Moreover, in addition to their small size, rodents possess a configuration of bony processes at the base of the skull which prevents use of sampling techniques such as those used in sheep (see Caraty *et al.*, Chapter 9, this volume), to measure neurohormone levels in hypophysial portal vessels of unanesthetized animals. Since anesthesia can dramatically alter endogenous pulsatility, alternatives to portal sampling approaches, such as push–pull perfusion (4, 5) and microdialysis (16, 17), have been devised and used to monitor endogenous pulsatile neurohormone release in unanesthetized rodents. Alternative methods have also been developed for administration of exogenous pulses; since the small size of rodents precludes use of self-contained pulse-infusion pump units like those designed for clinical use, more practical swivel, tether, and infusion system have been devised for chronic pulse administration studies in these species (18–20).

In this chapter we provide a single-source compendium of techniques for both sampling and administration of hormone pulses in unanesthetized, freely moving rodents. We first present methods for peripheral, intrahypophysial, and central sampling of pituitary hormones, neurohormones, and neurotransmitters, respectively. Methods for chronic pulse administration in behaving animals are then provided. Descriptions are given separately for each procedure, and additional information is included where appropriate on the combined use of two or more procedures. Where possible, applications in rats as well as seasonally breeding rodents, i.e., Syrian or Djungarian hamsters, are discussed.

Pulse Sampling Methods

General Considerations

Sampling parameters need to be chosen a priori based on published or preliminary data on pulsatility patterns in the particular experimental subject. Careful consideration is given to the technical limits of sampling intensity, sample recovery, and assay sensitivity (see Urban, Chapter 14 this volume). In general it is recommended that a sampling frequency should be at least three times the maximal endogenous pulse frequency, e.g., one sample collection every 20 min for an expected pulse frequency of 1 pulse/hr. In practice, however, higher sampling rates are almost always desirable, especially in

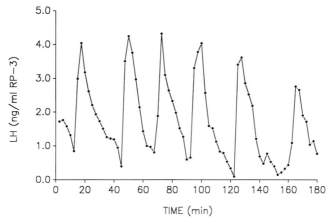

FIG. 1   Pulsatile LH secretion in a long-term ovariectomized rat. Blood samples (200 μl) were obtained via indwelling atrial catheters at 2.5-min intervals, and plasma was analyzed by LH RIA. During the experiment, a blood replacement mixture was infused back into the animal after alternate blood withdrawals. Note that after approximately 2 hr of this intensive sampling procedure, the LH profile shows subtle signs of oversampling, such as declining trough values, increased interpulse intervals, and reduced pulse amplitudes.

attempts to document relatively subtle changes in a pulse parameter following an experimental treatment.

In blood sampling, the choice of sampling frequency, total sampling duration, and sample size must also be made so that animals do not experience hypovolemia or other systemic stresses attendant to oversampling. In experiments lasting 5 hr or less, we have found that beyond replacement of more than 20% of total blood volume with physiological saline, or exchange of more than 80% of total blood volume with an erythrocyte–plasma mixture, ovariectomized rats can begin to exhibit a noticeable distortion of several endogenous LH pulse parameters (interpulse interval, pulse amplitude, trough levels). For each hormone and particular sampling regimen it is recommended that preliminary experiments be conducted in which pulse characteristics are compared among sampling time windows. Based on these observations, an empirical determination can be made as to the length of time that sampling can be conducted without the appearance of artifactual alterations in pulsatility. Figure 1 depicts such a preliminary experiment in which it was found that LH interpulse trough, pulse frequency, and pulse amplitude began to decline noticeably after approximately 2 hr of high-frequency (2.5 min) blood sampling. In some cases these types of sampling-induced artifacts can be manifest after intensive sampling *even* when a blood replacement mixture is used and hematocrit levels remain stable.

In microdialysis studies, by contrast, the duration of experiments is virtually unlimited, since fluid is not directly withdrawn from the animal and because the amount of neurohormone or neurotransmitter contained within a dialysate sample typically does not represent a significant proportion of the total neurochemical signal (17, 18). Sampling frequency, however, is typically limited by absolute recovery rates and the detectability of the substance in the assay employed. Microdialysates are usually collected as continuous, consecutive fractions and, thus, increased duration of each of these collection intervals yields greater absolute recovery rates. A suitable compromise must be reached, therefore, between the need for resolution of pulses through collection over shorter intervals and the requirement for sufficient detectability through collection over longer intervals. In some cases the limit on sample volume must also be considered; most sensitive radioimmunoassays can accommodate up to 200 μl of sample, while high-pressure liquid chromatography/electrochemical detection systems (HPLC/ECD) perform with greatest sensitivity when smaller sample injection loops (e.g., 25 μl) are utilized. In situations where sample size is limited, microdialysis flow rates can sometimes be adjusted to provide more concentrated dialysate samples and thereby maintain sufficient detectability.

Peripheral Blood Sampling in Rats

In rats, the simplest and least invasive method for monitoring peripheral hormone pulsatility is accomplished through repetitive blood sampling via indwelling atrial catheters. Radioimmunoassays are used to assay levels of the hormone of interest in plasma samples, and one of several pulse analysis programs, such as ULTRA (21), PULSAR (22), and Cluster Analysis (23), can be used to identify and analyze the patterns of pulsatility in a hormone data series.

A catheter is assembled by cutting a 15-cm length of polyethylene (PE 50) tubing (Intramedic Polyethylene tubing, Becton–Dickinson, Parsippany, NJ) and approximately 5 cm length of Silastic tubing (0.025 × 0.047 in.; Dow Corning Corporation, Midland, MI). Using an alcohol lamp, one end of the PE 50 tube is slightly melted to form a lip around the aperture. The Silastic tube is expanded by soaking in toluene and then slipped onto the end of the PE tubing and rinsed thoroughly with distilled water. The Silastic tube is then trimmed to leave an appropriate distance for the size of the animal. For Sprague–Dawley rats, the distance between the ridge formed by the end of the PE 50 and the tip of the Silastic tube is approximately 2.6 cm for a 200-g rat, 2.8 for a 300-g rat, and 3.0 for a 400-g rat. The tip of the Silastic tube is cut at a slight angle to facilitate insertion in the jugular vein. Before surgery, the free PE 50 end of the catheter is fixed to a blunted 23-ga needle on a 1-ml syringe containing heparinized (25 IU/ml), sterile 0.9% saline, and the catheter itself is flushed and left filled with this solution.

Catheter implantation surgeries are carried out using a sterile surgical technique. Instruments are soaked in Nolvasan solution (chlorohexadine diacetate, Fort Dodge Laboratories, Fort Dodge, IA), or some comparable disinfectant solution, removed, and returned to the solution as needed during procedures. A benchtop ventilation unit is used to direct anesthetic and dental acrylic solvent vapors away from the investigator. The following equipment and supplies are readied:

Catheter–syringe assembly
Anesthesia chamber
Nose cone (glass beaker) with absorbant cotton
Methoxyflurane anesthesia (Metofane, Pittman–Moore Corp., Munde-
 lein, IL)
Benchtop fume adsorber
Iris scissors, incision scissors
(2) fine-pronged, curved forceps
Hemostats
Cotton swabs, gauze
25 IU/ml heparin (Elkins-Sinn, Inc., Cherry Hill, NJ) in sterile 0.9%
 saline
3-O suture silk and needle
Plastic cuff (flange and 1-cm end of a 1-ml plastic syringe barrel)
Catheter plug (occluded and blunted 23-ga needle)
2.0% lidocaine hydrochloride solution (Bimeda Chemicals, Dublin,
 Ireland)
Dental acrylic cement (liquid acrylic and powdered resin, Lang Dental
 Mfg., Wheeling, IL)

The rat is placed in the anesthesia chamber on a grid stage which keeps the animal from having direct contact with a methoxyflurane-soaked pad beneath it. When the rat is sufficiently anesthetized, it is removed, shaved about the nape and the right side of the neck and chest, and secured on its back to an operating surface. The nose cone containing methoxyflurane-soaked cotton is used to maintain anesthesia during surgery. A rubber respirator tube is kept nearby to resuscitate animals in the event of overexposure to anesthesia. A 3-cm incision is made on the right side, starting 1 cm to the right of the clavicle and proceeding toward the head. Using a forceps, the external jugular vein is cleared and exposed from surrounding tissue. A drop of lidocaine can be introduced directly on the vein to induce dilation. A 16-cm section of suture is folded in two and the folded end is then tunneled under the vein with a forceps. The suture is cut at the fold leaving two 8-cm suture sections drawn to leave one-half of each section to either side. Surgical knots are fashioned with each thread and left loosely about the vein, the loops being left distal and proximal, respectively, to the heart. The distal suture is then tied tightly to prevent bleeding after the vein is cut. Iris scissors are used to make a small cut in the vein at a site in between the two suture loops, at a location approximately 1.0 cm above the level at which the vein disappears beneath chest muscles. Bleeding from the hole in the vein can be prevented by minimal tension being placed on the proximal suture loop. Using one prong of the curved forceps to expose the entry hole, the catheter is inserted into the vein until the PE 50 ridge just enters the vessel. Patency of the catheter is checked by slow withdrawal via the syringe. If necessary, the catheter is repositioned until operative. The proximal suture tie is then tightened about the vein below the ridge. An additional suture is then threaded under the vein and tied off above the ridge, thus securing the catheter tightly in place. Patency is again confirmed. The animal is flipped onto its abdomen and a 2-cm incision is made on the nape. Using a hemostat, the opposite end of the catheter (temporarily removed from the syringe) is tunneled underneath the skin and exteriorized through the dorsal incision. Patency is again checked. The ventral incision is closed with sutures or wound clips. The plastic cuff is slid down the catheter and the flange is inserted beneath the lips of the incision. The skin is then sutured up about the cuff. Patency is again checked. The catheter is cut to a 3-in. length, occluded with the plug, and stabilized within the cuff by the application of dental acrylic cement in the space between the catheter and the cuff.

For best results, sampling procedures should be carried out in as neutral and familiar an environment for the animals as is possible, e.g., in home cages with food and water available *ad libitum*. After at least 1 day of recovery from surgery, the rat is transported to the laboratory, the catheter plug is removed, and a disposable 1-ml syringe with a 23-ga blunted needle and extension catheter line (all filled with 10 IU/ml heparinized 0.9% saline) is connected via a short length of 23-ga stainless steel tubing to the catheter. The rat remains undisturbed for at least 2 hr before sampling. Just prior to sampling, the catheter is flushed with a small volume (200 μl) of the heparinized saline. To withdraw samples, fluid in the catheter is withdrawn slowly until undiluted blood appears in the flush syringe barrel. The flush syringe is removed and a fresh and empty sampling syringe attached and used to withdraw the desired volume of blood. An equal volume of heparinized saline plus the dead-space volume of the catheter is then slowly injected back into the animal. In more intensive sampling experiments where a blood replacement mixture is required, an equal or slightly greater volume of the mixture is slowly infused into the animal after a sample withdrawal and is followed by a flush infusion of a volume of heparinized saline just greater than the catheter dead space. Samples are dispersed into microcentrifuge tubes containing 5 μl of 50 IU heparinized saline and centrifuged. Wooden applicator sticks can be used to remove gelatinous blood components and facilitate maximum recovery of plasma. Plasma samples are stored at $-20°C$ until assay.

No matter how closely one adheres to the foregoing procedures, there will inevitably be a small percentage of rats in which catheters lose patency before sampling sessions. This is usually because (i) the catheter tip is not placed such that the aperture is within the atrium, (ii) the tip is slightly curled or otherwise deformed by peculiar apposition to the venous wall, or (iii) the tip has been covered or deformed by the formation of a fibrous clot. To minimize these occurrences, it is recommended that, before fitting an animal with an atrial catheter, the appropriate catheter dimensions and vein entry points be double-checked by autopsy of a littermate. If catheter patency is lost during experiments, flushing of the catheter with heparinized saline can sometimes restore use of the catheter. If all else fails, gentle manipulation of the animal into various postures can also restore patency. After any physical handling or other potential stress, however, the rat should be left undisturbed for an additional 1–2 hr before sampling is reinitiated.

In our experience, the use of tethers and swivels in manual blood withdrawal paradigms is unnecessary, since gentle handling and quiet surroundings on the day of experiments will yield a relatively inactive animal. Moreover, with only one tube extending from the animal, it is easy to keep the catheter from being twisted by the rat's movements or directly gnawed or mangled by the rat itself. Prehandling on days prior to experiments for a set period (e.g., 5 min on 3 different days) is also strongly recommended, as this conditions animals so they are less disturbed by initial attachment of the catheter attachment.

In experiments involving relatively intensive sampling, hematocrits should be checked midway through and toward the end of sampling sessions. When blood replacement mixture is used, the following procedure is employed to produce the mixture from washed rat erythrocytes and a commercially available, plasma-substitute solution. It is recommended that the blood replacement mixture be readied on the day before sampling experiments.

1. Assemble the following equipment, supplies, solutions, and donor animals; glassware and stir bars are autoclaved:

1000-ml, 250-ml, 100-ml, and 50-ml graduated cylinders

600-ml, 250-ml beakers

Two $2\frac{1}{2}$-in. and one 1-in. stir bars

Plasmanate plasma protein fraction (Cutter Biological Laboratories, Berkeley, CA)

Gentomycin (Gentocin; Shering Corp., Kenilworth, NJ)

25-mm filters (Product No. 4320, Gelman Sciences, Inc., Ann Arbor, MI)

Disposable, capped, plastic 15-ml centrifuge tubes

Hematocrit kit (Fisher Scientific, Itasca, IL)

Sterile, double-distilled H_2O (approximately 100 ml/2 donor rats)

Sterile, 0.9% saline (approximately 100 ml/2 donor rats)

3-ml syringes with 23-ga needles (6/donor rat)

Rack for centrifuge tubes

Anesthesia chamber

Methoxyflurane anesthesia

Ice bucket

Scissors, forceps

Pasteur pipettes bent 45°–90° with a bunsen burner

Vacuum aspiration apparatus

Citrate–phosphate–dextrose (CPD) solution, made from 5.28 g sodium citrate, 0.64 g citric acid, 5.12 g dextrose, and 0.44 g monosodium phosphate, diluted to 200 ml with sterile, double-distilled H_2O

Phosphate–dextrose (PD) solution, made from 1.28 g dextrose and 0.11 g monophosphate, diluted to 50 ml with sterile, double-distilled H_2O

Donor rats of the same sex, strain, and endocrine condition as the animals to be sampled

2. Aliquot 1 ml of the CPD solution into one 15-ml centrifuge tube for each donor rat. Flush each tube with the CPD solution. Put the filter in CPD solution in a beaker. Flush syringes with CPD solution, leaving 0.4 ml in each syringe. Place filter on top of first centrifuge tube with widest opening facing upward.

3. Deeply anesthetize first donor rat until it stops breathing, but heartbeat continues. Using large surgical scissors, open chest and expose the heart, taking care not to produce bleeding from the lungs or liver. Insert syringe needle into the right ventricle, withdraw blood, and transfer it through the filter and into a centrifuge tube (approximately 4 syringes/tube). Place tubes in ice bath. Sacrifice the anesthetized, donor animal by decapitation. Repeat these procedures in additional rats until sufficient amounts of donor blood have been obtained. Centrifuge the tubes at 700*g* for 8 min at 5°C.

4. Aspirate and dispose of serum. Reconstitute with approximately the same volume of sterile saline and wash cells by gently rocking the tubes.

Centrifuge again for 8 min. Aspirate, dilute, wash, and centrifuge erythrocytes a second time. Aspirate a third time, and add a volume of Plasmanate that equals approximately 60% of the volume of erythrocytes. Determine the hematocrit. Add 0.2 ml gentomycin solution to each 45 ml of mixture. The final hematocrit (50%) is reached by further diluting with PD solution.

5. Store in refrigerator for use within 3 days. The mixture should be warmed to 37°C before infusion into the recipient animal.

Peripheral Blood Sampling in Hamsters

Peripheral sampling of blood can also be accomplished via atrial catheters in the adult golden (Syrian) hamster (*Mesocricetus auratus*). The same procedures as those outlined above for rats can be used in golden hamsters, with some minor technical differences and some extra experimental considerations. For example, in adult male and female golden hamsters, weighing 120 to 200 g, a catheter tip length (PE 50 ''ridge'' to tip aperture) should be approximately 2.3 to 2.7 cm, respectively. Moreover, for implantation of catheters in this species, sodium pentobarbitol (80–100 mg/kg ip) is a preferred anesthesia. In the preparation of blood replacement mixture, blood is obtained from donor hamsters as described above for rats with the final hematocrit being 50 to 60%. Again, preliminary studies should be performed to empirically determine the optimum duration and frequency of sampling. As a starting point, we note that gonadotropin pulses in hamsters are successfully measured without eventual deterioration of pulsatility, by means of collecting 200-μl samples at 10-min intervals for 6 hr (24;blood replacement mixture was used in this study).

More diminutive hamsters, such as the Djungarian hamster (*Photopus sungorus*), do not avail themselves as well to pulse sampling experimentation, given their small jugular veins and small total blood volume. It should be noted, however, that basic sampling techniques have been successfully used to monitor LH pulsatility in mice, despite similar physical limitations (25).

Intrahypophysial Microdialysis in Rats

Intrahypophysial microdialysis (16, 26, 27) is a relatively new approach that we have found useful in monitoring neurohormone pulsatility (17). As for all microdialysis methods, the use of the system is based on the concept that exchange of solutes will occur across a semipermeable membrane which separates a relatively stationary pool and a moving pool of fluid. The direction and magnitude of the exchange for a particular factor is dependent on the concentration gradient which exists between the two pools. Thus, when a dialysis system is operated *in vivo*, exchange occurs across a dialysis membrane tube or cylinder, between a stationary extracellular pool of fluid and the moving pool of dialysis medium. All other factors remaining constant *in vivo*, it is the concentration of the substance in the extracellular fluid which determines the concentration gradient across the membrane. Changes in the interstitial concentration of the solute are therefore accompanied by proportional changes of the solute concentration in the dialysis medium. These fluctuations can be detected in continuously collected fractions by sensitive assays, and the original pattern of the interstitial fluid over time can be estimated. We have adapted this basic technique to the measurement of neurohormone levels in the extracellular fluid of the anterior pituitary gland. Using dialysis probes fashioned as cylindrical membranes affixed to concentric inflow and outflow tubes, we have found that the intrahypophysial microdialysis approach can be used to monitor neurohormone pulsatility in conscious, freely moving rats (16, 17, 27). Review of the advantages, disadvantages, and assorted applications of this technique can be found in previous articles (16, 27). Below we provide a working guide for the implantation and operation of an intrahypophysial microdialysis system, with particular focus on the measurement of pulsatile LHRH patterns. The reader is also directed to several reports which document the use of microdialysis for the measurement of other neuropeptides (28–36). For details on applications of related *in vivo* monitoring methods, such as push–pull perfusion, see for example descriptions for the rat by Levine and Ramirez (37) or Levine and Duffy (38), for the sheep by Levine *et al.* (5), and for the rhesus monkey by Terasawa (Chapter 10, this volume).

For measurement of neurohormone peptides, we strongly recommend that commercially available probes be used (e.g., CMA/10, 500 μm diameter, 2 or 4 mm tip length; Bioanalytical Systems, West Lafayette, IN). The membranes of these probes consist of a polycarbonate/polyether copolymer that optimally allows penetration of peptides. Moreover, the performance of these devices is remarkably consistent from probe to probe. It is also advised that preliminary *in vitro* tests of the dialysis system be performed as described below and that trial stereotaxic placements of probe cannulae be conducted in one or more of the animals from each litter and/or experimental condition, prior to surgical implantation in the experimental subjects.

The following materials are assembled for stereotaxic implantation of guide cannulae for intrahypophysial microdialysis probes.

> Basic stereotaxic apparatus for the rat (e.g., Radionics student model for rat and small animal, Part No. 3-0810, with three-way probe drive (Part No. 3-0018; Radionics, South Gate, CA)

Electric rodent clippers (Oster Corp., Milwaukee, WI)
Surgical scissors, forceps, hemostats, scalpel
3-O suture thread, needle
Nolvasan solution
Reusable thermal pad (No. 39DP, Braintree Scientific, Braintree, MA)
Atropisol opthalmic solution or ointment
Sterile 0.9% saline
Skull anchor screws (e.g., No. MF-5182, Bioanalytical Systems)
Jeweler's screwdriver
Rapid-dry, dental acrylic cement (methacrolate solvent and Jet acrylic
    powder; Lang Dental Mfg., Wheeling, IL)
Ketamine hydrochloride (Ketastat, 100 mg/ml; AVECO Fort Dodge, IA)
Xylaxine (1000 U/ml; Rugby Laboratories, Rockville Center, NY)
Buprenophine HCl (Buprenex: Norwich Eaton, Norwich, NY)
Plastic 1-ml syringes, 26-ga disposable needles
Plastic 3-ml syringes
Guide cannula and stylette (e.g., CMA/10 Intracerebral guide, No. MF-
    5166, Bioanalytical Systems) (see *Note* below)
Dental drill (Emesco engine, Teledyne Hanau, Buffalo, NY) and minia-
    ture bit (e.g., MF5176, Bioanalytical Systems)

Note: We have found that the distance from skull surface to ventral coordinate is greater than the distance from the hub to the guide cannula tip even
for CMA/10 guide cannulae. To overcome this problem, homemade guide
tubes can be fashioned from hypodermic needles, since these permit the hub
fitting of the stylette or dialysis probe to be positioned closer to the skull
surface, allowing further distance for ventral advancement of the tip. Alternatively, commercial manufacturers may be contacted to fashion special-order
dialysis probes and guide tubes of greater length.

Before surgery, a guide cannula is fitted with a stylette which extends
2 mm beyond the end of the cannula and mounted firmly to a guide clip on
the arm of a stereotaxic apparatus. The guide cannula should be checked
with a T square to ensure that it is straight and perpendicular in all planes.
The rat is then readied for surgery. All surgeries are performed on fully
anesthetized animals, using sterile surgical operating procedures. An adult
rat weighing 200 g or greater is anesthetized with injections of ketamine (100
mg/kg ip) and xylazine (0.1 mg/rat) and boosted with both drugs during
surgery if necessary. Ointment is applied to the eyes to prevent drying and
blistering which can appear as a side effect of ketamine. The animal's head
is shaved, secured in the ear bars, and centered in the stereotaxic frame
with its abdomen resting on the heating pad. The incisors are set taught over
the incisor bar, which is adjusted for the 0-horizontal plane. The nose bar

is also set firmly on the snout. Using a scalpel, a midline incision is made with a scalpel through the skin overlying the calvarium from midway between the ears to a point midway between the eyes. The skin and connective tissue are held in a retracted position with hemostats, and the bregma is visualized. This is facilitated by flushing with saline and drying of the skull surface with a stream of air. Four holes are drilled in the skull and the anchor screws are attached. Anchor screws should be placed at a sufficient distance from the stereotaxic target to avoid interference with lowering of the cannula. The guide cannula is lowered so the stylette tip touches bregma. From this point, the probe is raised and moved to the correct anterior–posterior and mediolateral coordinates, as indicated in a stereotaxic atlas. The guide cannula is lowered to skull, and dorsoventral coordinates are noted. A mark is made at the correct entry site and a hole is drilled, exposing the underlying dura mater. A sterile needle can be used to make a small opening in the dura. To stop any oozing or bleeding from the skull or meninges, a combination of flushing with saline, pressure with gauze, and drying with a stream of air is usually effective. We have found that patient use of these techniques can even be used to stop bleeding from the superior sagittal sinus. The stylette tip is then lowered to the previously noted dorsoventral coordinates, and the probe drive lowered the appropriate distance ventrally to desired dorsoventral coordinate; the correct positioning of the tip is such that the stylette traverses the anterior pole of the anterior pituitary, and the guide tube ends just dorsal to pituitary tissue. In our rats these coordinates are typically 1.0 mm lateral, 2.2 mm posterior to bregma, and 10.6 mm ventral to dura, skull in flat (0-plane) position. The dental acrylic and solvent is mixed in a disposable 3-ml syringe with a wooden applicator stick and directly applied about the anchor screws and hub of the guide cannula. After the dental acrylic dries, the skin is sutured up around the hub. The animal can be given a prophylactic injection of 10,000 IU of penicillin, im, and Buprenex administered (0.1 mg/kg sc q/12 hr for 24 hr). During arousal from anesthesia the rat should be monitored closely and prevented from bumping the headgear on the cage top, water bottle, or feeding tray. Rats are allowed to recover for at least 48 hr before experimentation.

For both *in vitro* exchange experiments and actual *in vivo,* intrahypophysial microdialysis experiments the following materials are assembled or prepared:

Microdialysis probe (e.g., CMA/10 Bioanalytical Systems)
Syringe microinfusion pump (e.g., Model 975, Harvard Apparatus, South Natick MA, or CMA/100 microinjection pump, Carnegie-Medicin, Solna, Sweden)

Inlet/outlet tubing (e.g., FEP polymer, No. MF-5164 Bioanalytical Systems)

Tubing connectors (e.g., No. MF-5163, Bioanalytical Systems)

Syringe selector/liquid switch (CMA-110, Bioanalytical Systems) (optional)

Gas-tight infusion syringe (No. 1002TLL; Hamilton Co., Reno, NV)

Single-channel fluid swivel device (e.g., 56-7479, Harvard Apparatus) (optional)

Collection tubes (microcentrifuge tubes)

Hot-water bath

Snap-freezing supplies (dry ice, metal tray, 95% EtOH)

Krebs–Ringer dialysis medium (See *NOTE* below) (123 mM NaCl, 4.8 mM KCl, 1.0 CaCl$_2$, 1.22 mM MgSO$_4$, 13.9 mM Na$_2$HPO$_4$, 2.45 mM NaH$_2$PO$_4$, 0.1 mM bacitracin, pH 7.4, filtered through 0.22-μm filter)

Stock solution(s) of radiolabeled or unlabeled peptide in Krebs–Ringer diluent

Note: For intracerebral microdialysis experiments in which biogenic amines and/or metabolites are monitored, a simpler medium is used to reduce interference with electrochemical detection, as described below.

The following procedures are used to ready the system for *in vitro* and *in vivo* use. The gas-tight syringe is fitted with a 23-ga, blunted needle, filled with medium, and mounted on the infusion pump. The inflow tubing is attached to the needle and fluid is pumped through it. With the pump switched off, the inflow tubing is attached to the inlet tube (short cannula) on the microdialysis probe. For new probes, the tip should be soaked in 70% ethanol for at least 30 min before use. After attachment of the inflow tubing, the probe is submerged in dialysis medium and the pump is switched on at a flow rate of 5 μl/min. The probe is flushed with the dialysis medium at this rate for at least 1 hr, and then the outflow tubing is also attached to the probe. We have found 1.5-ml microcentrifuge tubes can be adapted to hold and protect probes such that the tips remain immersed in fluid. The probes can be inserted and held securely in 1-mm-diameter holes through the screw caps on the microcentrifuge tubes, which in turn can contain either test solutions or fluid for longer-term protective storage. During *in vitro* exchange tests, the cap and probe inserted within it can be unscrewed from one microcentrifuge tube, lifted off, and screwed on securely to a microcentrifuge tube containing the next test solution. Optional components of the microdialysis system can include a syringe selector (liquid switch) which allows for switching to infusion mediums containing drugs or altered ion concentrations. A commercially available (Harvard Apparatus) or homemade (20) single-channel liquid swivel can also be placed within the infusion line to avoid tangling of the inflow and outflow tubing during experimentation with a relatively active animal.

Before conducting *in vivo* microdialysis experiments, *in vitro* exchange assessments are made to confirm the suitability of the probe and medium for collection of the neurohormone of interest and to select an appropriate flow rate. It is also necessary to establish that changes in peptide concentrations in the fluid surrounding the probe tip can be detected rapidly, so as to permit accurate resolution of peptide pulses *in vivo*. To determine the *in vitro* exchange rate, the pump is adjusted to one of several test flow rates (e.g., 0.5, 1.0, 1.5, 2.0, 4.0, and 5.0 μl/min). The volume of three to six fractions is measured and confirmed to be reasonably close to the expected value. The probe tip is then immersed in a solution containing a known concentration of radiolabeled or unlabeled peptide. Dialysate fractions of the desired duration are collected continuously for at least 1 hr and either counted in a gamma counter or stored for subsequent radioimmunoassay. The exchange or relative recovery rate is calculated as the percentage of the solute concentration in bathing solution which is determined in the dialysate. It should be confirmed that the relative recovery rate is (i) sufficiently high (above 2%) at a practical flow rate (0.5–5 μl/min), (ii) unchanged over time, viz. throughout several fractions, and (iii) the same for several test concentrations within the expected *in vivo* range of peptide levels in the interstitial fluid. Appreciable nonspecific binding of the peptide to the membrane or other components of the system can result in variable exchange rate values over time, or at different concentrations of the peptide. While in some cases addition of bovine serum albumin (0.5%) can prevent this from occurring, in other situations the variability or limited degree of peptide exchange can preclude experimental examination of the particular neurohormone. We have found, for example, that neuropeptide Y (NPY) exchanges at unsuitably low and variable rates, even with the use of the least adsorbant and most permeant commercial probes. The rapidity of exchange must also be confirmed for a particular peptide. For this test, it is recommended that probes be exposed to artificial "pulses" by alternate immersion in medium only and in medium containing a known concentration of peptide (Fig. 2). These tests should reveal nearly instantaneous attainment of the expected relative recovery in the peptide solution and a similar rapid decline following immersion in the blank solution.

To select an appropriate flow rate for *in vivo* experiments, the relative as well as absolute recovery (mass/time) at different flow rates should be considered. A pump speed should be chosen at which the relative recovery is sufficiently high and the absolute recovery is maximal. The relative recovery rate decreases with increasing speed, while the absolute recovery increases with increasing flow until an upper limit is reached where the concen-

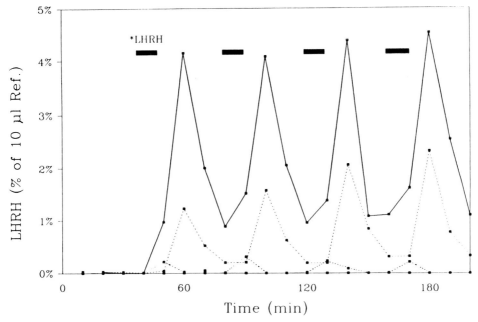

FIG. 2   Artificial LHRH pulse detection *in vitro*. Probes made of various tip materials
were alternately immersed in blank solutions and then for 5 min in a solution containing
radiolabeled LHRH. All probes allowed virtually instantaneous exchange of radiolabeled LHRH, although at differing rates of penetration. The greatest exchange was
obtained using CMA/10 probes, as shown by the top line (Bioanalytical Systems),
with polycarbonate/polyether tips. Less recovery was noted with homemade probes
fitted with tips made of polysulfone, as indicated by the lower two lines (100 and
50 kDa MW cut-off, respectively). [Adapted with permission from Meredith and
Levine (17)].

tration gradient across the membrane is maximized. At very high flow rates,
however, back-pressure within the dialysis tubing can become appreciable
and cause ultrafiltration to occur through the probe tip, thus interfering with
exchange and, hence, reducing absolute recovery. After considering all of
these factors, we have found that a 2.5 μl/min flow rate allows for suitable
relative recovery (4%) and optimal maximal recovery and does not approach
the flow rates at which pressure buildups can occur.

It is not necessary to repeat all of the foregoing tests for each individual
probe, or for each probe in between successive uses. We have found that
in using commercially available probes it suffices to check the relative recovery rate only. This is done before and after each experiment, using a standard

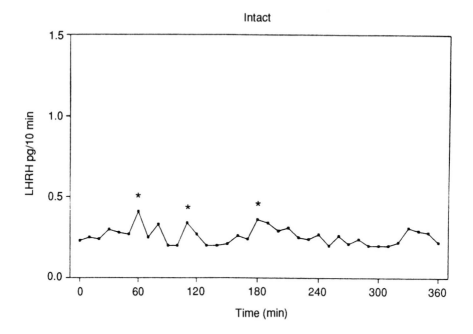

Intact

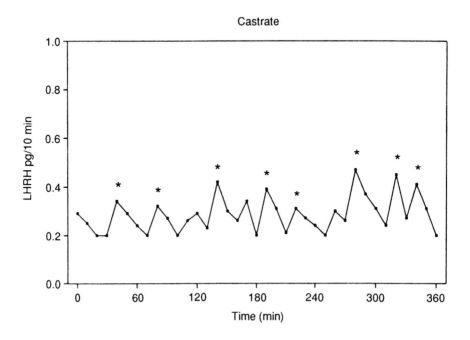

Castrate

peptide concentration. Probes which show deteriorating performance should not be reused.

In vivo microdialysis experiments are initiated by careful removal of the stylette from the guide cannula and insertion of the flushed microdialysis probe. If necessary, rats can be lightly anesthetized with methoxyflurane or ether vapors during this procedure. It should be confirmed, however, that such anesthesia does not interfere with subsequent pulsatility during the chosen sampling times. The pump is activated at the desired speed and the animal is left undisturbed for at least 2 hr. This time interval allows for behavioral acclimatization and for "washout" of somewhat higher levels of peptides in dialysates that can be produced artifactually by probe insertion (39). This time may also be used to make a final inspection of the system for leaks at all tubing connections, syringe seals, etc., and to reconfirm the consistency of the flow rate. To collect the experimental samples, the outflow tube is placed in a borosilicate tube suspended next to the cage. Fractions are collected over the desired time interval and processed as required for the particular peptide. In measurements of LHRH pusatility, we have used 5- or 10-min collection intervals to successfully monitor pulsatile release patterns in male rats (17). Dialysate samples containing LHRH are snap-frozen and stored at $-20°C$ for subsequent LHRH radioimmunoassay (RIA) (38). Figure 3 depicts pulsatile LHRH patterns that we have measured in the intrahypophysial interstitial fluid in an intact and a castrate male rat. Data such as these can be analyzed by one of several appropriate pulse analysis programs (see Urban, Chapter 14, this volume). In plotting and analyzing data obtained from microdialysis experiments, it is important to take into account the dead volume of the system, since this causes a delay between the time of an event during the session (e.g., drug administration, behavior, or correlative physiological activity) and the actual time of dialysate fraction collection. The dead volume for the system described here includes that within the probe (3 μl) and with outflow tubing (1.2 μl/100 mm). After the system is used in an experiment, double-distilled H_2O is thoroughly flushed through the system at 5 μl/min. The probe can be stored with its tip extending into a microcentrifuge tube, as described above, submerged in double-distilled H_2O. Standard histological procedures are used to carefully document the placement of dialysis probe tips and to assess the extent of

---

FIG. 3 Pulsatile LHRH patterns in intrahypophysial microdialysates obtained from a castrate and a testes-intact rat. Pulse frequency was analyzed by ULTRA analysis and found to be increased in castrate versus intact rats. [Adapted with permission from Meredith and Levine (17).]

tissue damage caused by implantation and operation of the dialysis system. Typically this damage is limited to an extremely thin layer of cells surrounding the area in which the probe tip is situated (17). The pituitary gland should also be inspected before sectioning, to confirm that significant bleeding from vessels of the Circle of Willis did not occur with cannula implantation.

Intracerebral Microdialysis in Rats

The development of microdialysis procedures for measurement of central neurotransmitters (29) actually predates their use in monitoring neuroendocrine peptide levels. The microdialysis approach, however, has only recently been exploited to examine pulsatility in central neurotransmitter systems (40). One major factor which has limited the use of microdialysis for measurement of pulsatile neurotransmitter release is the low level at which many synaptic transmitters are found to "overflow" into the extrasynaptic, extracellular compartment in brain tissue; this makes detection of neurotransmitter pulses in microdialysates problematic, given the short sampling intervals that are required in pulsatility measurements. A second factor that must be considered is that afferent systems which may control pulsatile neurohormone release may, or may not, themselves release their transmitter substances in a pulsatile fashion. Although some monoaminergic (41–43), amino acid (41), and peptidergic (44) transmitter cell groups have been shown to exhibit pulsatility in various experimental circumstances, it is not known how widespread this release mode is throughout transmitter systems in the hypothalamus and the rest of the brain. Regardless of whether afferent neurotransmitter systems convey pulsatile synaptic signals, the microdialysis approach can still be used as a powerful tool to study the hierarchy and functioning of neurotransmitter systems which can modulate the known pulsatile activity of neurosecretory cells. For example, we have used microdialysis to demonstrate that gonadal hormones may exert their negative feedback actions on the LHRH pulse generator via suppression of norepinephrine release in the preoptic area, and that opioidergic neurons appear to inhibit LH secretion independently of noradrenergic neurotransmission (45; Fig. 4).

The same basic operating procedures that are used in intrahypophysial microdialysis can also be used in intracerebral microdialysis, albeit with some important technical differences. In measuring neurochemical levels via microdialysis, some aspects of the method are actually simplified. For instance, there is no need for a specialized (longer) guide cannula. Moreover, the detectability of the transmitter at the site of the probe tip can be assessed immediately, instead of after collection of all samples and subsequent assay. Indeed, in some applications the mobile phase and detection system can

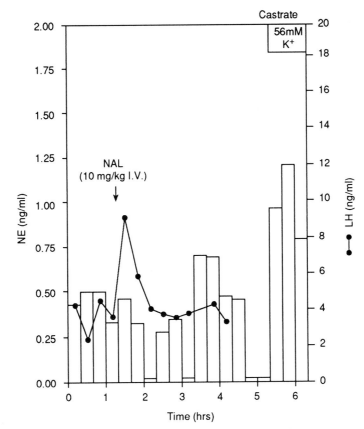

FIG. 4 Preoptic norepinephrine and peripheral LH patterns in a castrate male rat. Norepinephrine levels were monitored in consecutive microdialysates of the preoptic area by HPLC/ECD procedures. LH levels were measured in plasma samples taken concurrently through atrial catheters. Peripheral injection of the opiate receptor antagonist, naloxone, resulted in an increase in LH levels that occurred independently of any change in preoptic norepinephrine levels. Local dialysis with supraphysiological (56 mM) K$^+$ in the medium resulted in a significant stimulation of norepinephrine release, indicating proximity of the probe tip to viable noradrenergic terminals.

be adjusted such that virtual "on-line" measurements can be made. Other portions of the microdialysis approach, however, become more complex when used to analyze transmitter release. For catecholamines and indoleamines, microdialysis collection is most often coupled with HPLC/ECD for assay of the compound of interest. In these applications, it becomes critically important that the water and reagents used in preparing both the dialysis medium and the HPLC mobile phase be of the highest available purity. The sensitive detectors which are required for these measurements are operated at maximal amplification and are therefore subject to perturbation by even the slightest contaminant in the dialysis sample or mobile phase. It is recommended that a Milli-Q water purification system (Millipore Corp., Bedford, MA) be used to give ultrapure, 18-MΩ water for making these solutions. The following simplified microdialysis medium can be prepared for applications involving HPLC/ECD of catecholamines and indoleamines and their acid metabolites: 147 mM NaCl (No. 6406-1, Suprapur Chemicals, EM Science, Gibbstown NJ), 4 mM KCl (No. 4938-1, Suprapur Chemicals), 2.3 mM CaCl$_2$ 4H$_2$O (No. 2384-1, Suprapur Chemicals), filtered through a 0.22-μm filter.

When monitoring biogenic amines, several procedures need modification to protect the transmitter and permit its detection in most samples. It is recommended that samples be collected on ice and that a short outflow tube be used to convey dialysate to a microcentrifuge collection tube. These practices reduce the degree to which substances such as norepinephrine or serotonin are oxidized or otherwise degraded during sample collection. If tolerated by the ECD and necessitated by experimental conditions, the samples can be collected into sample tubes containing a small volume of 0.1 N perchloric acid. We have found that this acidification process, however, is unnecessary if samples are analyzed within 30 min of collection. This avoids interference in the elution and electrochemical detection of the amines. Since the sample size in these applications is limited by the size of the HPLC injection loop, it is also advisable to choose a flow rate and a collection interval which will (i) yield a sample in which the transmitter is sufficiently concentrated, (ii) yield a sample that is only slightly greater than the sample loop, thus allowing for injection of almost all of the sample, and (iii) permit adequate time resolution for measurement of endogenous aminergic fluctuations. In the measurement of norepinephrine release in the preoptic area (45) we have found that a 1.5 μl/min flow rate can be used with a 20-min collection interval and a 25-μl sample loop to ensure detection of norepinephrine in virtually all samples. When samples contain relatively high levels of norepinephrine, as is the case in microdialysates obtained from castrates, shorter collection periods can be used without loss of detectability in most samples.

An example is given below of a HPLC mobile phase which permits sufficient retention and detection of norepinephrine, a neurotransmitter which generally elutes quickly off of most reverse-phase chromatographic columns. Mobile phases which are preferentially used for assay of other oxidizable compounds which generally elute more slowly are described elsewhere (e.g., dopamine, Ref. 46; serotonin, Refs. 47, 48).

1. While stirring, add to 959 ml of Milli-Q H$_2$O 11 g sodium phosphate monohydrate (S-9638, Sigma Chemicals, St. Louis, MO)

2. Adjust pH to 2.75 with HPLC-grade phosphoric acid 85% (A260-500, Fisher Scientific, Fairlawn, NJ)

3. Add 219 mg octanesulfonic acid (1 mM; 0-8330, Sigma)

4. Add 1 ml of EDTA solution (29.2 mg/ml EDTA in Milli-Q H$_2$O; EDTA, No. 25-404-5, Aldrich Chemicals, Milwaukee, WI)

5. Vacuum filter through 0.22-μm, 47-mm nylon filter (No. N02SP04700, Micron Separations, Inc., Westboro, MA; high-pressure vacuum pump, Welch Vacuum Products, Skokie, IL). Stopper to degas by vacuum suction.

6. Add 40 ml HPLC-grade MeOH for a 4% v/v MeOH concentration (No. A452-4, Fisher Scientific)

An HPLC/ECD system consisting of the following components can be used to analyze catecholamines and indoleamines in microdialysates:

> ESA Model 420 HPLC pump (ESA, Bedford, MA)
> ESA Coulchem II electrochemical detector with Model 5011 high-sensitivity analytical cell
> PE Nelson Model 1020 integrator with accompanying software (Perkin-Elmer, Cupertino, CA)

While this chapter is not intended to serve as a detailed guide on all HPLC and ECD procedures, some practices and procedures for maintaining and using a HPLC/ECD system to assay microdialysates deserve note. First and foremost, the system must be dedicated to analysis of microdialysates or comparably "clean" samples *only*. Additional use of the system to measure amines or metabolites in tissue extracts makes it exceedingly difficult to maintain a low background current and thereby prevents electrochemical detection in the low picogram or subpicogram range. Use of the system to analyze tissue extracts can also shorten the functional lifetime of the HPLC column. Another beneficial practice is to recirculate the mobile phase, viz. from the outflow of the detection cell back into the mobile-phase-containing flask. This can actually reduce background currents by "cleansing" the mobile phase of oxidizable contaminants.

Before use in assaying microdialysates, the optimal electrode potential settings for detection of the compound of interest must be empirically determined by comparison of signals produced by a standard amount of amine at different electrode potentials. Using the foregoing system, we have found that sequential arrangement of oxidizing and reducing electrodes set at 300 and −350 mV, respectively, allow for optimal detection of norepinephrine. Others have described the use of somewhat similar settings (49) and even the use of a third electrode (50). Other preliminary procedures include injection of water blanks, blank dialysis medium, and dialysis medium or *in vivo* dialysates spiked with amine to confirm the elution time of the amine of interest.

A standard curve is then generated, and known amounts of amine are injected to confirm the accuracy of the extrapolated curve. The performance of individual columns can vary, and often "fine tuning" of the mobile phase is necessary to ensure that the chromatographic peak of interest elutes separately from other compounds and, in the case of rapidly eluting compounds such as norepinephrine, is not obscured by the deflections produced by the solvent front. Methanol and octane-sulfonic acid concentrations can be adjusted to retard and spread retention times.

The mobile phase is replaced after 1–2 weeks, depending on the intensity of usage. After replacement the system is allowed to equilibrate for 24 hr before injection of samples. In between uses, the mobile phase is circulated at a low speed. If the system is not used for very long periods, then it should be flushed and left filled with 20% methanol–H_2O (v/v). A mobile phase, or any fluid containing salts of any kind, should not be left stationary within the system for any appreciable length of time. Column cartridges are typically replaced after 4–6 months and piston seals are changed every 4–6 months, again depending on the intensity of usage. Other maintenance procedures include passivation of tubing with 6 N nitric acid (once before the first use of the system and thereafter only if required) and replacement of the precolumn filter at 4- to 6-month intervals. Further information on troubleshooting and other HPLC/ECD applications can be obtained from the various manufacturers.

Intracerebral Microdialysis in Golden Hamsters

We have used an adaptation of the microdialysis technique to monitor neurochemicals in intracerebral microdialysates obtained from golden hamsters. We have, for example, found that we can detect norepinephrine (Fig. 5) and other neuroregulators, such as prostaglandin E_2, in dialysates of the hamster preoptic area. There are some procedural details that are notably different when conducting microdialysis experiments in hamsters. In preparation for stereotaxic implantation of guide cannulae, for example, hamsters are preferentially anesthetized with 80–100 mg/kg of sodium pentobarbital given ip, as this drug produces effective anesthesia without respiratory complications in this species. Other procedural modifications must take into account the smaller size of adult golden hamsters (120 to 200 g). For instance, only two to three skull screws are used to anchor the stereotaxic headgear. Moreover, smaller diameter probes (e.g., 240-μm-diameter tip of CMA/11 probes, Bioanalytical Systems) are used to dialyze diminutive brain structures. As one would expect, however, these probes yield lower relative recoveries due to the reduced exchange surface area, and thus the detectability of the transmit-

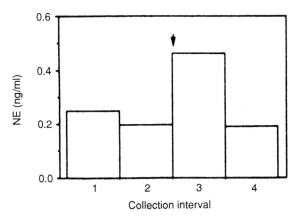

FIG. 5 Norepinephrine levels in preoptic microdialysates of the male golden hamster; arrow indicates the start of a 20-min dialysis period during which the medium contained 56 mM K$^+$. Samples were collected at 20-min intervals.

ter may have to be enhanced through the use of longer collection intervals. Atypical lighting conditions and midexperimental changes in room illumination are also a consideration when using hamsters in microdialysis studies. Hamsters are often used as experimental subjects in studies of photoperiod and seasonal breeding, and thus, extra modifications may be necessary to carefully control and provide a particular quality, intensity, and/or duration of illumination during experiments. It should be noted that the use of a standard LD 12:12 light cycle should in most cases not be used to house hamsters, since the daylength is interpreted as a "short day" and results in gonadal atrophy in this seasonally breeding animal. When experiments require collection of samples during the scotoperiod, infrared viewers can be used (e.g., FJW Optical Systems, Mt. Prospect, IL) to visualize the microdialysis equipment and experimental animal.

Concurrent Collection of Microdialysates and Peripheral Blood

With proper preparation, attention to detail, and careful execution of procedures, it is possible to collect sequential, peripheral blood samples through a jugular catheter while collecting intrahypophysial or intracerebral microdialysates. On the day before experimental sessions, rats or hamsters are fitted with atrial catheters as described, and blood replacement mixture is prepared. All materials and supplies for both sampling procedures are assembled. On the morning of experiments, the microdialysis system is readied and activated

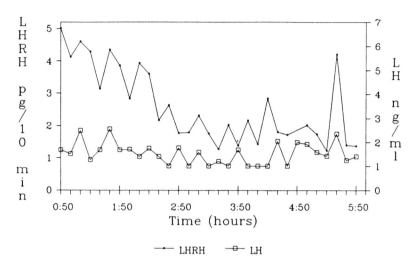

FIG. 6   Simultaneous measurement of pulsatile LHRH and LH patterns in a castrate male rat. LHRH was measured by LHRH RIA in consecutive intrahypophysial microdialysates and LH levels were determined by LH RIA in peripheral plasma samples. As in Ref. 38, pulses of the two hormones were found in almost all cases to be temporally associated.

first. Once the microdialysis system is operating smoothly and the animal is relatively quiet, the atrial catheter extension is attached and patency is established. If light anesthesia is used during initiation of these procedures, then several hours of recovery are allowed before sample collection. The blood sampling is performed at intervals which sufficiently lag the time of dialysate tube switching, so as to allow for unhurried blood sample collection, blood replacement, flushing, and, when necessary, dealing with troublesome catheters. Figure 6 depicts results from a successful experiment in which LHRH and LH patterns were determined simultaneously in a castrate male rat.

Pulse Administration Methods

In experiments which require short-term delivery of neuro- or peripheral hormone pulses, manual injections are administered at the appropriate times through catheters as described in a foregoing section. Many cellular and/or physiological processes, however, are regulated *in situ* by pulsatile signals which change in some characteristic over days, weeks, or even months. Seasonal breeding, for example, may be regulated under normal conditions by graded changes in the frequency of LHRH pulsatility over prolonged periods of time. Other cellular and/or physiological processes may not be regulated by graded changes in pulsatile stimuli over time, but nonetheless require prolonged exposure to a particular pulsatile stimulatory pattern before reaching a new homeostatic state. The rate of pituitary hormone gene transcription, for example, may be stimulated or inhibited by neuroendocrine pulses which are increased or decreased in amplitude or frequency, but prolonged exposure to the new pattern of neurohormone pulses may be required before expression reaches a new steady state (See Shupnik, Chapter 21, this volume). Experiments which address issues such as these can be facilitated, if not made feasible, by use of an automated pulse-infusion system. Described in the following sections are automated pulse-infusion systems that we have used to deliver pulsatile neurohormone stimuli in rats (18, 19) and in Djungarian hamsters (51). These systems were used successfully to identify direct negative feedback effects of steroids on the pituitary gland (18, 19), as well as to analyze the differential effects of LHRH pulse frequency modulation on LH and follicle-stimulating hormone (FSH) (51). In these experiments, as well as in other reports, we have examined the effects of exogenous pulsatile stimuli in animal models where the endogenous neurohormone pulsatility is blocked by barbiturates (52), reduced in frequency due to physiological inhibition (51), or absent due to transplantation of the target tissue (18–20). Below we describe only the basic pulse-infusion system, which can be used in an animal model of choice. For description of isolated pituitary paradigms, see Refs. 20, 51, and 52.

Automated Pulse Administration in Rats

A relatively simple and durable pulse-infusion system, consisting of a single infusion catheter, can be constructed from the following materials:

> PE 50 atrial catheter with Silastic tip, as described for peripheral sampling, except that it has a length of 50 cm
> Surgical and sampling supplies for implantation of catheters
> Spring tether (optional)
> Infusion syringe with 23-ga needle
> Peptide solution(s)
> Single-channel fluid swivel
> Syringe infusion pump (Model 975 Harvard compact infusion pump

for unvarying pulsatile stimuli, Model 2400-006 Harvard pump for computer-directed infusion paradigms, Harvard Apparatus)

Recycling interval timer (Dual Trol, Industrial Timer Corp., Waterbury, CT)

Computer (IBM compatible with free serial port, running BASIC software)

Cage with side-mount feeding bins and drinking tube

Cage top, washable stainless steel grid with center opening for exit of tubing from cage

The rat is anesthetized and fitted with an atrial catheter as described in a preceding section, the major difference in this procedure being the extended length of the catheter. This catheter is attached to a homemade or commercially available swivel extended over the cage. To protect the catheter and facilitate the action of the swivel, a spring tether can be slid over the catheter and attached by a small snap or Velcro pads to the plastic cuff which protects the exit of the catheter from the nape. The spring tether is attached at its other end to the swivel. Alternatively, a PE 90 sheath can be used in the same fashion and secured to the protective cuff on one end and the swivel on the other with epoxy. If necessary, connectors made from larger PE tubing or other inert material can be used to firmly connect the catheter and/or sheath or swivel to the swivel. PE tubing is also used to direct fluid from the syringe pump to the inflow tube at the top of the swivel. An older model, switch-activated compact syringe pump (Model 975, Harvard Apparatus) can be connected to a recycling interval timer which is programmed to activate the pump at appropriate intervals and for a specific period of time. This system can thereby deliver pulses of hormones at a fixed amplitude and frequency for unlimited periods, provided that the syringes are refilled daily with peptide solutions and that the peptide(s) in question do not degrade appreciably in 0.9% saline at room temperature. Occlusions or other problems with these infusion catheters are relatively rare, since the pulse infusions essentially flush them on a regular, intermittent basis. To make step changes in frequency, the recycling interval timer is reset manually in between pulses. A step change in amplitude is made by manually refilling the syringe with a new concentration of hormone, which is predetermined to give the appropriate amount of hormone in each pulse. For rats weighing over 200 g, it is advisable to limit the total amount of fluid delivered to 1 ml/hr and the rate of fluid infusion to 100 μl/min. Exceeding this latter limit, in particular, can produce tachycardia and behavioral stress. If air becomes accidently introduced into the inflow line at any time during pulse-infusion procedures, then the pump should be switched off immediately and a saline-filled syringe used to withdraw the air and completely refill the line with fluid. The system is then reactivated and the animal closely observed for any signs of cardiovascular distress. This system cannot be used to automatically change frequency or amplitude of pulses during experiments, as can the system described below.

Concurrent Pulse Administration and Pulse Sampling

In short-term experiments involving both delivery of pulses and withdrawal of samples from the peripheral circulation, a single catheter can be used to manually execute both procedures (e.g., Ref. 52). In longer-term experiments, however, it may be desirable to either automate sample collection (e.g., Ref. 53) or automate pulse infusions (18, 19). In either case, it is difficult to obtain samples and to deliver pulses over longer periods through a single catheter while ensuring the accuracy and timing of the pulse infusions. One alternative is to conduct sampling procedures and sample collections from catheters placed in different vessels. For example, we have successfully infused pulses through a carotid cannula and withdrawn samples from atrial catheters in short-term experiments (unpublished experiments). In longer-term experiments conducted over several days, however, a high percentage of atrial catheters can become inoperative from build-up of thrombi at their tips. Use of a catheter comprised of two concentric tubes can actually alleviate this problem even as it permits chronic infusion and collection; the automated pulse infusions serve to both deliver the desired pulsatile stimuli and also help maintain patency of the catheter. The infusion/withdrawal catheter consists of an inner PE 10 tube fitted within a section of PE 90 tubing. This catheter is implanted into a rat as described for a single PE 50 catheter and exteriorized, and the distal ends of the two tubes are made to diverge and attach to a special swivel apparatus as previously described (20). The infusions are administered through the PE 90 tubing, and blood samples are obtained via the free end of the PE 10 tubing.

Automated Pulse Administration in Djungarian Hamsters

We have used an automated pulse-infusion system to chronically deliver subcutaneous LHRH pulses in a small, seasonally breeding rodent, the Djungarian hamster (51). The Djungarian hamster is particularly useful in the study of seasonal reproductive processes, since photoperiodic effects on reproductive hormone levels in this species occur over a period of days, unlike the golden hamster, in which these responses can take weeks to be fully manifest (54). The infusion system is similar to that which we describe for the rat, except that smaller-sized catheter tubing (PE 20) is used to deliver pulses to the subcutaneous spaces of the nape. Before surgery, a 40-cm catheter is heated and molded into an elbow shape, leaving 1 cm length past the bend. The catheter is threaded through a steel tubing and washer unit up to the bent portion of tubing and then glued to the unit; the latter consists of a 5-mm-diameter aluminum washer, attached as a flange to the end of a 10-cm length of 16-ga stainless steel tubing. The washer–tube unit is thus used as a protective cuff at the exit of the catheter from the nape, just as the plastic syringe barrel is used in the rat (see above). This unit prevents the very active and very agile Djungarian hamsters from damaging the proximal end of the catheter. For implantation, the hamsters are anesthetized with methoxyflurane and the cranium is exposed. A 21-ga needle is passed through the scruff of the neck to emerge from the scalp incision. The distal end of the catheter assembly is attached to the needle. The needle is retracted, by drawing the catheter assembly under the skin to exit through the scruff until it is retained by the washer, which comes to rest subdermaly. A small amount of lidocaine is placed around the incision and the wound is closed with a silk suture. Following surgery, the catheters are connected to the infusion and swivel apparatus. The animals are thereafter housed individually and the catheter system and skin around the protective cuff are inspected daily. While animals receive chronic pulsatile stimuli of various characteristics, experimental variables such as coat color, weight, and estimated testes size can be noted. For parameters such as serum or tissue hormone levels, the animal is sacrificed after the desired period of pulsatile stimulation, terminal tissue and blood are obtained, and the appropriate assays are performed.

Computer-Directed Pulse Modulation

In some experimental situations it may be desirable to analyze the physiological effects of gradual changes in a pulse parameter over time. Indeed, it has been proposed that in many real, physiological situations alterations in endogenous pulsatility occur not as abrupt, steplike changes in pulse frequency or amplitude, but rather as gradual shifts in one or both of these pulse parameters. To model and assess the physiological nature of such changes in pulsatility, one needs a computer-directed pulse-infusion system, in which graded changes in the frequency or amplitude of pulsatile stimuli can be calculated and directed automatically. Such a program can be written for BASIC using any IBM-compatible computer with a free serial port. The computer can then be used to drive a Model 2400-006 Harvard Apparatus infusion pump. The frequency of activation of the pump controls the frequency of pulse infusion, and the amplitude of the pulse can be attained either by manual replacement of syringes at the appropriate time with a different concentration of peptide or in a totally automated fashion by programming the system to deliver infusions at different rates during the duration of the pulse infusion. In the Appendix which follows we describe a useful computer program which can be used to direct infusions or hormone pulses with constant features, or with a ramplike change frequency over a given time.

Summary

The direct study of pulsatility in smaller experimental animals is often avoided, due to the potential for technical difficulties in the use of approaches such as microdialysis or repeated blood sampling through conventional atrial catheters. In this chapter we have provided technical details of both conventional and relatively new methods for the study of neuroendocrine pulsatility in rodent animal models. This guide can be consulted when weighing the practical and scientific advantages of rodent animal models against the technical difficulties that accompany their use in the study of pulsatility. It is hoped that a reading of this chapter will tip the balance in favor of further study of this poorly understood neurosecretory phenomenon.

Appendix

```
10 REM PROGRAM ANDREW
20 KEY OFF:CLS
30 OPEN "COM1:1200,N,8,2" AS #1
40 PRINT #1, "STP" : GOSUB 620
50 PRINT #1, "CLT" : GOSUB 620
51 INPUT "ENTER SYRINGE DIAMETER (mm): ",DIAM
52 PRINT #1 ,USING "MMD ####.####";DIAM:GOSUB 620
53 IF RESPONSE$="" THEN GOSUB 140: GOTO 60
54 PRINT "ERROR-TRY AGAIN":GOTO 51
60  INPUT "ENTER PULSE RANGE (MLM,MLH,ULM, OR ULH): ",R$
70 IF R$="mlm" OR R$="mlh" OR R$="ulm" OR R$="ulh" THEN 100
80 IF R$="MLM" OR R$="MLH" OR R$="ULM" OR R$="ULH" THEN 100
90 PRINT "INVALID RANGE":GOTO 60
100 INPUT "ENTER PULSE RATE: ",PRATE
110 PRINT #1, USING R$+"####.####";PRATE
120 GOSUB 620 : IF RESPONSE$="" THEN 230
130 PRINT "OUT OF RANGE":GOTO 100
140 REM********************
```

```
143 REM GET DIAMETER RESPONSE SUBROUTINE
145 REM********************
150 PRINT #1, "DIA":GOSUB 620
160 PRINT "SYRINGE DIAMETER IS SET TO: ";RESPONSE$;"mm"
170 RETURN
230 INPUT "ENTER PULSE DURATION (MIN): ",PTIMEM
240 PTIME=PTIMEM*60
250 INPUT "ENTER INITIAL INTERVAL DURATION (MINUTES): ",IITIME
260 INPUT "ENTER FINAL INTERVAL DURATION (MINUTES): ",FITIME
270 INPUT "ENTER TOTAL RUNNING TIME (HOURS): ",TRTH
280 PRINT : PRINT "PRESS STOP/START ON PUMP TO INTERRUPT"
290 GOSUB 430
300 TIME$="00:00:00":PRINT #1, "RUN"
305 GOSUB 620
310 IF P$=">" THEN 330
320  PRINT "INTERRUPTED": PRINT : GOTO 40
330 IF TIMER<PTIME THEN 305
340 GOSUB 860
350 GOSUB 520
355 GOSUB 720
360 TIME$="00:00:00":PRINT #1, "STP"
365 GOSUB 620
370 IF P$=":" THEN 390
380 PRINT "INTERRUPTED":PRINT:GOTO 40
390 IF TIMER<ITIMS THEN 365
400 GOSUB 860
410 GOSUB 720
420 GOTO 290
430 REM ***********************************************
440 REM TIMER SUBROUTINE A- EXCECUTED ONCE A SECOND
450 REM ***********************************************
460 RATE=PRATE
480 PRINT #1, USING R$+"####.####";RATE
490 GOSUB 620
494 PRINT #1, "RNG" :GOSUB 620: RANGE$=RESPONSE$
495 PRINT USING "t=######    ####.### "+RANGE$;TTLTMS,RATE
500 PRINT #1, "KEY" : GOSUB 620
510 RETURN
520 PRINT USING "t=######          0 "+RANGE$;TTLTMS
530 RETURN
620 REM ****************************************
630 REM GET RESPONSE SUBROUTINE
640 REM ****************************************
650 S$="" : P$="" : RESPONSE$=""
660 WHILE P$<>":" AND P$<>">" AND P$<>"<" AND P$<>"*"
670 IF LOC(1) >0 THEN S$=S$+INPUT$(LOC(1),#1)
680 P$=RIGHT$(S$,1)
690 WEND
700 IF LEN (S$)>3 THEN RESPONSE$=MID$(S$,3,INSTR(3,S$,CHR$(13))-3)
710 RETURN
720 REM ****************************************
730 REM VARYING INTERVAL SUBROUTINE
```

```
740 REM *******************************************
750 TRTM=TRTH*60
752 IITIMS=IITIME*60
753 FITIMS=FITIME*60
754 TRTS=TRTM*60
760 IF IITIME>=FITIME THEN NCRMNTS=(IITIMS-FITIMS)/TRTS
770 IF IITIME<FITIME THEN NCRMNTS=(FITIMS-IITIMS)/TRTS
790 IF IITIME>=FITIME THEN ITIME=IITIME-(NCRMNTS*TTLTMS)/60
800 IF FITIME>IITIME THEN ITIME=IITIME+(NCRMNTS*TTLTMS)/60
805 ITIMS=ITIME*60
810 IF IITIME>FITIME THEN GOTO 830
820 IF ITIME>FITIME THEN GOTO 850
825 RETURN
830 IF ITIME<FITIME THEN GOTO 850
840 RETURN
850 PRINT #1, "STP":GOSUB 620 : PRINT S$
855 END
860 REM *******************************************
870 REM TOTAL TIME TALLY
880 REM *******************************************
890 TIMEA=TIMER
900 TTLTMS=TTLTMS+TIMEA
910 TIMEA=0:TIMEB=0
920 RETURN
```

Acknowledgments

The technical developments described in this chapter were supported by NIH Grants R01 HD20677, R01 HD09885, P01 HD31921, and P30 HD28048.

References

1. V. L. Gay and N. A. Sheth, *Endocrinology* **90,** 158 (1972).
2. D. J. Dierschke, A. N. Bhattacharya, L. E. Atkinson, and E. Knobil, *Endocrinology (Baltimore)* **87,** 850 (1970).
3. P. W. Carmel, S. Araki, and M. Ferin, *Endocrinology (Baltimore)* **99**(1), 243 (1976).
4. J. E. Levine and V. D. Ramirez, *Endocrinology (Baltimore)* **107**(6), 1782 (1980).
5. J. E. Levine, F. K-Y. Pau, V. D. Ramirez, and G. L. Jackson, *Endocrinology (Baltimore)* **111,** 1449 (1982).
6. I. J. Clarke and J. T. Cummins *Endocrinology (Baltimore)* **111,** 1737 (1982).
7. G. B. Ellis, C. Desjardins, and H. M. Fraser, *Neuroendocrinology* **37,** 177 (1983).
8. P. E. Belchetz, T. M. Plant, Y. Nakai, E. J. Keogh, and E. Knobil, *Science* **202,** 631 (1978).

9. I. J. Clarke, J. T. Cummins, J. K. Findlay, K. J. Burman, and B. Doughton, *Neuroendocrinology* **39**, 214 (1984).

10. R. C. Wilson, J. S. Kesner, J-M. Kaufman, T. Uemura, T. Akema, and E. Knobil, *Neuroendocrinology* **39**, 256 (1984).

11. F. Kimura, M. Nashihara, H. Hiruma, and T. Funabashi, *Neuroendocrinology* **53**, 97 (1991).

12. K. T. O'Byrne, M.-D. Chen, M. Nishihara, M., *et al. Neuroendocrinology* **57**, 588 (1993).

13. D. D. Nansel, M. S. Aiyer, W. H. Meizner II, and E. M. Bogdanove, *Endocrinology (Baltimore)* **104**, 524 (1979).

14. D. D. Nansel and D. F. Trent, *Endocrinology (Baltimore)* **104**, 532 (1979).

15. E. Knobil, T. M. Plant, L. Wildt, P. E. Belchetz, and G. Marshall, *Science* **207**, 1371 (1980).

16. J. E. Levine, J. M. Meredith, K. M. Vogelsong, and S. J. Legan, *in* "Microdialysis in the Neurosciences" (T. E. Robinson and J. B. Justice, Jr., eds.), pp. 305–325. Elsevier Science, Amsterdam/New York, 1991.

17. J. M. Meredith and J. E. Levine, *Brain Res.* **571**, 181 (1992).

18. F. J. Strobl, and J. E. Levine, *Endocrinology (Baltimore)* **123**(1), 622 (1988).

19. F. J. Strobl, C. A. Gilmore, and J. E. Levine, *Endocrinology (Baltimore)* **124**, 1140 (1989).

20. F. J. Strobl and J. E. Levine, *in* "Methods in Neuroscience: Cell Culture" (P. M. Conn, ed.), pp. 316–329. Academic Press, San Diego, 1990.

21. E. Van Cauter, M. L'Hermite, G. Copinschi, S. Refetoff, D. Desir, and C. Robyn, *Am. J. Physiol.* **241**, E355 (1981).

22. G. R. Merriam and K. W. Wachter, *Am. J. Physiol.* **243**, E310 (1982).

23. J. D. Veldhuis and M. L. Johnson, *Am. J. Physiol.* **250**, E486 (1986).

24. J. M. Swann and F. W. Turek, *Neuroendocrinology* **47**, 343 (1988).

25. M. J. Gibson, G. M. Miller, and A. J. Silverman, *Endocrinology (Baltimore)* **128**, 965 (1991).

26. M. K. Steele, K. N. Stephenson, J. M. Meredith, and J. E. Levine, *Neuroendocrinology* **55**, 276 (1992).

27. J. E. Levine and K. D. Powell, *in* "Methods in Enzymology" (P. M. Conn, ed.), Vol. 168, pp. 166–181. Academic Press, San Diego, 1989.

28. K. M. Kendrick, *in* "Methods in Enzymology" (P. M. Conn, ed.), Vol. 168, pp. 182–205. Academic Press, San Diego, 1989.

29. U. Ungerstedt, *in* "Measurement of Neurotransmitter Release In Vivo" (C. A. Marsden, ed.), pp. 81–105. Wiley, New York, 1984).

30. U. Ungerstedt and A. Hallstrom, *Life Sci.* **41**, 861 (1987).

31. N. Lindefors, Y.Yamamoto, T. Pantaleo, H. Lagercrantz, E. Brodin, and U. Ungerstedt, *Neurosci. Lett.* **69**, 94 (1986).

32. E. Brodin, B. Linderoth, B. Gazelius, and U. Ungestedt, *Neurosci. Lett.* **76**, 357 (1987).

33. K. M. Kendrick, E. B. Keverne, C. Chapman, and B. A. Baldwin, *Brain Res.* **442**, 171 (1988).

34. D. A., Morilak, M. Morris, and J. Chalmers, *Neurosci. Lett.* **94**, 131 (1988).

35. M. Takita, T. Tsuruta, Y. Oh-hashi, and T. Kato, *Neurosci. Lett.* **100,** 249 (1989).
36. F. Yamaguchi, T. Itano, O. Miyamoto, N. A. Janjua, T. Ohmoto, K. Hosokawa, and O. Hatase, *Neurosci. Lett.* **128,** 273 (1991).
37. J. E. Levine and V. D. Ramirez, *in* "Methods in Enzymology" (P. M. Conn, ed.), Vol. 124, p. 466. Academic Press, San Diego, 1986.
38. J. E. Levine and M. T. Duffy, *Endocrinology (Baltimore)* **122,** 2211 (1988).
39. K. M. Kendrick, *in* "Microdialysis in the Neurosciences" (T. E. Robinson and J. B. Justice, Jr., eds.), p. 327. Elsevier Science, Amsterdam/New York, 1991.
40. A. E. Herbison, C. Chapman, and R. G. Dyer, *Exp. Brain Res.* **87,** 345 (1991).
41. E. Terasawa, C. Krook, D. L. Hei, M. Gearing, N. J. Schultz, and G. Davis, *Endocrinology (Baltimore)* **123**(4), 1808 (1988).
42. H. Jarry, S. Leonhardt, and W. Wuttke, *Neuroendocrinology* **51,** 337 (1990).
43. H. Jarry, S. Leonhardt, and W. Wuttke *Neuroendocrinology* **53,** 261 (1991).
44. M. J. Woller, J. K. McDonald, D. M. Reboussin, and E. Terasawa, *Endocrinology (Baltimore)* **130,** 2333 (1992).
45. A. M. Wolfe, T. Porkka-Heikanen, J. R. Norgle, and J. E. Levine, "Society for Neuroscience Annual Meeting," Abstract #131.4, 1993.
46. D. E. Dluzen and V. D. Ramirez, *Neuroendocrinology* **52,** 517 (1990).
47. F.-C. Cheng, J.-S. Kuo, Y. Shih, J.-S. Lai, D.-R. Ni, and L.-G. Chia, *J. Chromatogr. Biomed. Appl.* **615,** 225 (1993).
48. M. Yoshioka, M. Matsumoto, H. Togashi, C. B. Smith, and H. Saito, *Brain Res.* **613,** 74 (1993).
49. E. D. Abercrombie and B. L. Jacobs, *J. Neurosci.* **9,** 4062 (1989).
50. E. D. Abercrombie and J. M. Finlay, *in* "Microdialysis in the Neurosciences" (T. E. Robinson and J. B. Justice, eds.), pp. 253–274. Elsevier, New York, 1991.
51. J. M. Meredith, F. W. Turek, and J. E. Levine, "22nd Annual Meeting of the Society for Neuroscience, Anaheim, CA," Abstract 90.5, p. 192, 1992.
52. A. C. Bauer-Dantoin, J. K. McDonald, and J. E. Levine, *Endocrinology (Baltimore)* **129,** 402 (1991).
53. H. F. Urbanski, D. Urbanski, and S. R. Ojeda, *Neuroendocrinology* **38,** 403 (1984).
54. F. W. Turek and E. Van Cauter, *in* "Physiology of Reproduction" (E. Knobil and J. Neill, eds.), pp. 1789–1830. Raven Press, New York, 1988.

[9] Sampling of Hypophyseal Portal Blood of Conscious Sheep for Direct Monitoring of Hypothalamic Neurosecretory Substances

Alain Caraty, Alain Locatelli, Suzanne M. Moenter, and Fred J. Karsch

Historical Perspective

The localized nature of the vascular link between the hypothalamus and the anterior lobe of the pituitary gland and the tremendous dilution of pituitary portal blood in the peripheral circulation have precluded the use of peripheral blood to assess the release of hypothalamic hormones that regulate anterior pituitary function. This led to a quest to develop procedures for sampling hypophyseal portal blood for the purpose of monitoring hypophyseotropic neuroendocrine signals. Initial success in developing a surgical procedure for gaining access to the portal vasculature was reported for the laboratory rat in the early 1970s (1), around the time that the pulsatile pattern of secretion of some of the anterior pituitary hormones was first being recognized (2). Subsequent developments led to the measurement of various hypothalamic hormones in portal blood of rats under differing physiological conditions, for example, the measurement of gonadotropin-releasing hormone on different days of the estrous cycle (3) and in response to treatment with gonadal steroids (4) and of growth hormone-releasing hormone and somatostatin in relation to the episodic release of growth hormone (5).

Although these early procedures for portal blood collection provided initial insight into the secretion of hypophyseotropic substances, the approaches were severely limited for a number of reasons. First, the terminal nature of the surgical procedure for gaining access to the portal vasculature required that samples be obtained from rats under anesthesia, which itself can alter hypothalamic neurosecretory activity. Second, the procedures involved either removing the pituitary gland or transecting its stalk, thereby precluding simultaneous measurement of hypothalamic and pituitary hormones in the same animal. Third, because only a brief sampling period was feasible, accurate assessment of pulsatile neuroendocrine activities was compromised. In the latter half of the 1970s, reports began to appear on the use of the portal blood collection approach in other species, such as the rhesus monkey (6, 7) and rabbit (8) in which more prolonged sequential sampling was feasible.

Methods in Neurosciences, Volume 20

Nevertheless, problems remained due to the necessity for anesthesia and the disruption of anterior pituitary function resulting from transection of the pituitary stalk.

In 1982, an important methodological advance was reported by Clarke and Cummins who developed a technique for prolonged sequential sampling of hypophyseal portal blood from fully conscious sheep (9). The key improvement over earlier methods was the surgical implantation of permanent guide tubes that provided access to the portal vasculature. After surgery, sheep were allowed to recover such that portal blood could be collected after the effects of anesthesia had worn off. In addition to this benefit, the pituitary gland remained intact and functional, such that both hypothalamic and pituitary hormones could be monitored simultaneously in the same animal. Several years later, this approach was refined by Caraty and Locatelli, who utilized an implantable collection apparatus making it possible to obain portal blood samples continuously for up to 24 hr (10, 11). This latter procedure has been continuously improved to the point that it currently allows remote sampling of portal blood from normally behaving undisturbed sheep at intervals as frequent as 30 sec (12) and for periods as long as 48 hr (13). This chapter describes this procedure as it is now used in our collaborative studies at the Institut National de la Recherche Agronomique (Nouzilly) and the University of Michigan (Ann Arbor).

The procedure is relatively easy to learn and, once mastered, can be performed with a success rate of nearly 100%. It involves surgical installation of the collection apparatus and the collection of blood after the animal has recovered from surgery. Thus far, the procedure has been used successfully in rams and ewes of three different breeds (Ile de France and Romanov in Nouzilly, Suffolk in Ann Arbor) and in animals ranging in age from 4 months (prepubertal) to several years (fully adult). (Methodologic details given here are for adult ewes in Ann Arbor; minor procedural differences exist in Nouzilly.)

Collection Apparatus

The collection apparatus is made prior to surgery by cementing a 12- and a 14-gauge, blunt-tip hypodermic needle (93 mm from needle tip to rim of hub) together with dental acrylic and affixing a plastic cup at one end (Fig. 1). The large needle (12 gauge) is used to introduce a stylet to cut portal vessels and as an air vent during sampling. The other needle (14 gauge) is used to aspirate portal blood. The cup is prepared from a conical, 1.5 ml polypropylene microcentrifuge tube (Labcraft) by cutting off the base of the tube so it fits over the two needles. A second cut is made such that the length of the

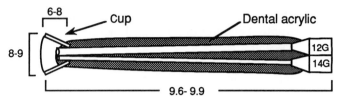

FIG. 1   Schematic cross section of collection apparatus consisting of two blunt-tip hypodermic needles cemented together with dental acrylic (shading) and a plastic cup affixed to the end. The numbers refer to dimensions referred to in text; 12G and 14G refer to needle sizes.

cup is 6 to 8 mm and its diameter is 8 to 9 mm. The cut is then placed over the tip of the needles and attached with dental acrylic. The total length of the apparatus, from rim of the needle hubs to brim of the cup, ranges from 9.6 to 9.9 cm; this length is measured and marked on the apparatus prior to surgery.

Surgical Preparation

Initial Approach

The approach for installation of the collection apparatus is illustrated in Fig. 2. Following treatment with antibiotic (long-acting penicillin) and restraint from feed and water for at least 24 hr, anesthesia is induced with sodium pentobarbital (17–20 mg/kg, iv) and maintained by inhalation of a mixture of halothane (1–2%) in oxygen : nitrous oxide (2 : 1). The head is secured in a custom-made frame (Fig. 3) such that lateral and vertical movement are prevented and the frontal and nasal bones are held at approximately a 45° angle relative to the surgical table; the table itself is tipped at an angle of approximately 30° with the head of the sheep elevated. The facial hair and wool are clipped and the skin is surgically prepared. The supraorbital foramina are palpated through the skin, and intradermal and subcutaneous injections of 5 to 10 ml of epinephrine (2.5 μg/ml saline) are made to promote vasoconstriction and minimize bleeding where the skin is to be incised. A triangular flap of skin is cut by first making a horizontal incision between, and 3 to 5 mm dorsal to, the supraorbital foramina; a second incision is then made rostrally from one end of the first incision to a point on midline approximately at the border of the facial and nasal bones (care being taken not to cut the facial vein). The skin flap is reflected laterally and the exposed triangular piece of frontal bone is removed using an osteotome and mallet,

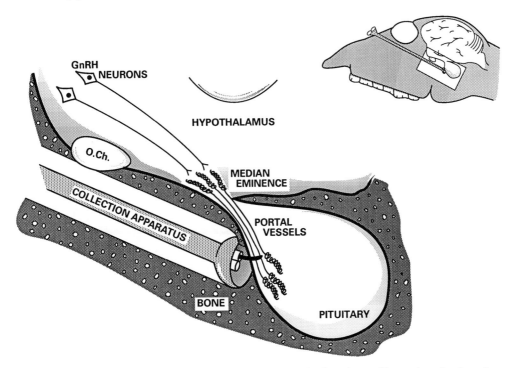

FIG. 2 Midsagittal section through the head of a sheep illustrating the location of the implanted collection apparatus in relation to the pituitary gland and portal vasculature. The stylet for cutting portal vessels is shown protruding from the upper needle of the collection apparatus. Inset in upper right illustrates position of collection apparatus implanted in head; rectangular box designates portion expanded below for detail. Modified with permission from Moenter *et al.* (14).

to reveal the dorsal nasal turbinates. (Sometimes cartilage remains after taking off the bone; this must be removed). The exposed turbinates are then cauterized to minimize bleeding on their removal. Using a bone rongeurs and suction, the exposed portion of turbinates and nasal septum are removed caudally to expose the cribiform plate of the ethmoid bone and then ventro-caudally to reach the posterior end of the nasal cavity. This exposes the face of the spenoid bone. Bleeding in the surgical field is controlled with pressure and electrocautery before proceeding to drill bone. Beyond this point, an operating microscope is used as needed to identify landmarks (Zeiss Operation Microscope, Model OPMI 99; lens magnifications of 12 and 19× and focal length of 22 cm are suitable).

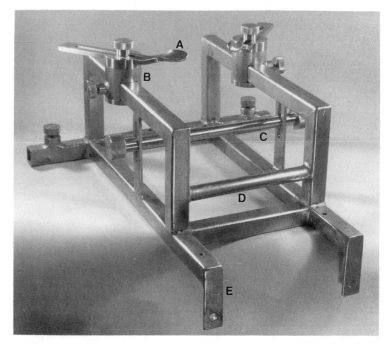

Fɪɢ. 3   Custom-made frame for securing head during surgery. The sheep's head ɪs locked in place by adjustable ear bars (A) held in a movable mount (B). The mandible is held firm by a horizontal bar (C) that adjusts vertically, and the mouth is positioned around a bite bar (D). The head frame is mounted onto the surgery table by means of a bracket (E). Design modified with permission from that of Dr. Iain J. Clarke, Melbourne.

Tunnel through Bone

The next step is to drill a tunnel from the rostral face of the sphenoid bone to the anterior face of the pituitary gland where the portal vessels are located. An Ototome high-speed bone drill with angled hand piece and a 6-mm burr is suitable for this purpose. The orientation of this tunnel at various planes between the rostral face of the sphenoid bone and the pituitary is illustrated in Fig. 4.

As an optional step to facilitate orientation in preparation of the tunnel, a small portion of the cribiform plate may be drilled away medial-laterally to expose dura mater covering part of the right and left olfactory bulbs. The tunnel is begun as illustrated in Fig. 4A using the remnants of the nasal septum for midline orientation, the dorsal tip of the widening of the septum

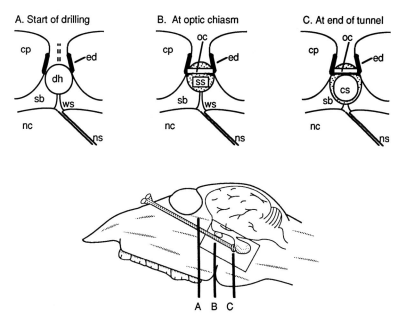

Fig. 4   Surgical landmarks for tunnel in sphenoid bone at three depths (A, B, C) as indicated in sagittal sketch of sheep head in lower portion of figure (rectangular box in sagittal sketch illustrates portion expanded for detail in Fig. 2). cp, Cribiform plate; cs, compact substance of sphenoid bone at end of tunnel; dh, drill hole at start; ed, exposed dura over olfactory bulbs; nc, nasal cavity; ns, nasal septum (dashed line is remnant of septum); oc, optic chiasm; sb, sphenoid bone; ss, spongy substance of sphenoid bone; ws, widening of nasal septum. Sagittal sketch of head modified with permission from Moenter *et al.* (14).

where it attaches to the sphenoid bone as the lower extent of the hole, and the dura that was exposed over the olfactory bulbs as the lateral margin. The tunnel is advanced through the spongy substance of the sphenoid bone until a portion of the optic chiasm is exposed as a white, nonvascular horizontal band approximately 2–3 cm beyond the entrance to the tunnel (Fig. 4B). The exposed optic chiasm serves as another marker for midline in that its ventral border slopes down slightly on either side. The tunnel is then widened ventrally so that the cup of the collection apparatus just fits under the optic chiasm.

Taking care to remain on midline, the tunnel is drilled caudally through the spongy substance of the sphenoid bone. The diameter of the tunnel should be slightly greater than that of the cup of the collection apparatus and frequent checks should be made to ensure that the collection apparatus fits, allowing the cup to make contact with bone at the base of the tunnel. Beyond the optic chiasm, the top of the tunnel should remain at the plane of the lower edge of exposed chiasm (see inset in Fig. 4). The distance between the exposed optic chiasm and the anterior face of the pituitary is 1–2 cm in the adult ewe. In some sheep, cartilage is encountered at the intrasphenoidal synchondrosis, located 50 to 75% of the distance between the optic chiasm and the pituitary. (Cartilage is especially prevalent in young sheep. In extreme instances, this cartilage may extend the remaining distance to the pituitary, in which case it must be picked rather than drilled away.) Beyond the cartilage (if present), the tunnel is extended caudally until the compact substance of the sphenoid bone proximate to the pituitary gland appears as a smooth nonvascular area (Fig. 4C).

To test for its goodness of fit, the collection apparatus is placed into the tunnel to ensure that it can be inserted up to the compact substance of the sphenoid bone; the tunnel is widened as necessary by additional drilling. Using extreme care not to drill into the pituitary, the compact substance is drilled until a small opening appears, or until the bone deflects slightly on application of gentle pressure. Beyond this point and assuming a good fit of the collection apparatus, use of the drill is not advised. Rather, any number of instruments may be used to chip the bone including a periosteal elevator, dental pick, or other instruments having a sharp rounded edge that can be introduced to the end of the tunnel. The remaining bone is chipped away to expose the dura mater adjacent to the anterior face of the pituitary gland; a small rim of bone is spared to form a seat for the collection apparatus. The cup should seat on bone, not the pituitary itself as this may compress the portal vasculature and reduce blood flow.

Distance to Pituitary and Removal of Dura Mater

Once the opening to the dura has been created, the collection apparatus is positioned such that the cup seats snugly against the rim of bone that remains at the end of the tunnel. The distance from the rim of the cup to the dura mater is determined by gently lowering a blunt probe through the upper (12-gauge) needle of the apparatus until slight resistance is encountered as the probe meets dura. The apparatus, with probe held in this position, is removed and the distance that the probe protrudes beyond the rim of the cup is measured. Ideally, the cup should seat against the bone 2 to 4 mm from the dura; if the distance is greater, additional bone should be chipped away to reduce this distance. The final distance from cup to dura, and the premeasured length of the collection apparatus (distance from rim of 12-gauge needle

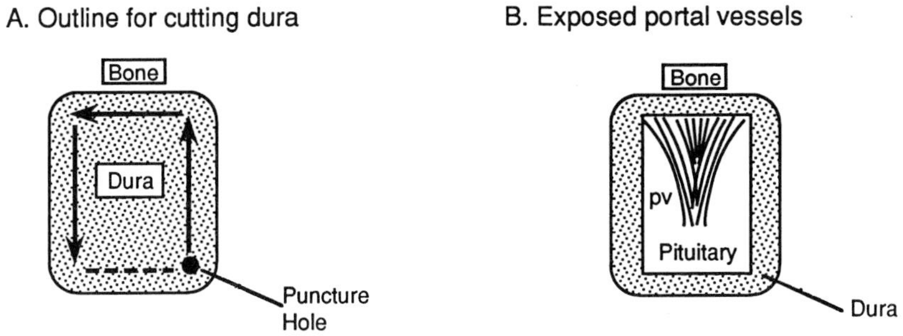

A. Outline for cutting dura

B. Exposed portal vessels

FIG. 5   Removal of dura mater on anterior face of pituitary gland to expose portal vessels. (A) Position of puncture hole and direction of dural incision (arrows). Dashed line indicates where dura is cut with scissors and reduced by electrocautery. (B) Exposed portal vessels (pv) on anterior face of pituitary after removal of dura.

hub to brim of cup) are recorded for subsequent reference when cutting portal vessels.

The densest array of portal vessels is located at midline along the anterior face of the pituitary gland just beyond the exposed dura mater, which next must be removed. In removing the dura, extreme care must be exercised to avoid damage to the portal vasculature. An 18-gauge needle is used to puncture a small hole in one ventrolateral corner of the exposed dura, an area with relatively few portal vessels (see Fig. 5A). It is helpful to attach the hub of this needle to a probe, which can serve as a handle. Using a hook and/or barbed microdissecting knife with cutting edge on the inside position (e.g., Roboz RS-6215), the dura is cut dorsally from the puncture hole, then laterally across midline, and finally ventrally to end in the lower corner of exposed dura opposite the puncture hole (Fig. 5A). This creates a dural flap that can be removed by cutting along its ventral border with a scissors. Any remaining fragments of dura are removed or reduced by electrocautery (taking care not to cauterize portal vessels).

Depending on the preparation, the exposed portal plexus appears either as individual vessels or as a dense red vascular bundle, often in the shape of a triangle situated over the creamy colored pituitary (Fig. 5B). Immediately following completion of surgery, the location and appearance of the exposed portal vasculature are sketched for subsequent reference to determine the placement of the cut when beginning the collection. It should be noted that the portal vasculature is exposed along the anterior face of the pituitary, not along the pituitary stalk.

Placement of Collection Apparatus and Closure

Once bleeding from the dura and bone has ceased, all clots and fragments of bone are removed by irrigation and suction. The collection apparatus is placed into its final position such that the cup fits snugly to form a water-tight seal on the bone at the end of the tunnel. In fitting the apparatus, the 12-gauge needle is positioned dorsally and aimed at the portal vessels, whereas the 14-gauge needle is positioned ventrally. Plugs are inserted loosely into the needle hubs and a mixture of dental acrylic is poured into the surgical site to fill the tunnel and ventral portion of the exposed nasal cavity. Care must be taken not to pour acrylic that is too liquid as this may pass around the brim of the cup and seal it shut. Once the acrylic has hardened, the plugs are removed and saline is flushed through one needle to ensure that fluid exits from the other needle and that there are no leaks (dead space in properly positioned apparatus usually ~0.7 ml). (If saline cannot be pushed through the apparatus, the cup has likely been sealed shut with dental acrylic and the preparation will not be useful for portal blood collection.) After again closing the needle hubs with plugs, the remainder of the exposed nasal cavity is filled with dental acrylic and the surface smoothed in the same contour as the frontal bone.

The skin incision is next closed with interrupted sutures; a small piece of skin is removed around the needle hubs to enable even closure adjacent to the collection apparatus. If the apparatus is of proper length (usually 9.6–9.8 cm for an adult Suffolk ewe), the distal portion of the hubs is all that is exposed beyond the skin (collection apparatus in final position illustrated in inset in Fig. 2). The animal is allowed to recover and is maintained on antibiotics until sampling of portal blood, performed at least 1 week after surgery to allow ample time for healing of the surgical field. In some instances, sampling has been performed as long as 50 days after surgery. To maintain patency between surgery and sampling, the collection apparatus is flushed daily with 3 to 5 ml of sterile physiological saline to prevent build-up of clots and debris. The apparatus is filled with saline between flushings unless excessive formation of clots prevents easy flushing, in which case the collection apparatus is filled with heparinized saline (100 U/ml). Between flushings, the needles are closed with plugs.

Collection Procedure

Collection Area and Preparation of Sheep

The collection site consists of a sheep holding area and a collection room separated by a wall with an observation window; one type of arrangement

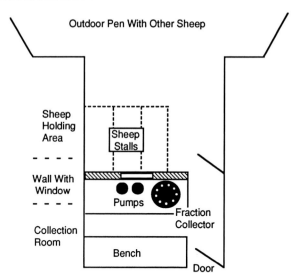

FIG. 6   Collection area showing room with peristaltic pumps and fraction collector separated by a wall with observation window from the sheep holding area.

is shown in Fig. 6. The sheep holding area contains adjacent sheep stalls (0.5 × 1.5 m) and may open to an outdoor pen so experimental animals are not deprived of visual, auditory, and olfactory exposure to other sheep. The collection room contains two peristaltic pumps (Gilson Minipuls 2, Rainin Instruments, Woburn, MA) and a fraction collector for dispensing samples into tubes contained in an ice bath. This arrangement permits remote sampling from animals that appear unstressed and undisturbed, yet it allows visual monitoring of the animals through the observation window. One peristaltic pump is used to obtain portal blood; the other is used for the simultaneous withdrawal of jugular blood and infusion of heparin. Portal blood may be collected from two to six sheep at one time, the number depending on sampling frequency and the related practical constraints of processing large numbers of tubes. For example, two sheep are usually collected together if the sampling interval is 1 to 10 min, whereas more sheep may be collected together if hourly samples are taken. To prevent the stress of social isolation, a single animal should not be sampled in the absence of other sheep.

One day before sampling, animals are moved to the collection stalls to allow acclimation. A Teflon catheter (14-gauge, 13.3-cm, Becton–Dickinson) is inserted into each jugular vein, filled with heparinized saline (100 U/ml), and closed with an injection cap. One jugular catheter is used for subsequent withdrawal of peripheral blood and the other is for infusion of heparin. On the day of collection, heparinization of the animal is initiated by an intrave-nous bolus of sodium heparin (25,000 U) via jugular catheter ~60 min prior to cutting portal vessels; this treatment is repeated every 30 min until portal flow is established. After the first heparin bolus, it is convenient to attach extension tubing connecting one of the jugular catheters to a three-way stopcock in the adjacent room, allowing subsequent heparin to be adminis-tered without disturbing the sheep. Prior to cutting portal vessels, the collec-tion apparatus is flushed as during the routine daily maintenance and filled with saline. The portal collection line that leads through one of the peristaltic pumps is connected to the hub of the lower needle of the collection apparatus by means of an adapter. The pump is then turned on to determine the time required for fluid to move from the collection apparatus to the sample tube in the fraction collector (usually 2–4 min). This allows subsequent alignment of hormone values in portal and jugular blood. The pump remains turned on in order to check for bleeding prior to cutting portal vessels (usually negligi-ble). After the third half-hourly bolus of heparin, the animal should be suffi-ciently heparinized to cut the portal vessels.

Establishing Portal Blood Flow

For cutting portal vessels, a stylet is prepared by slightly bending the end of a 17-gauge needle so that it forms a small arc when inserted into the upper needle of the collection apparatus and rotated 180° (see Fig. 2 for tip of stylet in position to cut portal vessels). The distance that the stylet can be introduced into the upper needle is set by a movable collar around the shaft of the stylet, locked at the desired position by means of a set screw. The initial distance is set to be the length from the tip of the needle hub to the pituitary gland (calculated from the surgical notes as the length of the collection apparatus plus the distance from the cup to the dura). With reference to the surgical notes indicating the location of portal vessels and with the peristaltic pump running, the stylet is lowered through the upper needle of the collection apparatus. A series of hits of the collar against the hub of the needle is made in the general shape of a semicircle and the stylet is removed (it is helpful to straddle the sheep while performing this procedure). If portal vessels are cut, blood appears in the collection line after ~10 sec. Additional cuts, increasing progressively 1 mm in depth, are made by adjusting the position of the movable collar and repeating the above procedure until a portal blood collection rate of 1.0 to 2.0 ml/10 min is established. This collection rate is usually achieved with a cut 2 to 3 mm into the pituitary gland. It is often observed that, within a few minutes after cutting the portal vascular, blood flow decreases, probably due to the constriction of portal vessels, and then increases spontaneously after 30 to 60 min. Patience is thus required to avoid cutting too many portal vessels.

Once portal flow has started, it is advisable to reduce the heparin dose by terminating the 25,000-U boluses and beginning constant infusion of heparin via the second peristaltic pump at the dose of ~8500 U/hr (640 U/ml physiological saline infused at a rate of 2.2 ml/10 min). (Although this dose of heparin is suitable for most sheep, it is important to stress that considerable variation exists among animals such that modified doses are sometimes required.) Once the appropriate portal collection rate has been achieved, the remaining jugular catheter is attached to an extension tube leading through the second peristaltic pump, allowing withdrawal of jugular blood at the same rate as the heparin infusion (2.2 ml/10 min). The heparin and jugular lines are run in opposite directions through the pump head to provide simultaneous infusion of heparin and withdrawal of jugular blood. The time required for jugular blood to travel through the collection line (usually ~14 min) is determined to permit subsequent alignment of hormone values in portal and jugular samples.

It is important to note that portal vessels are not cannulated; rather they are cut. (Portal vessels are much too small to cannulate individually with this procedure.) Blood flowing into the cup of the collection apparatus is aspirated via the lower needle. By adjusting the rate of draw on the pump to be slightly greater than the rate of flow of portal blood into the cup, portal blood traverses the collection line as a series of small blocks separated by air that enters the system via the upper needle. (This blocking of blood is a distinct benefit when evaluating moment-to-moment secretory dynamics of hypothalamic substances, see below.) Further, it is important to cut only a portion of the portal vasculature such that the anterior pituitary is not deprived of hypophyseotropic support. A sampling rate of 0.1 to 0.3 ml/min is ample for most applications, yet does not appear to compromise pituitary function. (The optimal collection rate, however, depends on the desired sampling frequency, the number of neurosecretory substances to be monitored, and the sensitivity of the assay for the hormone to be measured.)

Sampling and Processing

Detailed procedures for collection and processing blood samples vary with the interval between samples and stability of the hypophyseotropic substance(s) to be measured. The procedure now described is for samples obtained at 10-min intervals for measurement of gonadotropin-releasing hormone (GnRH). Because the procedure is automated by the use of peristaltic pumps and a fraction collector, most animals require relatively little attention; one person can generally handle both the collection and processing (including extraction) of samples obtained at 10-min intervals from two sheep. The sheep should be monitored periodically to check that the collection lines remain patent and are not becoming tangled.

Tubes containing 0.5 ml of 3×10^{-3} M bacitracin (to inhibit activity of proteolytic enzymes in blood) for collection of portal samples, and matched tubes without bacitracin for jugular blood, are loaded into the ice bath of the fraction collector. The timer on the fraction collector is set to dispense samples, which are being continuously withdrawn by the peristaltic pumps, into 10-min pools. The rate of withdrawal of peripheral blood via the jugular catheter is constant, as determined by pump speed, whereas the rate of withdrawal of portal blood varies according to the rate of its flow into the cup of the collection apparatus. Thus, the volume of portal blood in each 10-min sample is measured to the nearest 0.1 ml, to allow correction for dilution of portal plasma with bacitracin. Variation in volume between adjacent samples is usually no more than 10 to 20% but, in some cases, a progressive increase in volume of the portal sample is observed during the course of collection. During the collection, hematocrits of both portal and jugular blood are determined hourly to monitor blood loss, to assess the volume of plasma in portal samples, and to determine the extent to which portal blood may be contaminated with cerebrospinal fluid (almost always negligible). On at least four occasions during the collection, a jugular sample is taken into bacitracin, processes as a portal sample, and assayed for GnRH as a procedural blank.

At all times during collection and processing, samples must be kept cold (4°C) to minimize degradation of GnRH. At hourly intervals, the samples accumulated in the fraction collector are removed and centrifuged (15 min, 1500 g, 4°C) to separate cells from the mixture of plasma and bacitracin. A 750-μl aliquot of each portal sample is dispensed into a tube for extraction and assay. This aliquot, plus the remainder of each portal sample (for reassay back-up), and the jugular samples are snap-frozen in an ethanol–dry-ice bath and stored at −20°C. Portal samples should be extracted within a few weeks of collection as GnRH activity decreases over time, even when the samples are stored frozen. In view of this and in the interest of efficiency, the above processing procedure may be modified such that the 750-μl aliquots of portal samples are dispensed directly into tubes containing 2.0 ml methanol, allowing extraction on the day of collection. These tubes are vortexed and centrifuged as above, and the supernatant containing extracted GnRH is decanted and dried in a vortex evaporator.

Autopsy

Unless the sheep is to be sampled at a later date (see below), the animal is killed with an overdose of barbiturate and the calvaria opened to remove the brain. The pituitary is excised, inspected carefully, and sectioned coronally, and the extent and depth of the lesion are recorded.

Applications of the Procedure: Benefits

The portal blood collection procedure as described here enables hypophyseotropic signals to be monitored directly as they travel to the pituitary of animals that are fully conscious and relatively undisturbed. A sufficient volume of portal blood is obtained not only to permit assay and reassay of a hormone in duplicate, but also to measure multiple hormones in the same sample. In addition to these benefits, the procedure has numerous other attributes that permit multiple applications. Illustrative examples based on our studies of secretion of GnRH and luteinizing hormone (LH) are now provided.

Simultaneous Monitoring of Hypothalamic and Pituitary Hormones

Because the procedure does not compromise pituitary function, it is readily possible to monitor GnRH and LH in the same animal. This is illustrated in Fig. 7, which presents the patterns of GnRH and LH in samples obtained at 10-min intervals from a ram orchidectomized several days previously. It is clear that GnRH is secreted episodically and that each burst of secretion is coupled to a pulse of LH. Simultaneous measurement of hypothalamic and pituitary hormones is possible because the pituitary is not removed, nor is its stalk severed. Rather, only some of the portal vessels are cut along the anterior face of the pituitary gland; those that remain are sufficient for continued hypophyseal function.

Prolonged Sampling

Another benefit of the technique is the capacity to obtain portal blood continuously for at least 48 hr. Fluctuations in hypophyseotropic hormones may thus be monitored as an animal undergoes a change in its physiologic state.

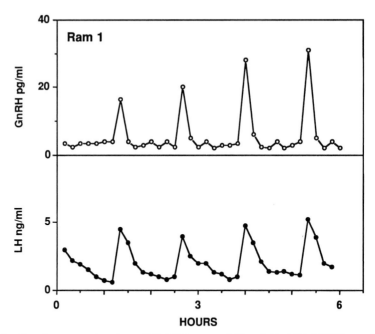

FIG. 7   Simultaneous patterns of GnRH in portal blood (top) and LH in peripheral blood (bottom) obtained at 10-min intervals for 6 hr from a ram orchidectomized several days previously. Note coincidence of pulsatile pattern of the two hormones. Modified with permission from Caraty and Locatelli (10).

It has been possible, for example, to monitor GnRH secretion and LH every 10 min for most of the follicular phase of the estrous cycle of the ewe. As illustrated in Fig. 8, GnRH pulses become lower in amplitude as the cycle progresses from the early to the midfollicular phase; these pulses then give way to a massive GnRH surge that begins with and continues well beyond the preovulatory LH discharge. Such prolonged observations in the same sheep can provide substantial insights into physiological regulatory mechanisms. The actual limit to the duration of continuous sampling has not been determined but it is likely that, if red blood cells were replaced to compensate for blood loss, periods even longer than 48 hr would be feasible. In addition, portal blood collection can be interrupted, if necessary, for short periods (e.g., 30 min) by disconnecting the sampling lines and plugging the collection apparatus and jugular cannulae. This permits animals to be removed temporarily from their pens for special procedures, such as checking estrous behavior.

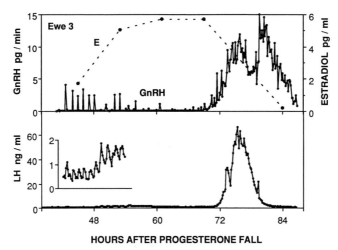

FIG. 8   Patterns of GnRH in portal blood (top) and LH in jugular blood (bottom) in samples obtained from one ewe at 10-min intervals for approximately 48 hr during the follicular phase of the estrous cycle. Concentrations of estradiol (E) determined at less-frequent intervals are shown in upper panel. Inset in lower panel depicts pulsatile pattern of LH otherwise obscured by scale. Adapted with permission from Moenter *et al.* (13).

Repeated Sampling

Another attribute of the method is the capability of collecting portal blood on separate occasions from the same animal, as portal flow can be reinitiated after one sampling is completed simply by introducing the stylet into the collection apparatus to recut portal vessels. As illustrated in Fig. 9, nearly identical pulsatile patterns of GnRH secretion were observed in an ovariectomized ewe sampled on three occasions spanning a period of 36 days. Such repeated sampling provides the potential for monitoring hypophyseotropic hormones in the same individual during long-term changes in physiological state, such as during transitions between the breeding and nonbreeding seasons. However, caution must be exercised with this application because, in most animals, the amplitude of GnRH pulses was found to be reduced in the subsequent samplings.

Moment-to-Moment Changes in Neuroendocrine Activity

Another important benefit of the procedure is that it can provide a direct accurate description of the true moment-to-moment secretory dynamics of

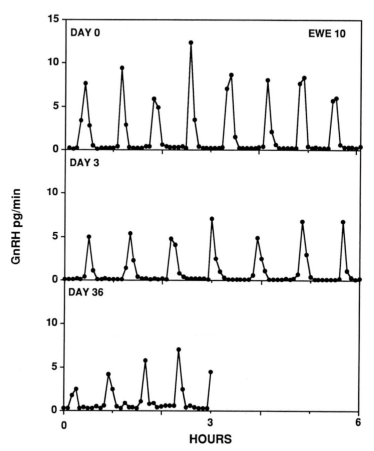

FIG. 9   Patterns of GnRH in portal blood obtained at 5-min intervals from an ovariec-tomized ewe on three separate occasions: Day 0, 3, and 36 (sampling on Day 36 terminated for reasons other than technical difficulties). Note the nearly identical pattern of GnRH release on all three occasions. From F. J. Karsch and D. L. Foster, unpublished.

hypophyseotropic substances, provided samples are obtained with sufficient frequency. This is in contrast to the measurement of pituitary hormones in peripheral circulation, which reflects integration of three processes: secretion, mixing in the periphery, and metabolic clearance. There are two reasons why this technique allows direct assessment of the actual secretory event. First, the method detects GnRH on its one and *only* pass down the portal vessels. This is so because there is no detectable recirculation of GnRH from the periphery (even during the massive GnRH surge) due to its rapid

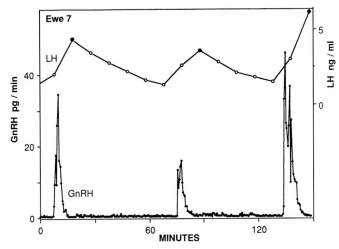

FIG. 10   Patterns of GnRH in portal blood sampled every 30 sec for 2.5 hr from a ewe ovariectomized several days previously. Concentrations of LH in samples of jugular blood obtained at 10-min intervals are shown at top. Note explosive nature and different characteristics of each GnRH pulse, as well as the extremely low baseline between pulses. Adapted with permission from Moenter *et al.* (12).

metabolism and dilution in the relatively vast volume of peripheral blood. Thus, for GnRH to be detected in a given sample, it must be released while the sample is actually being collected. The second reason the procedure accurately discloses the dynamics of neurosecretory processes relates to the mechanics of the collection system. As described previously, portal blood enters the collection line in such a way that blocks of blood (5–20 μl) are separated by air that enters the system via the upper needle of the collection apparatus. This virtually eliminates mixing of blood and dispersion of neuro-secretory signals during their transit from the portal vessels to the collection tube.

The moment-to-moment secretory pattern of GnRH during a pulse in an ovariectomized ewe from which portal blood was sampled every 30 sec for 2.5 hr is illustrated in Fig. 10. Individual pulses of GnRH were found to consist of an explosive burst, rising from undetectable to peak values in as little as 60 sec, maintenance of elevated secretion for about 5 min, and a precipitous drop back to baseline almost as abruptly as the rising edge of the pulse. Studies in which GnRH pulses of known shape were generated *in vitro* by a computer-driven pump and delivered into the collection system verified that the pattern of GnRH illustrated in Fig. 10 is a true representation of the pattern actually released into the portal vasculature (12). We have utilized this application of the method to evaluate the secretory dynamics of GnRH in response to various stimuli and have gathered evidence that the contour of GnRH pulses is physiologically regulated (N. P. Evans and F. J. Karsch, unpublished). Further, we have found that GnRH release is not strictly episodic in all circumstances, for example, during the preovulatory GnRH surge when the concentration of this hormone in portal blood is continuously elevated for many hours (15).

Other Applications

The procedure can be readily adapted for use in immature sheep by shortening the needles used in the collection apparatus, by reducing the diameter of the cup, and by making minor modifications to the surgical approach (16). This permits evaluation of developmental changes in the secretion of hypophyseotropic hormones. The procedure has also been used to assess the secretory dynamics of hormones released by the anterior pituitary gland (17). In this regard, the concentrations of pituitary hormones in portal blood, which is near the site of secretion, are some 100-fold greater than those in the peripheral circulation. The influences of dilution, recirculation, and metabolic clearance are thus minimized, facilitating determination of moment-to-moment changes in pituitary hormone release. A practical benefit of the procedure is that samples can be obtained anytime between 1 and 7 weeks after surgical installation of the collection apparatus. The investigator thus has the option of performing all surgeries for a large experiment prior to sampling, maximizing efficient use of resources and personnel.

Limitations and Problems

Although learning the procedure is not difficult, many types of technical problems can arise (more than can easily be listed here). Learning to troubleshoot the system to rectify such problems comes best with experience. Beyond technical problems, a number of limitations are noteworthy. First, it is difficult to control the number of portal vessels that are cut; the percentage of the total portal blood flow diverted into the collection system has thus far not been determined. Although some alteration in pituitary function would be expected to result from reduced hypophyseotropic support, available data indicate such an alteration must be rather small. Yet, this is difficult to quantify. Compromised pituitary function may be more of a problem with repeated samplings of the same animal due to damage and necrosis of pituitary tissue resulting from previous collections. Although separate samplings of the same sheep are possible, the animals must eventually be killed to determine the suitability of placement of the collection apparatus and to visualize the site where portal vessels were cut.

It is difficult to assess the degree of stress associated with the surgical and sampling procedures, and the extent to which this may influence the specific neuroendocrine function that is being investigated. Yet, it is important to note that sheep behave normally and appear to be undisturbed during the recovery and sampling periods. Further, we have found that the pattern of cortisol secretion over a 48-hr collection period exhibited occasional small rises, but no sustained large increase as is observed during acute stress (18). Nevertheless, the best way to assess any potential complication of stress is to characterize the neuroendocrine response of interest in terms of pituitary function prior to undertaking portal collection experiments and to determine if this response is altered by the portal sampling procedure.

Additional problems arise from systemic delivery of the large doses of heparin required to prevent clotting and blockage of the collection system. Heparin can initiate bleeding from the surgical site and, in the case of prolonged collections, can initiate internal hemorrhage. Bleeding from the surgical site can be eliminated by extending the interval between surgery and sampling (e.g., 2 to 4 weeks), but in this case continued regular flushing of the collection apparatus is necessary to prevent fibrin and debris from accumulating within the cup. Although heparin-related problems are not generally an issue during short samplings (e.g., 6 to 12 hr), they can be limiting to long-term collections (e.g., 48 hr).

Suitability for Other Species

The procedure should be adaptable to species other than sheep, given certain anatomical features of the pituitary and its vasculature. In this regard, four features of the sheep make it especially well suited. The first is the angle of the pituitary (see Fig. 2). The anterior face of the pituitary of most adult sheep hangs nearly perpendicularly from the base of the brain, such that the densest array of portal vessels is readily accessible with the surgical approach described here. Second, the sheep has a well-formed diaphragma sella, a thick dural fold that separates the pituitary from the brain (the pituitary stalk extends through a small opening in this fold). The diaphragma sella acts as a barrier to prevent cerebrospinal fluid from draining into the site of portal blood sampling. Third, in sheep there is no vasculature along the anterior face of the pituitary other than the portal system, making it possible to obtain portal blood that is not contaminated with blood from other sources. Fourth, the size of the sheep is ideal in that the skull is readily amenable to the surgical approach; the rate of portal blood flow is ample to obtain enough sample for assay and reassay of hormones in duplicate; and the total blood volume is sufficient for serial sampling over prolonged periods. Those species that share these anatomical features should be suitable for the portal blood collection method described here.

Summary: Future Perspectives

The chapter describes a procedure for remote continuous sampling of hypophyseal portal blood of sheep. The procedure offers advantages over earlier methods for portal blood collection because it allows both hypothalamic and pituitary hormones to be monitored for prolonged periods from animals that are fully conscious and apparently undisturbed. Although the procedure is not without problems and limitations, it has many applications and it has allowed hypothalamic neurosecretory signals to be characterized to a degree that is unparalleled by other approaches.

Many future developments should be possible, including adaptation of the technique to other species and the simultaneous monitoring of multiple neurosecretory substances in the same samples. Additional exciting new applications should arise by combining the procedure with other techniques used in neuroendocrine investigation, for example, electrical stimulation and recording as well as the local delivery of regulatory substances to discrete neuroendocrine centers implicated in the control of anterior pituitary function.

Acknowledgment

We acknowledge Drs. Iain J. Clarke and James T. Cummins (Melbourne) for initial development of the portal blood collection technique in sheep and thank them for teaching it to one of us (F.J.K.). We appreciate the extensive critical comments of Dr. Neil P. Evans in the preparation of the manuscript. This work was supported by the National Institutes of Health (HD-18337 and HD 18258) in the United States and the Institut National de la Recherche Agronomique in France.

References

1. J. C. Porter, R. S. Mical, I. A. Kamberi, and Y. R. Grazia, *Endocrinology (Baltimore)* **87,** 197 (1970).
2. D. J. Dierschke, A. N. Bhattacharya, L. E. Atkinson, and E. Knobil, *Endocrinology (Baltimore)*, **87,** 850 (1970).

3. D. K. Sarkar, S. A. Chiappa, and G. Fink, *Nature (London)* **264,** 461 (1976).

4. D. K. Sarkar and G. Fink, *J. Endocrinol.* **80,** 303 (1979).

5. P. M. Plotsky and W. Vale, *Science* **230,** 461 (1985).

6. P. W. Carmel, S. Araki, and M. Ferin, *Endocrinology (Baltimore)* **99,** 243 (1976).

7. J. D. Neill, J. M. Patton, R. A. Dailey, R. C. Tsou, and G. T. Tindall, *Endocrinology (Baltimore)* **101,** 430 (1977).

8. R. C. Tsou, R. A. Dailey, C. S. McLanahan, A. D. Parent, G. T. Tindall, and J. D. Neill, *Endocrinology (Baltimore)* **101,** 534 (1977).

9. I. J. Clarke and J. T. Cummins, *Endocrinology (Baltimore)* **111,** 1737 (1982).

10. A. Caraty and A. Locatelli, *J. Reprod. Fertil.* **82,** 263 (1988).

11. A. Caraty, A. Locatelli, and G. B. Martin, *J. Endocrinol.* **123,** 375 (1989).

12. S. M. Moenter, R. M. Brand, A. R. Midgley, Jr., and F. J. Karsch, *Endocrinology (Baltimore)* **130,** 503 (1992).

13. S. M. Moenter, A. Caraty, A. Locatelli, and F. J. Karsch, *Endocrinology (Baltimore)* **129,** 1175 (1991).

14. S. M. Moenter, A. Caraty, and F. J. Karsch, *Endocrinology (Baltimore)* **127,** 1375 (1990).

15. S. M. Moenter, R. C. Brand, and F. J. Karsch, *Endocrinology (Baltimore)* **130,** 2978 (1992).

16. J. M. Manning, C. G. Herbosa, C. R. Friedman, and D. L. Foster, *Soc. Neurosci. Abstr.* **18**(1), 191 (1992).

17. K. McFadden, V. Padmanabhan, and A. R. Midgley, Jr., *Biol. Reprod.* **46** (Suppl. 1), 175 (1992).

18. A. Caraty, M. Grino, A. Locatelli, V. Guillaume, F. Boudouresque, B. Conte-Devolx, and C. Oliver, *J. Clin. Invest.* **85,** 1716 (1990).

[10] *In Vivo* Measurement of Pulsatile Release of Neuropeptides and Neurotransmitters in Rhesus Monkeys Using Push–Pull Perfusion*

Ei Terasawa

Introduction

Direct measurements of the release of neuropeptides, neurotransmitters, and neuromodulators in the stalk–median eminence or portal circulation in animals are essential for neuroendocrine research. However, because of the anatomical characteristics of primates and ethical considerations for animal experimentation, direct collection of portal blood from unanesthetized monkeys is not feasible. Accordingly, we have modified the push–pull perfusion method described for the rat by Levine and Ramirez (1) to collect samples from the stalk–median eminence of the rhesus monkey (*Macaca mulatta*). Our modifications are characterized by permanent implantation of a stainless steel chamber on the skull, providing repeated access to the stalk–median eminence, and by the use of ventriculography for visualization of key brain structures (2–4). This modified method allows (i) the cannula to be inserted into the desired location within the stalk–median eminence with great accuracy, (ii) samples to be collected repeatedly from a single animal on several occasions under different physiological conditions, (iii) samples containing neurohormones and neurotransmitters to be collected in an amount sufficient for detection with various assays, and (iv) neuroactive substances to be applied directly to the sampling location *in vivo*.

Although the push–pull perfusion method has some weaknesses (see below), when used carefully the method provides a powerful tool for neuroendocrine research and investigation into the pulsatility of neurohormone release in particular. The basic principles of sample collection by our modified push–pull perfusion method are similar to those of the push–pull perfusion methods utilizing permanently implanted cannulae which have already been described for rats, sheep, and monkeys (5–9).

---

* All experiments presented in this article were performed following the standards established by the Animal Welfare Act and the documents entitled "Principles for Use of Animals and Guide for the Care and Use of Laboratory Animals."

Methods in Neurosciences, Volume 20

Stereotaxic Brain Surgery with Ventriculography

We have developed a method by which a push–pull cannula is inserted into the stalk–median eminence a few days prior to perfusion and removed between experiments, since permanent implantation of a cannula could cause damage to neuroterminals and induce an extensive gliosis. Our procedure not only decreases scar formation, thus increasing the recovery rate of neurohormones from the tissue, but also allows multiple experiments in a single monkey.

To permit insertion of a push–pull cannula into the stalk–median eminence when an experiment takes place, permanent implantation of a stainless steel chamber onto the skull is necessary. The chamber implantation surgery is performed stereotaxically with the aid of X-ray ventriculography which was originally reported by Hume and Ganong (10) and modified by Slimp *et al.* (11). The third ventricle is visualized by injection of radioopaque material into the foramen of Monro (Fig. 1A). The ventriculographs obtained during this initial surgery are later used to accurately position the tip of the push–pull cannula in the stalk–median eminence (12, 13). Since the stalk–median eminence is located ventral to the infundibular recess and dorsal to the sella turcica, and since the skull structures of primates exhibit considerable variation, the use of the ventriculogram yields greater accuracy than the use of the skull radiograph alone.

Procedure for X-ray Ventriculography

Prior to the initiation of surgery, a sterilized stainless steel needle (20 gauge, 12 cm in length) is placed in the stereotaxic apparatus and the three coordinates of the ear bar zero are recorded. Sterility of the needle is maintained.

The monkey is tranquilized with ketamine (10 mg/kg im, Aveco Co., Inc., Fort Dodge, IA), intubated, and then anesthetized and maintained during the surgical procedure with a mixture of 60–70% N_2O, 30–40% O_2, and 1–2% halothane administered by spontaneous respiration. The head is shaved and fixed in a stereotaxic apparatus (Model 1730, David Kopf Instruments, CA) modified to accept X-ray film cassettes. Lateral and dorsoventral skull radiographs are taken for verification of correct head position and for initial calculation of the anterior–posterior (AP) and vertical coordinates of the caudal edge of the sphenoid bone (Fig. 1A). The head is then prepared and draped for aseptic surgery. A midline rectangle ($\sim$6 $\times$ 10 mm, long dimension for AP direction) of the parietal bone is removed and an incision is made in the dura mater $\sim$2 mm lateral to the sagittal sinus.

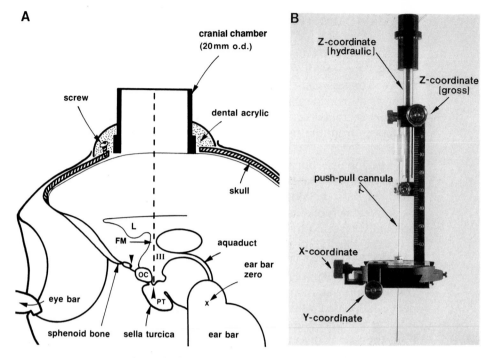

A

cranial chamber
(20 mm o.d.)

screw

dental acrylic

skull

L

FM

aquaduct

III

ear bar
zero

OC

eye bar

PT

x

sphenoid bone   sella turcica   ear bar

B

Z-coordinate
[hydraulic]

Z-coordinate
[gross]

push-pull cannula

X-coordinate

Y-coordinate

FIG. 1   (A) A schematic from lateral radiographs illustrating the monkey skull with a cranial chamber, ear and eye bars, key bone structures, and the ventricle system. The small arrowhead indicates the caudal edge of the sphenoid bone, the coordinates of which are used for the calculation of the foramen of Monro (FM) to inject a radioopaque material. The large arrowhead indicates the infundibular recess of the third ventricle (III), visualized by ventriculogram and necessary for the later placement of a push–pull cannula. The dotted line indicates the center of the cranial chamber placed directly over the infundibular recess (see text for details). Other abbreviations: L, lateral ventricle; OC, optic chiasm; PT, pituitary gland. (B) A photograph of a hydraulic microdrive unit with a push–pull cannula.

The stereotaxic location of the foramen of Monro of the rhesus monkey is estimated by the following regression equations:

For adult females

AP coordinate $Y_1 = 0.708\ X_1 + 0.970$
Vertical coordinate $Y_2 = 0.621\ X_2 + 9.841$

For adult males

AP coordinate $Y_1 = 0.767\ X_1 - 0.773$
Vertical coordinate $Y_2 = 1.017\ X_2 + 5.769$

For juvenile females

$$AP \text{ coordinate} \qquad Y_1 = 0.851\, X_1 - 2.453$$
$$Vertical \text{ coordinate} \qquad Y_2 = 0.663\, X_2 + 10.206$$

X_1 represents the AP coordinate of the caudal edge of the sphenoid bone and Y_1 the AP coordinate of the foramen of Monro; X_2 is the vertical coordinate of the caudal edge of the sphenoid bone and Y_2 the vertical coordinate of the foramen of Monro. The above equations were derived from analysis of the ventriculographs of 70 female and 17 male adult rhesus monkeys as well as 80 juvenile (10–60 months of age) female rhesus monkeys at the Wisconsin Regional Primate Research Center. Correlation coefficients ($r = 0.656$ to 0.979) are all highly significant ($p = 0.0001$). Similar formulas are available for the cynomolgus monkey (*Macaca fascicularis*) (14).

The needle in the stereotaxic apparatus is positioned on the midline between the cerebral hemispheres at the estimated AP coordinate. The dura mater is retracted with forceps, and the needle is lowered slowly into the foramen of Monro at the estimated vertical coordinate. One-tenth of a milliliter of iothalamate meglumine (Conray, Mallinckrodt Pharmaceuticals, St. Louis, MO) is injected into the foramen of Monro over a 15-sec period. Lateral and dorsoventral radiographs are then taken. Because clearance of the radioopaque substance from the ventricular system takes place more quickly in juvenile than in adult monkeys, radiographs should be taken immediately after injection in juveniles, and 15–30 sec after injection in adults.

Cranial Chamber Implantation

For optimal positioning of the push–pull cannula prior to perfusion experiments, the center of the cranial chamber should be placed on the skull directly over the infundibular recess (Fig. 1A) and the top of the chamber should be implanted exactly parallel to the horizontal axis of the stereotaxic frame. For rhesus monkeys we use a stainless steel chamber of 20 mm outer diameter.† (A small cranial chamber with an outer diameter of 5 mm is also available for small animals such as marmoset monkeys and guinea pigs.)

---

† Although for many years we have used a chamber with three pedestals, with which the chamber can be fastened onto the skull by using bolts and nuts, balancing the chamber at the desired position is difficult and requires a substantial amount of time. Therefore, we have altered our approach by using a chamber with deep grooves, which catch the dental acrylic, available through Crist Instrument Co., Inc. (Damascus, MD) and Narishige Scientific Instrument Lab (Tokyo, Japan).

Following ventriculography, the needle for the Conray injection is removed from the electrode holder, and a positioning rod with a pointer (Crist Instrument Co., Inc.) is attached to the holder. The tip of the pointer is placed above the skull opening and aimed at the infundibular recess at the midline using the lateral and dorsoventral ventriculographs. The exact positioning is confirmed by additional radiographs. The pointer is removed from the positioning rods, and a positioning ring (Crist Instrument Co., Inc.) holding the cranial chamber is attached. The holder with the chamber is lowered until the chamber reaches the skull. The outer line of the cranial chamber is marked, and the skull is removed along the mark using a dental drill. Several screws are placed around the chamber as anchors, and the chamber is fixed to the skull with dental acrylic (Fig. 1A). Use of the positioning ring attached to the stereotaxic apparatus ensures that the cranial chamber is centered over the infundibular recess and that the top of the chamber is parallel to the two horizontal axes.

Before the completion of surgery, a microdrive unit (Model M095B, Narishige Scientific Instrument Lab, Tokyo, Japan, Fig. 1B), which is conventionally used for electrophysiological recordings (13), is outfitted with a cannula and stylet assembly and mounted on the chamber. The cannula is subsequently inserted into the brain aiming for the dorsal part of the hypothalamus, at which X, Y, and Z coordinates are recorded. Lateral and dorsoventral radiographs are taken for future reference during cannula insertions. The cannula is withdrawn from the brain, and the cortical surface is treated with a small amount of chloromycetin ointment (Parke Davis, Morris Plains, NJ). The cranial chamber is then filled with 1% silver sulfadiazine ointment (Boots Pharmaceuticals, Inc., Lincolnshire, IL) and covered with a cap. The skin incision around the chamber is closed with sutures. Antibiotics (Crystiben/penicillin, Solvay Veterinary, Inc., Princeton, NJ) and dexamethasone (American Regent Laboratories, Inc., Shirley, NY) are given as prophylactics at the completion of the surgery.

Postsurgical Care and Maintenance of Monkeys Implanted with Cranial Pedestals

On the third postsurgical day, the cap is removed from the cranial chamber, and the cranial chamber is cleaned with hydrogen peroxide and filled with 1% silver sulfadiazine. It is necessary to keep the chamber open thereafter to prevent anaerobic bacterial growth. For protection from chronic infection around the chamber opening, the monkey is treated twice weekly with hydrogen peroxide and 1% silver sulfadiazine. With such maintenance, the chamber remains on the skull and is functional for several months to more than 3 years.

The chamber-implanted monkey lives in its home cage with a compatible companion. After the initial surgery, animals are allowed to recover fully (at least 1 month) before push–pull perfusion experiments are begun. Animals are rested for at least 1 month between two push–pull perfusion experiments.

Adaptation of Monkeys to the Researchers and Experimental Situation

The adaptation of monkeys to the researchers and to the experimental situation prior to push–pull perfusion is one of the most important elements for success of the push–pull perfusion, since (i) neuroendocrine data should be obtained under normal physiological conditions and (ii) jerky movements due to inadequate adaptation to the experimental situation breaks the balance of push and pull flow rates. Our adaptation procedures are as follows: (i) The researcher establishes familiarity with a monkey by hand feeding in its home cage. (ii) He/she restrains the monkey in a primate chair, which is well padded with soft material such as sheepskin, for a few hours at a time in the beginning, gradually increasing the time to an entire working day and then several days at a time. Three to 5 weeks are spent on this adaptation procedure. (iii) The final week before the push–pull perfusion, the monkey is completely equipped for the experiment except for insertion of the cannula. During the entire experiment food and water are provided *ad libitum*. When the monkey is completely adapted to the experimental condition, it is relaxed during the entire procedure, eats and drinks well, and does not show aggressive behavior toward the researcher. If a new researcher is assigned to a monkey that has already been adapted, it is necessary to begin the adaptation procedure over to establish familiarity with the new researcher.

Push–Pull Perfusion

Specifications of the Push–Pull Cannula

For rhesus monkeys we use a push–pull cannula specially produced by Plastics Lab (Roanoke, VA). The cannula consists of an outer (pull) cannula, 0.8 mm in diameter (20 gauge) and 98.3 mm in length, and an inner (push) cannula, 0.35 mm in diameter (28 gauge) and 98.8 mm in length. The stylet is 0.41 mm in diameter (27 gauge) and 98.8 mm in length. These dimensions can be altered along with the purpose and setup. For good perfusion, it is extremely important that the tip of the inner cannula is extruded only 0.5–0.7 mm from the tip of the outer cannula. Similarly, to prevent additional tissue damage on insertion of the inner cannula, the length of the stylet should be identical to that of the inner cannula.

Implantation of Pull Cannula and Stylet

Prior to cannula implantation, calculations for the desired location of the three coordinates are made using ventriculographs and the final radiographs taken during chamber implantation surgery. Since nonhuman primates have a relatively large median eminence and stalk, it is possible to insert the cannula repeatedly into different locations within the structure for multiple experiments in a single animal.

Three days before push–pull perfusion, the monkey is anesthetized with ketamine hydrochloride (10 mg/kg) and 0.1 ml (2 mg) of xylazine im (Mobay Corp., Shawnee, KA) and placed in the stereotaxic apparatus. All instruments that contact the brain are sterilized. The inside of the cranial chamber is carefully cleaned with hydrogen peroxide, and Keflin (Eli Lilly & Co., Indianapolis, IN) is applied. Due to regeneration of the thickened dura mater after a piece of skull has been removed, the dura mater in the center area of the chamber must be perforated with a sharpened stylet. A microdrive unit (Model M095B,‡ Narishige Scientific Instrument Lab, Tokyo, Japan) outfitted with an outer cannula and an inner stylet is then attached to the chamber using the stereotaxic apparatus for alignment. The cannula and stylet are lowered 30 mm, and a set of radiographs is taken to visualize cannula placement. The three coordinates of the microdrive are adjusted to achieve the desired cannula placement, additional radiographs are taken to verify cannula placement, and the cannula is subsequently lowered further to reach its final position. A set of final pictures is taken for the record. With this procedure an adjustment of 200 μm difference can be accomplished. Placement of the cannula in the third ventricle is not desirable because of the difficulty in balancing push and pull flow rates during perfusion.

Following cannula insertion, the monkey is removed from the stereotaxic apparatus and placed in a primate chair, to which the animal was well adapted prior to the study (3). Although the animals are restrained, they are fully conscious and able to take food and water voluntarily throughout the experiment. The cannula and stylet are left in place for 3 days (or a minimum of

---

‡ The company has developed a new model, which is smaller in size and lighter in weight than the M095B. This new model is more useful for push–pull perfusion experiments than the conventional model.

2 days)§ to allow clearance of cellular debris and avoid potential blockage of the tubing during perfusion.

Push–Pull Perfusion

On the day of perfusion, the stylet is replaced with an inner cannula. Both push and pull cannulas are respectively connected to peristaltic pumps via polyethylene tubing (Fig. 2). A modified Krebs–Ringer phosphate buffer solution (artificial cerebrospinal fluid; 123 mM NaCl, 4.8 mM KCl, 1.22 mM MgSO$_4$, 13.9 mM Na$_2$HPO$_4$, 2.45 mM NaH$_2$PO$_4$, 1 mM CaCl$_2$, pH 7.4) with 58 μg/ml bacitracin (Sigma, St. Louis, MO) is infused at 20 μl/min through the inner cannula using the peristaltic pump. Perfusate is collected through the outer cannula by an identically calibrated pump in 10-min fractions on ice using a fraction collector. Each sample is aliquoted for duplicates or different assays, frozen on dry ice immediately, and stored at −70°C.

Application of Our Push–Pull Perfusion Technique

An example of luteinizing hormone-releasing hormone (LHRH) release in a female ovariectomized rhesus monkey measured using the push–pull perfusion method is shown in Fig. 3. LHRH release is pulsatile, and interpulse intervals in adult ovariectomized female and orchidectomized male monkeys are 35–65 min (3, 15). The interpulse interval in early (23–28 months of age) and midpubertal (33–45 months of age) monkeys is similar to that in adults, but the interpulse interval is longer (~80 min) in prepubertal monkeys (4, 16–18). Ovariectomy in pubertal monkeys increases mean LHRH release, pulse amplitude, and basal LHRH release; it does not cause these changes in prepubertal monkeys (18). Estrogen injection in ovariectomized pubertal monkeys suppresses mean LHRH release, pulse amplitude, and basal LHRH release during the period 2–24 hr after treatment, but it does not cause these changes in ovariectomized prepubertal monkeys (19). LHRH release, pulse amplitude, and pulse frequency are all increased during an LH surge, which is induced in ovariectomized monkeys by either a large dose of estrogen (20) or a small dose of estrogen followed by progesterone (21).

Because our method allows for multiple experiments within a single animal, we analyzed variations in LHRH release within individual monkeys as well as between monkeys (3). Pulse frequency (expressed as interpulse interval)

---

§ Based on our experience, the best results can be obtained 3 days after insertion of the pull cannula–stylet assembly. However, the experiment can be done 2 days after insertion.

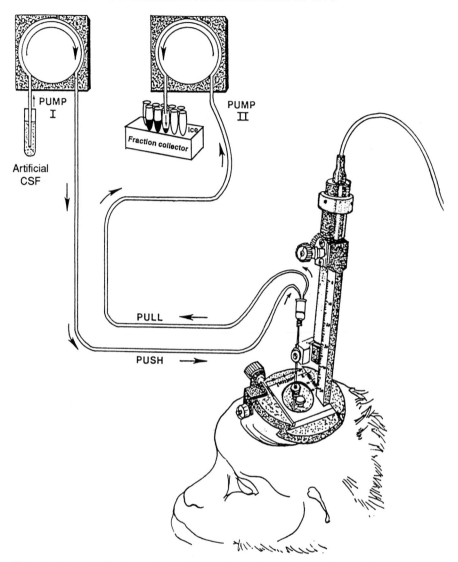

FIG. 2   A schematic illustration of the push–pull perfusion method and experimental setup in the rhesus monkey. A hydraulic microdrive unit is attached to the cranial chamber on the monkey's head. The tip of the push–pull cannula is placed in the stalk–median eminence. Artificial cerebrospinal fluid (modified Krebs–Ringer phosphate buffer) is continuously infused into the stalk–median eminence by pump I, while perfusates are collected by identically calibrated pump II in vials on ice using a fraction collector. [Modified with permission from Terasawa *et al.* (2).]

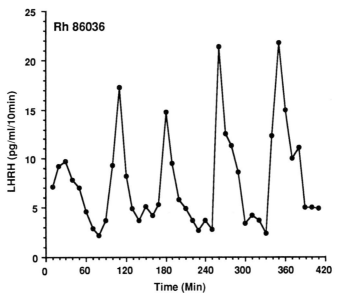

FIG. 3 An example of LHRH release in an ovariectomized monkey measured by the push–pull perfusion method. Samples are obtained at 10-min intervals for 7 hr.

is quite consistent among experiments conducted on a single animal, suggesting that each animal has a characteristic LHRH pulse frequency as long as the animal is under similar physiological conditions. In contrast, other parameters of LHRH release (mean release, basal release, and pulse amplitude) vary greatly with cannula location in the stalk–median eminence. Our analysis further indicates that mapping of the amount of LHRH release during push–pull perfusion reflects the distribution of LHRH neuroterminals in the rhesus monkey (3), i.e., mean LHRH release is highest when the cannula tip is placed in the caudal portion of the median eminence, where the zona externa is located, presumably due to a high density of LHRH neuroterminals in that region. Moderate LHRH release is observed when the cannula tip is placed dorsal to the pituitary stalk and ventral to the infundibular recess of the third ventricle. Mean LHRH release is lowest in areas of the median eminence which are rostral or caudal to the infundibular recess. Mediolaterally higher LHRH release is observed in placements within 1 mm of the midline than in more lateral placements (1–2 mm from the midline). Again these findings parallel the distribution of LHRH neuroterminals; a band of LHRH-positive fibers in the zona externa of the median eminence courses along the caudal aspect of the infundibulum toward the

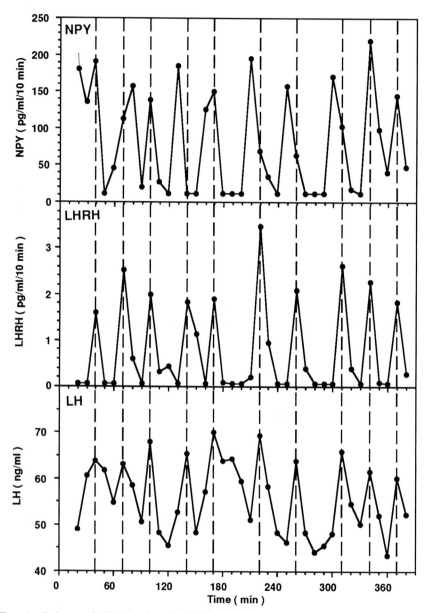

FIG. 4   Release of NPY (top) and LHRH (middle) measured in aliquots of the same push–pull perfusate samples collected from the stalk–median eminence of an adult castrated monkey. LH levels (bottom) in blood samples collected simultaneously with perfusates were also monitored. The release of NPY, LHRH, and LH was

pituitary gland (22, 23). This relationship between mean LHRH release and cannula placement is not affected by the sequence of cannula placements in animals undergoing multiple experiments (3).

The interpulse interval of LHRH release obtained using the push–pull perfusion method is consistent with previous reports of LHRH release measured by other methods in several species (24–27), with the estimated value obtained from monitoring LH pulsatility (28–33), and with the estimated interval between bursts of multiple-unit firing activity (34–36). LHRH release is correlated with LH release when measured over a short period (3). However, blood sampling during several hours of push–pull perfusion of the stalk–median eminence results in gradually decreasing LH and/or LHRH levels, possibly due to compounded stress as described below. Despite the fact that we do conduct the push–pull perfusion experiments almost exclusively in conscious monkeys, we have done one LHRH/LH correlation experiment under Saffan sedation (Glaxo Labs., Greenford, Middlesex, UK). In this experiment we observed a perfect synchrony between LHRH and LH pulses (Fig. 4) (15).

To estimate the perfusion area around the cannula tip, [³H]progesterone (NEN Products, Boston, MA) dissolved in modified Krebs–Ringer phosphate buffer solution was infused into the stalk–median eminence of a monkey. The infusion rate was adjusted to 20 μl/min, and a total 0.2 μCi of [³H]progesterone was infused for a period of 10 min, the time required for the radioactive solution to pass through the push–pull perfusion system. The perfusion was terminated immediately and pentobarbital sodium 30/mg/kg body weight (Abbott Laboratories, Chicago, IL) was injected into the animal. A block of the basal hypothalamus with the stalk–median eminence was carefully dissected and kept frozen ($-40°C$) until thin sections were made to determine the distribution of radioactivity. The unfixed hypothalamic block was cut into 10-μm sections on a cryostat in a dark room. The individual sections were mounted on microscope slides coated with photographic emulsion, NTB 3 (Eastman Kodak, Rochester, NY), and stored for 2 months in a dark room. The slides were then developed photographically and the sections were counterstained with cresyl violet. Diffusion of progesterone was determined microscopically on the autoradiogram. Heavy labeling was found in a restricted area of 500–800 μm (mean 700 μm) around the push cannula, which

---

pulsatile. Pulses of NPY occurred simultaneously with or 10 min preceding LHRH pulses, and peaks of LHRH and LH release occurred synchronously. Dotted lines are coincident with pulses of LHRH reported by the PULSAR algorithm. [Modified with permission from Terasawa and Gore (39); Woller *et al.* (15).]

was located in the rostral median eminence. These results suggest that the area infused by a push–pull cannula is quite localized in the stalk–median eminence.

Advantages of the Push–Pull Perfusion Method

The push–pull perfusion method is a powerful tool for direct measurement of neurochemical substances in the hypothalamus in fully conscious animals. It is advantageous to collect neuropeptides and neurotransmitters at the site of release where the neuroterminals are concentrated. Using the method described in this article, we are able to measure, in samples collected from the stalk–median eminence, LHRH and other neuropeptides, such as neuropeptide Y (NPY), β-endorphin, corticotropin-releasing hormone, somatostatin, and growth hormone-releasing hormone, by radioimmunoassay (RIA); neurotransmitters, such as γ-aminobutyric acid (GABA), glutamate, norepinephrine, epinephrine, dopamine, and serotonin and their metabolites (dihydrophenyl glycol, methoxyhydroxyphenyl glycol, dihydroxyphenylacetic acid, homovanillic acid, and 5-hydroxyindoleacetic acid), by high-performance liquid chromatography with electrochemical detection; and other substances such as prostaglandin E_2 and cyclic adenosine monophosphate (cAMP), by RIA (2, 15–19, 37, 38). As new assays are established or as assays improve, this list could increase further. Interestingly, the release of many of these neurochemical substances is pulsatile (2, 15, 39, 40).

The second advantage of our push–pull perfusion method is its application in measuring more than one neuropeptide and/or neurotransmitter simultaneously. In our observations, norepinephrine pulses precede or occur simultaneously with LHRH pulses, although norepinephrine pulses occur almost twice as frequently as LHRH pulses (2). NPY release also precedes LHRH release by 10 min or occurs simultaneously with LHRH release (Fig. 4) (15). The coupling of LHRH and NPY pulses does not change when pulse frequency increases during the LH surge induced by estrogen and progesterone (21).

The third strength of the push–pull perfusion method is that it allows application of neuroactive substances locally while perfusates are continuously collected from the extracellular space where the neuroterminals are concentrated. This method not only provides some of the advantages of *in vitro* perfusion experiments, such as bypassing the blood–brain barrier, but also allows testing of the effects of neuroactive substances in a restricted area of the hypothalamus *in vivo* under physiological conditions without anesthesia. Moreover, the method of direct application of a neuroactive substance to the stalk–median eminence is superior to injection of the substance into the third ventricle, a technique commonly used in neuroendocrine studies, since a substance injected into the third ventricle may diffuse over large areas where facilitatory as well as inhibitory neurons responding to the substance are distributed. For instance, it was found that infusion of NPY into the stalk–median eminence stimulated LHRH release in a dose–responsive manner in ovariectomized monkeys (41), and estrogen priming of ovariectomized monkeys shifted the dose–response curve to the left, indicating the sensitization of neurons in the brain with estradiol (42). In contrast, the results of NPY infusion into the third ventricle and the median eminence were inconsistent, dependent on the infusion site as well as on the hormonal milieu of ovariectomized monkeys (43), presumably due to the diffusion of NPY into diverse areas of the brain after third ventricular infusion. In addition to NPY, direct infusion of potassium, norepinephrine, methoxamine (an α_1-adrenergic stimulant), endothelin, neurotensin, angiotensin, prostaglandin E_2, or bicuculline (a GABA-A antagonist) into the stalk–median eminence generally stimulates LHRH release (3, 44, 45), while infusion of prazosin (an α_1-adrenergic antagonist), GABA, β-endorphin, or antiserum to NPY generally suppressed LHRH release (3, 15, 37, 41).

Because nonhuman primates have a large-size stalk–median eminence relative to the area of infusion ($\sim 700 \mu$m), several push–pull perfusion experiments (up to a dozen) can be performed in a single monkey. This is enormously advantageous for studies of nonhuman primates, since they are a scarce resource. In addition, the push–pull perfusion method can be combined with electrical stimulation as we have shown in prepubertal and pubertal monkeys (4), coupled with recording of multiple- or single-unit activity, and accompanied with *in vivo* voltammetric analysis of oxidizable neurochemical substances.

The use of the microdialysis method also provides a powerful approach to neuroendocrine research with minimum trouble during perfusion (see Chapter 8 by Levine *et al.*, this volume). However, the microdialysis approach may not be as useful as the push–pull perfusion method in nonhuman primates for several reasons: (i) The recovery rate of neuropeptides, but not catecholamines, through the microdialysis membrane is not as good as that using the push–pull perfusion, so that detection of neuropeptides in perfusates with the available RIA is often difficult. (ii) Because of the long length of the microdialysis probe to increase the recovery rate, sample collection will not be restricted within the stalk–median eminence and is likely to include samples from other parts of the medial basal hypothalamus. (iii) Sampling from the pituitary is difficult; because the diaphragma sellae consists of hard bone in primates, the insertion of a cannula into the anterior pituitary gland can only be done through a small hole, the pituitary fossa. Therefore, the procedure would cause pituitary infarction.

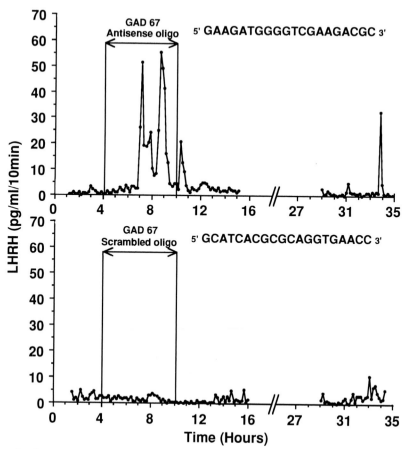

FIG. 5 An example of the effects of antisense oligodeoxynucleotide for GAD67 mRNA on LHRH release in a prepubertal monkey measured by a push-pull perfusion method. After 4 hr of control samplings, antisense oligo (top) or scrambled oligo (bottom) was infused for 6 hr, while perfusates were continuously collected. The sample collection was continued for an additional 6 hr and 14 hr later the sampling was resumed for another 6 hr. Note that infusion of the antisense oligo, but not the scrambled oligo, resulted in an increase in LHRH release (D. Mitsushima *et al.*, unpublished observations).

Finally, push–pull perfusion can be used as an aid in molecular and cellular studies. In addition to the points made above, synthesis, cleavage, and degradation can be estimated by measurements of precursor peptides (if they are released from the terminals), cleavage fragments, and degradation enzymes. We observed that the ratio of the release of gonadotropin-associated peptide (GAP), a fragment of the proLHRH molecule, to the release of LHRH in perfusates obtained from the stalk–median eminence was approximately 1 to 1 in pubertal monkeys, as was reported for the portal circulation in sheep (46). The push–pull perfusion method will also be powerful when employed in combination with molecular biological approaches. For instance, infusion of antisense oligodeoxynucleotides for genes encoding a neuropeptide/neurotransmitter or its receptor or its enzyme through the push cannula may suppress the release of the neuropeptide or neurotransmitter obtained through the pull cannula, since the oligodeoxynucleotide can be taken into the cells and hybridized with the specific mRNA of interest.

We have already confirmed that this can be done: Infusion of antisense oligodeoxynucleotides for glutamic acid decarboxylase (GAD67 and GAD65) mRNAs into the stalk-median eminence in prepubertal monkeys resulted in an increase of LHRH release within 3 hr of infusion, by reduction of GAD synthesis and presumably by the reduction of GABA release (Fig. 5, 47). GABA is an inhibitory neurotransmitter restricting LHRH release before the onset of puberty (45).

Problems and Concerns

Despite the many advantages of the push–pull perfusion method, the use of this technique has some drawbacks. (i) Occlusion of the polyethylene tubing or the cannula is the most significant difficulty of the method. This can occur as a result of suction of tissue fragments and debris in the pull pathway, but it can also be caused by salt precipitation in the push pathway. However, careful preparations of the cannula, the push and pull cannula assembly, and the polyethylene tubing can help to prevent potential occlusion. In fact, an experienced researcher can readily collect perfusate samples for more than 15 hr without any problem. When a partial occlusion occurs anywhere in the system, the balance of push and pull pressure is not maintained and the volume of perfusate collection becomes reduced. This leads to tissue damage, and the value of the neurohormone in the sample of reduced volume becomes abnormal. (ii) Tissue damage is a great concern for this method. Although our approach using short-term cannula placement does not cause the extensive gliosis associated with permanent placement of the cannula, it does cause some gliosis. In addition, infusion must cause tissue damage; the second insertion of a cannula at the identical coordinates results in reduced levels of neurohormones in the perfusate, although the amount of neurohormone released is stable for more than 15 hr or as long as perfusion continues. Nevertheless, it appears that damage is not extensive and that some regeneration of the capillaries occurs, since we can conduct an average of seven or eight push–pull perfusion experiments per single monkey and up to a dozen per juvenile monkey during the course of its sexual maturation. Notably, many ovarian-intact animals used in push–pull perfusion experiments and then returned to the breeding colony subsequently had normal pregnancies, deliveries, and nursing. (iii) There are limitations on the simultaneous collection of frequent blood samples. Despite the fact that serial blood sampling alone or push–pull perfusion alone yields stable levels of a hormone or neurohormone, respectively, for many hours, the combination of both procedures results in the decline of either or both substances 2–4 hr after the initiation of simultaneous sampling. We interpret this problem to mean that each procedure produces a minimum stress, but the combination of both procedures precipitates a visible stress effect. Although serum cortisol levels and β-endorphin levels in perfusates during push–pull perfusion are not particularly elevated (3, 35), a minimum stress component should be allotted for this procedure.

Conclusions

The push–pull perfusion method described in this article is not limited to the use of large animals such as rhesus monkeys and baboons. In fact, in our Primate Center this method has been successfully applied to marmoset monkeys (*Callithrix jacchus*), which weigh ~350 g, by miniaturization of the skull chamber and microdrive unit, for the study of neuroendocrine changes due to social dominance (48). Many refinements, including use of push–pull perfusion without chair restraint, are expected in the future. We believe that our method and its application to other species will be useful also for the study of pulsatile release of neurohormones and neurotransmitters. Moreover, the method can be applied for other neuroendocrine studies as well as for the study of mechanisms underlying behavior, such as studies of feeding and drinking behaviors.

Acknowledgments

This technique is established under the auspices of NIH Grants HD11355, HD15433, and RR00167. The author expresses sincere appreciation to former postdoctoral research fellows (Drs. Marla Gearing, Sukumal Chongthammakun, Lee Claypool, Gen Watanabe, and Nancy Schultz-Darken), graduate students (Michael Loose, Andrea Gore, and Michael Woller), and a specialist (Cathy Krook) who helped to establish this difficult method and make it workable, and to former undergraduate students (Erik Alexander and Paul Palmer) for analysis of the ventriculographs to derive the equations reported in the manuscript. The protocol for this study was reviewed and approved by the Research Animal Resource Center, University of Wisconsin. This work (#32-039) is filed at the Wisconsin Regional Primate Research Center.

References

1. J. E. Levine and V. D. Ramirez, *Endocrinology (Baltimore)* **107,** 1782 (1980).
2. E. Terasawa, C. Krook, D. L. Hei, M. Gearing, N. J. Schultz, and G. D. Davis, *Endocrinology (Baltimore)* **123,** 1808 (1988).
3. M. Gearing and E. Terasawa, *Brain Res. Bull.* **21,** 117 (1988).
4. L. E. Claypool, G. Watanabe, and E. Terasawa, *Endocrinology (Baltimore)* **127,** 3014 (1990).
5. J. E. Levine and V. D. Ramirez, in "Methods in Enzymology" (P. M. Conn, ed.), Vol. 168, p. 466. Academic Press, San Diego, 1986.
6. N. W. Kasting and J. B. Martin, in "Methods in Enzymology" (P. M. Conn, ed.), Vol. 103, p. 176. Academic Press, San Diego, 1983.
7. J. E. Levine, K.-Y. F. Pau, V. D. Ramirez, and G. L. Jackson, *Endocrinology (Baltimore)* **111,** 1449 (1982).
8. J. E. Levine, R. L. Norman, P. M. Gliessman, T. T. Oyama, D. R. Bangsberg, and H. G. Spies, *Endocrinology (Baltimore)* **117,** 711 (1985).
9. P. M. Gliessman, K.-Y. F. Pau, J. D. Hill, and H. G. Spies, *J. Appl. Physiol.* **61,** 2273 (1986).
10. D. M. Hume and W. F. Ganong, *Electroencephalogr. Clin. Neurophysiol.* **8,** 136 (1956).
11. J. C. Slimp, B. L. Hart, and R. W. Goy, *Brain Res.* **142,** 105 (1978).
12. E. Terasawa, J. J. Noonan, T. E. Nass, and M. D. Loose, *Endocrinology (Baltimore)* **115,** 2241 (1984).
13. R. R. Yeoman and E. Terasawa, *Endocrinology (Baltimore)* **115,** 2445 (1984).
14. K. Crawford, E. Terasawa, and P. L. Kaufman, *Brain Res.* **503,** 265 (1989).
15. M. J. Woller, J. K. McDonald, D. M. Reboussin, and E. Terasawa, *Endocrinology (Baltimore)* **130,** 2333 (1992).
16. G. Watanabe and E. Terasawa, *Endocrinology (Baltimore)* **125,** 92 (1989).
17. A. C. Gore and E. Terasawa, *Endocrinology (Baltimore)* **129,** 3009 (1991).
18. S. Chongthammakun, L. E. Claypool, and E. Terasawa, *J. Neuroendocrinol.* **5,** 41 (1993).
19. S. Chongthammakun and E. Terasawa, *Endocrinology (Baltimore)* **132,** 735 (1993).
20. E. Terasawa, C. Krook, G. Watanabe, and W. E. Bridson, *Endocrinology (Baltimore)* **118** (Suppl.), 256 (1986).
21. M. J. Woller, D. M. Reboussin, and E. Terasawa, *Biol. Reprod.* **44,** (Suppl.), 95 (1991).
22. P. C. Goldsmith and T. Song, *J. Comp. Neurol.* **257,** 130 (1987).
23. A. J. Silverman, J. L. Antunes, G. M. Abrams, G. Nilaver, R. Thau, J. A. Robinson, M. Ferin, and L. C. Krey, *J. Comp. Neurol.* **211,** 309 (1982).

24. P. W. Carmel, S. Araki, and M. Ferin, *Endocrinology (Baltimore)* **99,** 243 (1976).
25. I. J. Clarke and J. T. Cummins, *Endocrinology (Baltimore)* **111,** 1737 (1982).
26. D. A. vanVugt, W. D. Diefenbach, E. Alston, and M. Ferin, *Endocrinology (Baltimore)* **117,** 1550 (1985).
27. A. Caraty and A. Locatelli, *J. Reprod. Fertil.* **82,** 263 (1988).
28. D. J. Dierschke, A. N. Bhattacharya, L. E. Atkinson, and E. Knobil, *Endocrinology (Baltimore)* **87,** 850 (1970).
29. A. R. Midgley and R. B. Jaffe, *J. Clin. Endocrinol. Metab.* **33,** 962 (1971).
30. S. S. C. Yen, C. C. Tsao, F. Naftolin, G. Vandenberg, and L. Ajabor, *J. Clin. Endocrinol. Metab.* **34,** 671 (1972).
31. E. Knobil, *Recent Prog. Horm. Res.* **36,** 53 (1980).
32. E. Terasawa, C. Krook, S. Eman, G. Watanabe, W. E. Bridson, S. A. Sholl, and D. L. Hei, *Endocrinology (Baltimore)* **120,** 1808 (1987).
33. M. Gearing and E. Terasawa, *Am. J. Physiol.* **25,** 23 (1991).
34. J. C. Thiery and J. Pelletier, *Neuroendocrinology* **32,** 217 (1981).
35. M. Kawakami, T. Uemura, and R. Hayashi, *Neuroendocrinology* **35,** 63 (1982).
36. R. C. Wilson, J. S. Kesner, J.-M. Kaufman, T. Uemura, T. Akema, and E. Knobil, *Neuroendocrinology* **39,** 256 (1984).
37. M. Gearing and E. Terasawa, *Brain Res.* **560,** 276 (1991).
38. E. Terasawa and S. Chongthammakun, ''Proceedings of the 21st Annual Meeting of the Neuroscience Society,'' No. 361.1, 1991.
39. E. Terasawa and A. C. Gore, *in* ''Modes of Action of GnRH and GnRH Analogs'' (W. F. Crowley, Jr., and P. M. Conn, eds.), p. 256. Springer-Verlag, New York, 1992.
40. A. C. Gore, D. Mitsushima, and E. Terasawa, *Neuroendocrinology* **58,** 23 (1993).
41. M. J. Woller and E. Terasawa, *Endocrinology (Baltimore)* **128,** 1144 (1991).
42. M. J. Woller and E. Terasawa, *Neuroendocrinology* **56,** 921 (1992).
43. A. H. Kaynard, K.-Y. F. Pau, D. L. Hess, and H. G. Spies, *Endocrinology (Baltimore)* **127,** 2437 (1990).
44. M. Gearing and E. Terasawa, *Neuroendocrinology* **53,** 373 (1991).
45. D. Mitsushima, D. L. Hei, and E. Terasawa, *Proc. Natl. Acad. Sci. U.S.A.,* **91,** 395 (1994).
46. I. J. Clarke, J. T. Cummins, F. J. Karsch, P. H. Seeburg, and K. Nikolics, *Biochem. Biophys. Res. Commun.* **143,** 665 (1987).
47. D. Mitsushima, F. Marzban, D. L. Hei, T. G. Golos, and E. Terasawa, ''Proceedings of the 23rd Annual Meeting of the Neuroscience Society,'' No. 258.1, 1993.
48. W. Saltzman, D. H. Abbott, N. J. Schultz-Darken, and E. Terasawa, *Biol. Reprod.* **48** (suppl. 1), 65 (1993).

[11] *In Vitro* Systems for Modeling Target Tissue Responses to Secretory Pulses of the Islet Hormones: Glucagon and Insulin

Charles J. Goodner

Background

The hormones of the Islets of Langerhans are secreted as discrete pulses with pulse intervals ranging from 5 to 15 min in mammalian species (1, 2). This secretory pattern has been documented for insulin, glucagon, somatostatin, pancreatic polypeptide, and the C-peptide of proinsulin. In the original observations made in fasting unanesthetized rhesus monkeys, secretory pulses of insulin and glucagon were synchronous with a small oscillation of the fasting blood glucose suggesting that the hormonal events were imposing a time-dependent effect on their target tissues (1). It was subsequently demonstrated in the same *in vivo* model that a large oscillation in hepatic glucose production was occurring synchronously with the islet hormone secretory pulses and fully accounted for the observed oscillation in the fasting glucose concentration (3).

The intrapancreatic origin of hormonal pulses was established by the demonstration that insulin, glucagon, and somatostatin were spontaneously secreted as large pulses from the isolated perfused dog pancreas (4). The pulses remained robust for 3 hr even with perfusion of media at a constant glucose concentration. In later work it has been documented that spontaneous electrical events (5) and synchronous changes in the intracellular calcium concentration in islet cells (6–8) are coupled to the episodic secretory behavior of the islets and that both may originate in spontaneous cyclic glycolytic pathways in these cells (9). The fact that secretion of the more than one million individual islets appears as a large coherent pulse in hormone concentration in the portal blood draining the pancreas indicates that there must be a mechanism for interislet coordination of individual secretory events. The major candidate for this communication network is an intrapancreatic ganglionic neural network (10). Pharmacologic studies in the perfused dog pancreas suggest that peptdergic neurotransmitters mediate coordination of secretory activity. In addition to the intrinsic pancreatic coordination of secretory activity there are data to suggest that these events can be modulated by other systems in the whole animal. For example the pulse interval is consistently shorter

Methods in Neurosciences, Volume 20

by 20–30% in the perfused pancreas preparation compared to the interval observed in the same species *in vivo* (11). It has also been demonstrated that imposition of exogenous glucose cycles can, within limits, alter the islet secretory rhythm (12). This capacity for modulation by nutrients is even more pronounced for a lower frequency ultradian secretory cycle that appears to be superimposed on the higher frequency pulses described above (13, 14). It is of considerable interest that at either the higher or the lower ultradian frequency spontaneous insulin pulses appear to be abnormal in patients with diabetes (15–17).

Another area of investigation is the functional relationship between the several endocrine cell types within the islets, relationships that might be relevant to the question of an islet pacemaker. Work on the anatomy of the islet microcirculation and on local endocrine regulation has established a sequence for blood flow within the islets from the central core of B-cells (insulin secreting) to the peripheral mantle of A-cells (glucagon secreting) and then to the mantle D-cells (somatostatin secreting) (18–22). It is clear that this B–A–D sequence is of physiologic importance for regulation of glucagon secretion via insulin inhibition of glucagon secretion within the intraislet microcirculation. Somatostatin seems to affect neither B- nor A-cells via a local endocrine route but the possibility remains that it could operate via a paracrine mechanism. These relationships would theoretically permit the B-cells to act as a pacemaker for episodic secretion by the A- and D-cells; however evidence suggests that each cell type is capable of independent, spontaneous episodic secretory behavior (11). This relationship is physiologically important since the liver is a major target tissue for insulin and essentially the only target tissue for glucagon. Insulin pulses reaching the peripheral circulation would be expected to act on the major insulin-sensitive tissues, skeletal muscle and adipose tissue.

A number of factors contribute to the complexity of studying the impact of islet secretory events on target tissues. First, the amplitude of the hormone pulses in hepatic portal blood is two- to three-fold higher than that in the peripheral circulation. This presents a problem in selecting the appropriate dose range for *in vitro* studies. Again, as in the neuroendocrine case, multiple hormones impinge on a single target tissue in a short period of time providing the potential for physiologically important hormonal interactions, the modeling of which presents additional experimental complexity. The liver portal sinusoids possess a fenestrated endothelium that readily admits insulin and glucagon to the cell-surface receptors. Insulin is significantly cleared from plasma (by about 50%) during first passage through the hepatic portal circulation. This provides the potential for control of overall hormone metabolism by modulation of pulse amplitude since the rate of clearance of insulin is nonlinear with respect to concentration over short periods of time. The hepatic clearance of insulin also acts a damper on the amplitude of insulin pulses reaching the peripheral target tissues, tending to reduce the impact of the primary secretory pulses.

Limitations of in Vivo Models for Investigating Target Responses to Hormone Pulses

The need for *in vitro* models to fully study the impact of pulsed vs continuous hormone secretion on target tissue response stems in part from the inherent limitations of *in vivo* methods for studying insulin and glucagon action. These limitations include the difficulty of separating primary responses from secondary events in the highly interrelated fuel regulatory systems. Thus pulses of insulin administered to the whole organism will affect hepatic pathways for glucose production and storage while at the same time affecting the supply of precursors for these pathways derived from insulin-sensitive peripheral tissues. In addition, unless special steps are taken such as administration of islet-inhibiting doses of somatostatin, exogenous pulses of hormone will be intermixed with and superimposed on spontaneous endogenous pulses. If the goal is to examine the effects of pulses on hepatic pathways, the hormone would ideally be introduced into the hepatic portal circulation. Although technically feasible, this route complicates the experimental model particularly for rodent models. The need to administer exogenous pulses can be avoided by simply observing time-dependent correlations of target pathways with spontaneous endogenous pulses. However, as in neurophysiologic studies, correlations in time of spontaneous episodic effector events with putative responses do not necessarily prove a causal relationship. It is only possible to deduce a causal relationship when unambiguous, timed signals can be delivered to the system and the time-dependent response measured, as in the classic use of evoked potentials. For example, in our study showing synchrony between cyclic changes in hepatic glucose production and spontaneous pulses of insulin and glucagon, the presence of a temporal correlation by itself could not discriminate between a primary role for one or the other hormone; it is possible that both are acting in concert or for the operation of some unknown indirect pathway (3). For all of these reasons *in vitro* models are necessary to establish the physiologic role of islet secretory pulses.

The liver is the first target tissue of interest for addressing the question of the potential physiologic importance of a pulsatile pattern of islet secretion. Glucagon acts exclusively on the liver where it is the major hormone that stimulates pathways for increased production of glucose. Glucagon acts through its surface receptor to activate adenylate cyclase and increase the synthesis of cyclic AMP (cAMP). The pathway of gluconeogenesis is accelerated through activation of key regulatory enzymes by a cascade of phosphorylation–dephosphorylations and at the genomic level by stimulating the transcription of the gene for the enzyme phosphoenolpyruvate decarboxylase (PEPCK) (23), the first committed step in the gluconeogenetic pathway. Insulin potently opposes this action of glucagon. Glucagon also stimulates the pathway for mobilization of the hepatic glycogen store. Insulin also opposes this action of glucagon and stimulates synthesis of the glycogen store. In the physiologic setting these opposing actions of glucagon and insulin regulate the flow of fuels between the liver and the periphery (24). The classic studies from which these concepts were developed have relied on experiments employing steady-state conditions or simple step changes in the concentration of hormones and substrates. The question raised by the new knowledge of a pulsed pattern of hormone secretion is whether unique control information is carried by this pattern, and, if so, what are the mechanisms responsible?

Factors Important in the Selection of in Vitro Models

A useful system must be capable of generating measurable responses to the test hormone at rates rapid enough to be synchronized with the pulse frequency found *in vivo*. It must permit delivery of a coherent hormonal signal that exposes the test cells to a reasonable facsimile of the physiologic hormone pulse traversing the tissue capillaries *in vivo*. The best approximation of these conditions is provided in a perfused organ preparation with an intact microcirculation. Whereas, models employing perifused isolated cells or cultured cells do not provide the normal barrier function of the microcirculation and limit conclusions regarding time constants for measured hormone response rates. For a tissue with fenestrated endothelium such as the liver (or in the case of the neuroendocrine system, the anterior pituitary) this limitation is less critical than that for tissues such as skeletal muscle or adipose tissue where the capillary transit times of hormones, such as insulin, may be quite slow (25, 26). These considerations are of much greater concern for modeling systems with higher pulse frequency, while systems with low-frequency hormone pulses may not be greatly influenced by transport delays or slow rates of response.

The choice of an *in vitro* model is also often influenced by the extent to which responsive pathways survive the necessary preparative aspects of the model. Perfused organ preparations, such as the perfused rat liver, require special consideration for adequate oxygenation of the tissue at desirable media flow rates. Slower flow rates are less likely to impose pressure artifacts on the tissue such as swelling and exudation of extracellular fluid from the capsule. Slower flow rates also facilitate measurements of organ extraction rates or production rates by widening the concentration difference for precursors or products between inflowing and outflowing media. Maintenance of adequate oxygenation at slower flow rates usually requires addition of erythrocytes which may complicate interpretation of results. Even the most elaborate perfusion models display a progressive loss of integrity in the barrier functions of the microcirculation and in metabolic rate over a period of hours, limiting the duration of experiments. Methods using isolated cells also have limitations. The method of isolation usually requires treatment of the donor organ with proteolytic enzymes such as collagenase. Cell separation also requires low-speed centrifugation, often in the presence of an unphysiologic density gradient medium. Tissues vary greatly in their ability to maintain normal hormonal responsiveness during isolation procedures. Of two insulin-responsive tissues isolated, adipocytes generally retain hormone responsiveness while isolated hepatocytes lose many metabolic responses including the ability to respond normally to insulin. However, isolated heptocytes respond vigorously to glucagon and may be used for studies of pulsed delivery of this hormone. As a substitute for freshly isolated hepatocytes, the rat hepatoma cell line, H_4IIEC3, has become the classic *in vitro* model in which to study the hepatic effects of insulin. This line is easily cultured under conditions that provide large numbers of cells highly responsive to insulin. In H_4IIEC3 cells insulin actively regulates expression of the gene for PEPCK. Unfortunately these cells lack glucagon receptors and therefore cannot be used to study the interaction of pulses of insulin and glucagon per se. When insulin effects are studied with this cell line, analogs of cAMP are used to mimic the effect of glucagon.

The system should be capable of resolving a series of pulses into separate or nearly separate signals over the physiologic range of frequencies to be examined. These considerations generally dictate that the perfusion system be an open or one-pass system as opposed to a recirculating system. Second, as a general principle, the hormone entry port should be introduced into the flowing stream of oxygenated medium as close upstream as possible to the test organ or cells. This location limits the mixing of the signal in the medium stream before reaching the target cells (27).

When the hormone stream flow is stopped the concentration or hormone decreases exponentially as washout occurs. As the signal achieves a steady state during initiation of the pulse, the curve of rising concentration is a mirror image of the concentration curve of washout. The shapes of these curves and, therefore, the discrete nature of the signal depend on the flow rate of the moving medium stream and the volume of the test system exposed to the stream, higher flows and lower volumes yielding the sharper peaks of signal concentration. The use of a column filled with a supporting matrix of gel as provided by polyacrylamide beads limits the volume of mixing and greatly enhances the coherence of a hormone pulse traversing the column. The upper limit on flow is set by the resistance to flow of the system. In perfused organs this is a function of the size and status of the microcirculation. In other systems the filter serving to confine the test cells is usually the point of resistance to flow. Increasing perfusion pressure to increase flow is accompanied by an undesirable degree of sheer stress on cells or the microcirculation. In order to minimize transient changes in overall flow rate, the rate of flow of the hormone delivery stream should generally be kept as low as is compatible with good solubility of the signal molecule.

To summarize, selection of conditions of flow for a given system is often a matter of compromise to best achieve the experimental goals. Higher flows yield sharper signal transients and better oxygenation. Lower flows magnify changes in concentration when measurement of rates of tissue uptake or production is the goal. High rates of flow are often limited by undesirable pressure within the system. Low rates of flow may cause undesirable smearing of signal pulses at the pulse frequency being modeled. In our experience, to resolve repeated pulses at intervals near 10 min the ratio of system volume (ml) to flow rate (ml/min) should be 3 or less.

In Vitro Models

Perfused Liver Preparations

This established model has been used (28) to compare the effects of pulsed vs continuous delivery of both insulin and glucagon on hepatic glucose production. It has been shown that the effect on hepatic glucose production of pulsatile administration of glucagon as well as of insulin, depending on the applied time interval of hormone exposure, is equipotent or even superior to the respective hormones' continuous infusion even if the hormone load is significantly reduced. Hepatic glucose production by isolated perfused rat livers has been monitored in response to glucagon and insulin infusion, using a nonrecirculating perfusion system. Further description of current methodology for liver perfusion is beyond the scope of this chapter. The method described by Komjati and co-workers (28) is a good starting place for the interested reader.

Perifused Hepatocyte Models

To facilitate more detailed studies of dose–response relationships, kinetic events, and biochemical mechanisms for differential effects of pulses we developed an isolated hepatocyte model (29, 30). We adapted the model from the system developed by Smith and Vale (31) for superfusion of rat anterior pituitary cells. In this system test cells are supported in a matrix of microscopic carrier beads held in a column configuration. The coherent linear flow through such a system minimizes the first-order effect of mixing thereby permitting sharper resolution of transient metabolic events at any given perifusate flow rate.

Hepatocytes are isolated from the livers of 180- to 220-g Sprague–Dawley rats essentially as described by Berry and Friend (32). Perfusion and washing buffers are formulated as described by Seglen (33). Livers are first perfused with a total of 250 ml of calcium-free buffer at a rate of 25 ml/min. Oxygenation is provided by a Silastic tubing "lung" (34). A recirculating perfusion is then established with 100 ml buffer containing calcium and collagenase at 0.05%.

After 16 to 18 min the livers are gently disrupted, filtered through coarse (437 μm) then fine (105 μm) polypropylene mesh, and washed in physiological buffer. Separations are done at very slow spin rates (50 rpm) to avoid mechanical cell damage. The cells are resuspended in basal medium Eagle (BME, Gibco) with added 1% bovine albumin, 0.1 mM sodium pyruvate, 1 mM sodium lactate, 100 U/ml penicillin, 100 μg/ml streptomycin, and glucose at the concentration dictated by the experimental protocol. The cells are incubated in this medium with gentle shaking at 37°C under a 95% O_2/5% CO_2 atmosphere for 30 min. After a final filtration (105 μm) cells are washed 3× in BME. Cell count, wet weight determination, and trypan blue exclusion testing are then performed. In our studies, mean trypan blue exclusion was 86 ± 5% (SD), $n = 49$. The yield of viable cells is 2–3 g wet weight from a single donor rat. Perifusion columns are loaded with 300–400 mg wet weight hepatocytes depending on the experimental goal. For some studies we have been able to load five identical columns containing 380 mg cells derived from the same donor. The typical column contains 4.5 × 10^6 viable cells at the start of an experiment.

Columns are made from 10-ml plastic syringes. Prior to loading, each column is clamped vertically and fitted with a 105-μm mesh retaining filter at the bottom (outflow) end of the syringe. A suspension of presoaked polyacrylamide gel beads (Bio-Gel P-2 or P-4, 100–200 mesh, 0.75 g dry weight, Bio-Rad, Richmond, CA) is added and allowed to settle onto the mesh. This layer of beads serves as a barrier filter to limit loss of cells during loading and initiation of medium flow. For each column the desired wet weight of test cells is gently slurried with 1.5 g dry weight beads in cold oxygenated buffer. With the outflow clamped, the slurry of cells and beads (6 ml) is added to the column and allowed to settle. When complete the cell layer in the column occupies about 5 ml. Operations up to this point are performed in a cold environment with solutions and cells at 4°C.

The column is then removed to the perifusion system and the plunger containing the inflow port (a 16-gauge needle) is fitted. The head space is reduced to 1 ml. The inflow and outflow lines are fitted and the column is submerged in the warm bath while perifusion is started immediately at a rate of 2.25 ml/min per column. This procedure is repeated for each column until all are loaded and being perifused with warm, oxygenated media. The perifusate medium is pumped (via a multichannel peristaltic pump) from a reservoir through individual channels of Silastic lung to the head of each column. The columns, the multichannel lung, and the connecting tubing are submerged in a stirred constant temperature bath. Each column receives a hormone entry port entering the medium line just as the stream reaches the head space. Hormone solutions or control fluids are introduced via a second peristaltic pump at the rate of 0.05 ml/min.

Outflow from each column is directed past a Clark oxygen electrode for continuous measurement of oxygen consumption before diversion to a fraction collector or other analytical device. To accomplish oxygen monitoring in multiple medium streams without altering rates of flow or introducing long delays, we fabricate a manifold out of Plexiglas. A block of plastic is bored and threaded to accept standard Yellow Springs O_2 electrodes. The bore hole is made to extend 3 mm past the tip of the electrode thus creating a small volume chamber (about 0.2 ml). The diameter of the bore is just sufficient to admit the O ring securing the membrane of the electrode tip as a press fit.

The small chambers are then accessed by three small holes drilled through the plastic and fitted with stainless steel needle stock and tubing. Two are used for inflow and outflow of medium, the third is used to aspirate any bubbles that might lodge in the chamber during an experiment. The whole assembly is mounted so that the block, electrodes, and tubing can be submerged in the water bath. A system of valves is employed to permit calibration by directing freshly oxygenated media to the electrodes while shunting medium past the array. The electrodes are connected to an electronic interface that permits the signal to be captured in memory, displayed, and analyzed with the aid of a small computer. The ability to measure oxygen consumption provides a ready index of the metabolic status of the cells on the columns. This is particularly important during the developmental phases of the work. We have also found that rapid changes in oxygen consumption during response to a glucagon pulse are highly correlated with other events and can be used to monitor the kinetics of hormone responses. On line measurement of oxygen consumption may not be needed for other systems. Cell viability and degree of oxygenation can usually be estimated indirectly by measuring other metabolic events such as the rate of active uptake of indicator molecules, release of intracellular enzymes, or production of anaerobic products. For some systems the cell mass may be small relative to the oxygen capacity of the medium thereby removing any concern about adequate oxygenation.

Multiple columns (35) are particularly useful when designing experiments to compare patterns of hormone delivery. In our simplest protocol we use paired columns to compare the same dose of glucagon delivered continuously or as a series of pulses. By repeating the experiment many times at graded doses we can construct two directly comparable dose–response curves, one for each mode of administration (30). The availability of multiple columns also permits kinetic studies to be conducted in which the key analysis required measuring a variable in intact cells harvested from the column. This was the case for a kinetic study of the effect of insulin pulses on the number of cell-surface receptors (36). In this study we employed five matched columns in an experiment. The kinetic analysis of metabolic events during perifusion experiments can be conducted by analyzing the concentration of a substance on-line in the moving stream, or by collecting timed samples and analyzing them separately to reconstruct a kinetic event. For example, in our studies of glucagon-stimulated glucose production by perifused hepatocytes we directed a portion of the outflow stream through an automated glucose analyzer (Technicon Autoanalyzer, ferrycyanide method). The remaining outflow stream was directed to a fraction collector. Timed samples of media were then available to measure the concentration of other products such as cAMP or radiolabeled glucose synthesized from labeled lactate contained in the perifusion medium. Figure 1 presents a schematic of the basic perifusion system.

General Features of Perifusion Protocols

We have tested the stability of the preparation. In preliminary studies we have found that freshly isolated cells display evidence of metabolic stress during the first 30–60 min after perifusion is started. For example oxygen consumption is higher at the start and declines to reach a steady state by 45 min. The release of the enzyme lactate dehydrogenase (LDH) is also highest at the start and rapidly falls to steady low levels after 30 min. For these reasons we routinely allow a 60-min recovery period during which basal medium is perifused before an experimental protocol is started. The total duration of experiments is usually under 3 hr although we determined that the preparation is relatively stable for periods up to 4 hr. Stability is determined in three ways. First, basal oxygen consumption can be directly monitored and displays on average a gradual cumulative fall of 8% over 240 min. Second, hepatocyte uptake of labeled ouabain is an excellent measure of viable cell

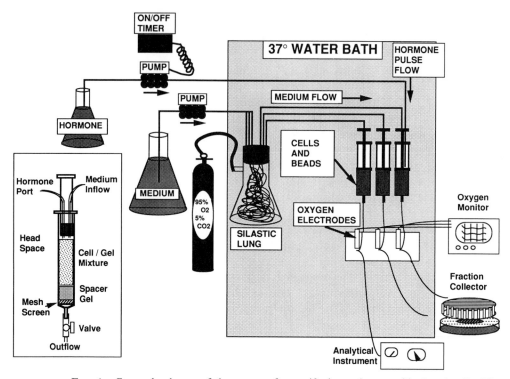

FIG. 1   General scheme of the system for perifusing columns of isolated cells. The inflowing medium was warmed by passing through tubing submerged in a stirred, constant temperature water bath. The columns and a manifold holding oxygen-sensing electrodes were also submerged in the bath. Oxygenation of media for each column was accomplished by individually pumping medium through Silastic tubing coiled in a warmed jar filled with an oxygen/CO_2 mixture. Hormones or other signals were introduced at the top of each gel column via a separate peristaltic pump that was controlled by a timer when appropriate. Outflow from the columns was collected in fraction collectors and/or routed through analytical instruments. The inset depicts the configuration of individual columns after loading of the gel–cell mixture.

mass (37). We determine fractional cellular uptake of ouabain by infusing a test bolus of [^{3}H]ouabain and [^{14}C]sucrose (to serve as a marker of extracellular space) at intervals during perifusion. The fractional uptake is determined from the ratio of ^{3}H/^{14}C in outflow media during passage of the test bolus over the column. There is a 9% decline in ouabain uptake between 1 and 4 hr of perifusion. A third test of cellular metabolic integrity is the ability of succinate to stimulate oxygen consumption. Viable hepatocytes largely exclude extracellular succinate and therefore do not display a change in respiratory control when exposed to this intermediate. The ratio of basal oxygen consumption to consumption during exposure to succinate was found to be 1.06 ± 0.01 (SEM) after 300 min of perifusion. The respiratory control ratio determined during exposure to the uncoupling reagent dinitrophenol (DNP) was $1.37 \pm .08$ (29).

Suitable Indices of Active Cellular Mass for Quantifying Metabolic Events

We count the total number of cells in aliquots of the washed cell solution in a standard hemocytometer chamber under high power. The percentage of viable cells at the outset is easily determined by counting the percentage of cells that exclude the dye trypan blue in the same chamber. To determine wet weight of cells we place aliquots of the cell suspension in tared microcentrifuge tubes, centrifuge at high speed, decant the supernatant media, and reweigh the tubes. These data are useful for loading multiple columns with equal cell mass and for standardizing cell masses from experiment to experiment. For a more precise guide to the active cell mass one can measure the uptake of labeled ouabain by each column at the end of an experimental period. Data relating ouabain uptake to a unit mass of cells can be obtained in pilot studies done with typical cellular preparations.

The other measure that proves useful is to analyze the total DNA in the cells harvested from the columns at the end of experiments by one of two methods (38, 39). The later simpler method is preferred. Total cellular DNA provides a reasonable index of remaining intact and presumably viable cells, since lysed cells lose their DNA during perifusion. Again, in pilot studies we determined the mass of DNA per mass of viable cells from cells prepared in the standard fashion. From these data we could assign a value for cell number in an experimental column or in aliquots of cells taken for analyses based on the relatively simple DNA analysis (38, 39). Examples of these quantitative relationships taken from our studies are presented in Table I.

Assessment of Signal Characteristics and the Kinetics of a Unit Response

All of our work with column systems has utilized a square wave hormone signal, i.e., the hormone infusion pump is turned on at a constant rate for a finite period and then turned off. The hormone delivery tube is prefilled before the first pulse to ensure that hormone enters the flowing medium

TABLE I   Quantitative Relationships in Column Preparations of
Isolated Hepatocytes[a]

Quantity	Units	Mean	SE	n^d
Wet weight per column	mg	380		30
DNA content per column	μg	103±	1.3	30
Cell number per column	10^6	4.48		30
Trypan blue exclusion: before[b]	percentage	93±	1.8	30
Trypan blue exclusion: after[c]	percentage	84±	1.5	30
Q_{O_2}				
After 60 min	$\mu M \times min^{-1} \times g^{-1}$	3.94±	0.2	22
After 120 min	$\mu M \times min^{-1} \times g^{-1}$	3.92±	0.3	30

[a] Columns were 10-ml plastic syringes. The nominal volume of cells and gel was 6 ml per column.
[b] Measured in cells before columns were loaded.
[c] Measured in cells harvested after a total of 3 hr perifusion.
[d] Number of experiments.

stream instantaneously on turning on the pump. The distance (therefore volume) between the hormone entry port and the target cells is held to a minimum to reduce the mixing volume for the signal. For each unique perifusion system, we examine the kinetics of the signal by infusing a trace-labeled test signal and collecting fractions of outflow for analysis. The diameter of outflow tubing is kept small (1.19-mm id polyethylene tubing; dead space, 1.0 ml) to minimize hydrodynamic signal distortion. The general shape of the signal created by a 3-min square wave infusion is depicted in Fig. 2. For studies involving multiple pulses at different frequencies we routinely perform a control experiment employing labeled pulses to actually observe the degree of separation of pulses to be expected at the test frequencies. An example of this analysis is given in Fig. 3. It is clear that in this system, clean separation of individual pulses begins to degrade when the pulse interval is reduced below 10 min. For most protocols such simple visualization of the system kinetics is sufficient to interpret the results.

The data from tracer analyses of the signal can also serve for more definitive kinetic analysis of unit responses to a single hormone pulse using the technique of deconvolution. Deconvolution is a mathematical method for separating the contribution of the physical system (the head space volume, gel volume, and outflow tubing) from the total response to better estimate parameters of the biological response (27; see also Veldhuis *et al.*, Chapter 15, this volume). We used this technique to study the kinetics of hepatocyte responses to glucagon pulses (40), as illustrated in Fig. 4. The data showed that metabolic responses to glucagon fell into fast and slow kinetic families. Glucagon stimulation of hepatic glucose production decayed with $t_{1/2}$ of

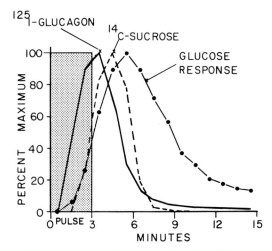

FIG. 2   The shape of a square wave hormone pulse eluted from a perifusion column. A column of isolated hepatocytes was exposed to a 3-min square wave pulse of labeled glucagon and sucrose. The effluent was collected in 0.5-min fractions. The shape of the elution curves for glucagon and sucrose (as an extracellular marker) and response of the cells to glucagon (as increment in glucose) are displayed. The hormone and sucrose pulses have largely cleared the cells by 3 min after the end of the signal infusion while the cellular response is obviously prolonged. [Reproduced with permission from D. S. Weigle, D. J. Koerker and C. J. Goodner (41).]

3 min while glucagon stimulated ketogenesis and generation of cAMP decayed with $t_{1/2}$ less than 1 min. These differences in relaxation time for unit responses to a hormone pulse became the key parameter in a model we developed that largely accounts for the ability of pulsed glucagon administration to yield greater integrated hepatic glucose production than the same amount of glucagon administered as a continuous signal (41).

Modifications for Studying the Kinetics of Rapidly Changing Cellular Events

To study the change in number of cell-surface insulin receptors during the response of hepatocytes to a pulse of insulin we have modified the basic system as follows (36). The problem requires collecting viable cells at frequent intervals during and after exposure to an insulin pulse. At the time interval of interest further processing of the surface receptors has to be stopped without disrupting the cells. These goals have been accomplished

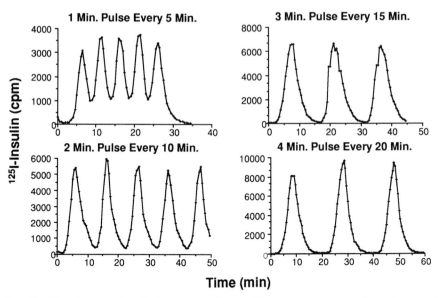

FIG. 3   The shape of the elution curve after multiple square wave pulses at several frequencies. In this experiment brief pulses were repeated at intervals from 5 to 20 min. The pulse duration was always ⅕th the interpulse interval. Labeled insulin was the test signal and the columns were loaded with cultured rat hepatoma cells attached to microcarrier beads. At the highest frequency, washout of individual pulses began to smear into the next pulse such that the hormone concentration remained constantly above baseline. [Reproduced with permission from H. C. Harrison Jr., C. J. Goodner, and M. A. Berrie (45).]

by including five identically prepared columns in each experiment. This permits protocols in which five different time intervals can be compared. To achieve the second goal we arrange the system to permit very rapid cooling of the media traversing an individual column of cells. Cooling to below 10°C is known to completely inhibit the active processes responsible for receptor internalization. A short glass coil is placed in the inflow line just upstream from each column. The columns are also mounted so that they and this segment of inflow line can be quickly moved to and submerged in beakers of iced water. The delay time for media to flow from the cooling coil to the column is predetermined (30 sec). At each experimental time interval the termination sequence for the designated column is as follows. At the delay interval before the experimental time (−30 sec) the glass heat exchanger is moved to the ice bath. At the designated time the column is also moved to the bath. The rapidity of cooling is judged by monitoring oxygen consumption

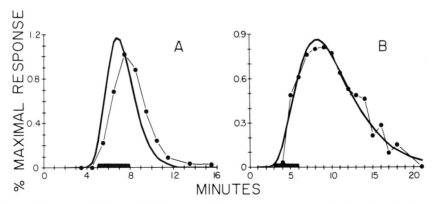

FIG. 4   Deconvolution applied to two different responses to a single pulse of gluca-gon. The solid lines, no symbols depict the shape of response after deconvolution has been applied to the data. The lighter lines with symbols are the original data. (A) Curve for release of cAMP from perifused hepatocytes exposed to a 3-min pulse of glucagon (1500 pg/ml). (B) Curve of release of glucose in the same experimental circumstances. In the case of the more rapid response (A), by correcting for system variables such as mixing delays, deconvolution led to appreciation of a significantly faster rate of relaxation than is apparent in the raw data. For the slower response (B) deconvolution made no apparent difference. [Reproduced with permission from D. S. Weigle, I. R. Sweet, and C. J. Goodner (40).]

by columns undergoing the procedure. We have found that oxygen uptake falls to within 5% of baseline in 0.9 ± 0.1 min. Flow is continued for 12 min, at 4°C. At this time the column is disconnected from all flow and the cells are harvested into cold media. This sequence is repeated for each column. The 12-min cold perfusion serves as an extensive wash to remove any extra-cellular insulin from the system. The cold-harvested cells are then studied with conventional methods to determine surface-binding characteristics.

Summary of Results Obtained with Perifused Isolated Hepatocytes

We described the basic phenomenon of pulse-enhanced hepatic response to glucagon using a system of perifused isolated hepatocytes in a paired column system. Dose–response curves for delivery of the same time-averaged amount of glucagon differed markedly between.pulsed and continuous admin-istration. Below 1000 pg/ml glucagon, the curve for pulsed hormone was shifted to the left and the EC_{50} was 186 vs 884 pg/ml for pulsed vs continuous glucagon. In the dose range equivalent to the concentration in portal plasma, pulsed glucagon enhanced hepatic glucose production twofold. This phenomenon was not due to differential desensitization of the glucagon response. The degree of desensitization was comparable for both modes of administration. The dose–response curves for glucagon administered in the two modes are shown in Fig. 5.

We developed a mathematical model to describe the output of hepatocytes to a series of pulses. The model is based on the kinetics of a single response to a glucagon pulse. This model reproduced the characteristics of the observed dose–response curves for pulsatile and continuous delivery of glucagon over a 90-min experiment. Both the left shift for pulsed glucagon administration at mid dose ranges and the greater maximum response to continuous delivery of glucagon at the higher dose range were replicated by the model (Fig. 6). The key determinant of the enhanced response to pulses proved to be the rate of decay of the hepatocyte response to a single pulse of glucagon. The above model also predicts that the optimal frequency (30) of a series of pulses to enhance the integrated response will also be a function of the rate of decay or relaxation of the response to a single pulse. We tested this hypothesis by increasing the time-averaged dose of glucagon achieved by increasing pulse frequency compared to the same dose delivered continuously. As predicted by the model, pulses delivered in the physiologic frequency range achieved the optimum pulse enhancement. We point out that the optimal interpulse interval is equal to two to four response decay halftimes and that this relationship can probably be generalized to other pulsing hormonal systems such as GH and the gonadotropins. We suggest that ultradian endocrine secretory frequencies have evolved to match the decay time of the target tissue response, since this arrangement tends to optimize the overall response achieved by a given amount of hormone synthesis and release.

Because the kinetic characteristics of the response to a hormone pulse play such an important role in our model, we examined in some detail the rates of onset and relaxation of individual components of response of hepatocytes to a glucagon pulse. Net glucose production, gluconeogenesis, ketogenesis, and the oxidative burst were measured and compared to the release of cAMP and residence time of labeled glucagon during a single glucagon pulse. The rates of decay of the responses fell into a rapid and a slower group. Release of intact ^{125}I-glucagon from the column, release of cAMP, and formation of β-OH butyrate were rapid with a decay $t_{1/2}$ of 0.85–1.03 min. For net glucose production and increased respiration the decay $t_{1/2}$ were 3.25 and 4.75 min, respectively. Relaxation of gluconeogenesis (conversion of [^{14}C]lactate to [^{14}C]glucose) was intermediate, decay $t_{1/2}$ of 1.96 min. When hepatocytes were stimulated by cAMP alone or with glucagon plus IBMX, a phosphodiesterase inhibitor, the rate of relaxation of the stimulated net glucose production was the same as that for glucagon

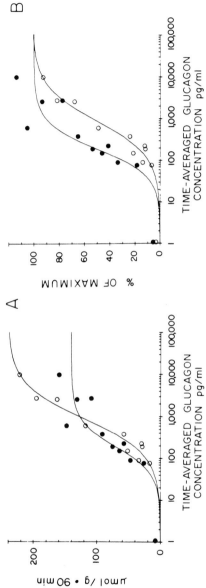

FIG. 5 Dose–response relationships for total glucagon-stimulated glucose production versus time-averaged glucagon concentration in isolated perfused hepatocytes. In a series of experiments glucagon was administered as six 3-min pulses every 15 min to one of a pair of columns while the same amount was administered continuously to the other. This format was repeated over a wide range of total glucagon dose and the depicted dose–response relationships were generated. (A) Total glucose produced versus glucagon dose. (B) Percentage of maximum response for each mode. The open circles are data from continuous glucagon administration, the solid circles are data from pulsed administration. Both sets of curves demonstrate a shift to the left of the relationship during pulsed administration. Panel A also demonstrates that at high doses the response to continuous glucagon exceeds that to pulsed hormone and eventually reaches a higher maximum. Within the physiological concentration range for glucagon in portal blood (between 100 and 1000 pg/ml) pulsatile administration results in a twofold increase in hepatic response. We have termed this effect pulse enhancement [Reproduced with permission from D. S. Weigle, D. J. Koerker, and C. J. Goodner, *Am. J. Physiol.* **247**, E564 (1984).]

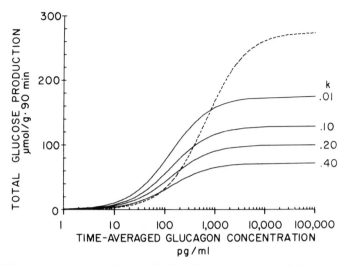

FIG. 6   The dose–response relationship for glucagon-stimulated glucose production derived from a mathematical model. A model was developed based on the general shape of the unit response to a single pulse and to a continuous infusion of glucagon. It was determined that the parameter describing the rate of relaxation of the response to a single pulse was the critical determinant of the dose–response relationship for the pulsed mode. The family of curves depicted were generated by the model when several rate constants were applied. At a rate of relaxation near that observed in the biological system (0.13 min^{-1}) the shapes of the curves faithfully mimic the experimental data. Both pulse enhancement at intermediate doses and the higher maximum for continuous glucagon at high doses are reproduced by the model. The central feature of the model, i.e., the critical importance of the rate of relaxation of a unit response, may probably be generalized to other episodic effector systems. [Reproduced with permission from D. S. Weigle, D. J. Koerker, and C. J. Goodner (41).]

alone. These data indicate that the rate-limiting steps are at steps distal to the cAMP cascade. The finding that the rate of decay of the ketogenesis response to glucagon is more rapid than that for glucose production raises the possibility that different degrees of pulse enhancement for these two categories of response would be induced at a given pulse frequency. The optimal frequency for ketogenesis would be more rapid than the physiologic pulse frequency seen under normal basal conditions. We postulate that this might be a mechanism for limiting stimulation of ketogenesis while providing an effective stimulation of hepatic glucose production in the overnight fasted animal (40).

Because the first steps in hormone stimulation of the target tissue are

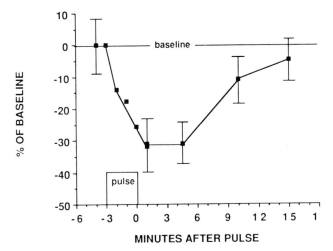

FIG. 7   The response of the population of surface insulin receptors to a single pulse of insulin. Five matched columns of perifused hepatocytes were exposed to pulses of insulin. Columns were harvested at timed intervals by exposing them to a cold medium stream designed to stop further receptor movement. The cells harvested from columns were then assayed for surface receptor binding. In a series of experiments the kinetics of receptor internalization and recycling back to the surface was reconstructed as shown. The rapidity of these events is such that hepatocytes undergo a nearly complete processing cycle during each of a series of pulses delivered at the physiological pulse interval. In studies not shown the same changes depicted here were seen following the sixth of a series of similar pulses [Reproduced with permission from C. J. Goodner, I. R. Sweet, and H. C. J. Harrison (36).]

receptor binding, activation, internalization, and processing, we tested the hypothesis that the early events in the receptor-processing cycle could be entrained to pulses of insulin at the physiologic pulse interval (36). To test this question we modified our system to permit simultaneous perifusion of five columns of hepatocytes from the same donor rat. The columns were exposed to pulses of insulin and the cells harvested at intervals thereafter for determination of surface insulin binding. The population of surface receptors declined rapidly after a single 3-min pulse of insulin, reaching a nadir between 1 and 5 min after the end of the pulse. The surface population then returned to baseline between 10 and 15 min after the pulse (Fig. 7). The percentage reduction of surface receptor number was dose related to the amplitude of the pulse, reaching a maximum reduction of 45%. The ED_{50} for reduction was 251 μU/ml insulin. The affinity remained unchanged throughout. After a series of five pulses at 15-min intervals the behavior of surface binding to a sixth pulse was identical to that after a single pulse. These data indicate that a large proportion of the population of surface insulin receptors may be cycled from the surface to the interior and back to the surface of the hepatocyte during each pulse of islet secretion. The timing of these events is such that each arriving pulse of insulin would encounter a full complement of newly recycled surface receptors. We suggest that the intrinsic timing of the receptor-processing cycle serves to optimize the sensitivity of the liver to insulin pulses that arrive within the physiologic range of secretory pulse frequency.

Kinetic Studies of Gene Regulation Using Perifused Cultured Hepatoma Cells

Background

Our work has focused on developing models and methods to investigate the impact of islet hormone pulses on long-term regulation of hormone-sensitive genes in the liver. In other endocrine systems displaying an ultradian rhythm, the mechanisms for the differential effects of pulses are through changes in the degree of desensitization and the expression of hormone-sensitive genes in the respective target tissues (42). Because the gonadotropin-releasing hormone (GnRH)–gonadotropin system has appreciably longer interpulse intervals than the islets, it is easier to accept the concept of pulse-related effects on gene regulation. Could pulses of insulin or glucagon at 10- to 15-minute intervals differentially affect gene expression given the measured time course of overall stimulation of these events? For certain insulin- and glucagon-sensitive enzymes, the published kinetics of events in gene expression are fast enough to make the hypothesis tenable. If one examines the array of genes known to be regulated by insulin and/or glucagon, there is a spectrum of rates for effects on transcription, turnover of mRNA, and translation and turnover of the product enzyme itself (23). Transcription of the following enzyme genes is affected by insulin: PEPCK, fatty acid synthase, pyruvate kinase, glucokinase, glyceraldehyde-P-dehydrogenase, glycerol-P-dehydrogenase, glucose-6-P-dehydrogenase, tyrosine aminotransferase, and 6-phosphofructo-2-kinase/fructose-2,6-bisphosphatase. Among the more rapidly responding genes (with respect to transcription) are ones that control key steps in hepatic glucose metabolism (PEPCK and glucokinase). The most detailed kinetic information is available from the extensive study of PEPCK by Hanson and co-workers and Granner and his co-workers (23, 43). The first specific step, initiation of transcription (measured in a nuclear runoff assay), is most rapidly inhibited by insulin with a $t_{1/2} = 12–15$ min.

Subsequent steps have progressively slower kinetics, $t_{1/2}$ = 22, 28, and 24 min for decline in the primary 6.8-kb nuclear transcript, the 3.2-kb nuclear transcript, and the 3.2-kb cytoplasmic transcript, respectively. There was also a 20-min lag between the nuclear and cytoplasmic phases of the process. When the overall rates of decline in mRNA^{PEPCK} and active PEPCK were examined, they were equal, with the $t_{1/2}$ = 20–30 min. The rate of stimulation fo PEPCK transcription by analogs of cAMP was equally rapid, increasing ninefold within 30 min. Thus the stimulation of transcription by cAMP-dependent processes and its opposition by insulin are very complex, but rapid, time-dependent processes (44). To test the effect of exposing this system to peaks of the opposing regulators, glucagon mimetics, and insulin at 10- to 15-minute intervals we established a three-column system for perifusing cultured H$_4$IIEC3 hepatoma cells (45).

Tissue Culture and Microcarrier Attachment

The H4IIEC3 cell line was generously provided by D. Granner of Vanderbilt University Medical Center (Nashville, TN). The cells are maintained in α-MEM supplemented with 5% FBS, 2.5% NBCS, 2.5% DCS, and Pen/Strep. In preparation for cell attachment, Cytodex-3 microcarriers are weighed out dry into 50-ml Falcon tubes in aliquots of 300 mg. These are allowed to swell in phosphate-buffered serum (PBS) for at least 2 hr, washed with two changes of PBS, and then autoclaved. On the morning of attachment, the beads are washed with two changes of warmed, serum-supplemented culture medium and resuspended in 50 ml of the same medium. Then each aliquot is transferred to a sterile, 500-ml, polycarbonate Erlenmeyer flask (Corning) and placed in the 37°C incubator with 5% CO$_2$ atmosphere for at least 30 min.

For cell attachment, we use a modification of the protocol used by Agius *et al.* (46). One culture flask (150 cm^2, Corning) of cells grown to confluence is used to inoculate each Erlenmeyer flask of microcarriers. The cells are removed from the culture flask with trypsin/EDTA, pooled, resuspended in medium, and then inoculated in equivalent aliquots into the Erlenmeyer flasks with the microcarriers. These flasks are gently swirled for 15 sec at inoculation and every 30 min thereafter for at least 3 hr. At the end of 3 hr approximately 98% of the cells are attached to the beads, when examined microscopically, and they appear 100% viable by trypan blue exclusion. At approximately 6 hr after inoculation, each aliquot of microcarrier-attached cells is transferred from the Erlenmeyer flask to a sterile, 50-ml Falcon tube. The attached cells are allowed to settle, the serum-containing medium is removed, and the cells are washed with two changes of serum-free α-MEM supplemented with 1% human albumin. One wash is also used to rinse the Erlenmeyer flasks. The attached cells are then resuspended in 50 ml of the same albumin-supplemented medium and transferred back to the 500-ml Erlenmeyer flasks. These are returned to the 5% CO_2 incubator and left overnight without stirring. Immediately prior to the beginning of an experiment the following morning, each flask of attached cells is transferred by pipette to a perifusion column fitted with a stopcock at the bottom and a flow adapter at the top. The flow adapter is adjusted so that its terminus rests at the top of the settled beads and attached cells.

Perifusion Column System

Our previous column methods are adapted to long-term culture as follows. To maintain sterility, the perifusion columns and tubing are gas-sterilized and sterile tissue culture media are used. The new system consists of three siliconized (Sigmacote, Sigma, St. Louis, MO.), gas-sterilized, low-pressure chromatography columns (Bio-Rad, 8 ml volume, 1.0 cm I.D.) perifused in parallel with oxygenated medium, warmed to 37°C. All columns receive medium supplemented with 0.1 mM 8-CPT-cAMP and 0.5 μM dexamethasone. One column, designated "stimulated," receives no insulin. The second column, designated "continuous," receives insulin-supplemented medium. The third column, "pulsatile," receives an equivalent time-averaged amount of insulin delivered intermittently via a small, primed hormone tube that passes through the medium channel and terminates immediately above the bed of attached cells. The pulsatile insulin is driven by a separate peristaltic pump (SAGE) that is connected to a programmable intervalometer/timer (Cole-Parmer). In our experiments, the average medium flow rate was 1 ml/min, and the hormone flow rate was 0.08 ml/min. Each experiment lasted 3 hr but cultured hepatocytes have been satisfactorily maintained for several days in this system. At the end of the perifusion experiment PBS is perfused to wash out media, then the flows are interrupted and the columns inverted over siliconized RNase-free beakers.

Quantitation of mRNA^{PEPCK}

The attached cells and beads from each column are immediately expressed with a syringe of PBS from the column into a sterile 50-ml tube. The cells and beads are twice allowed to settle ($\sim$1 min) and then are washed with

PBS. Following the second wash, TNA is extracted according to McKnight *et al.* (47), only with an additional phenol/chloroform extraction. The TNA pellet is resuspended in $0.1\times$ SET [$1\times$ SET = 10 nM Tris(pH 7.5), 5 mM EDTA, 1% sodium dodecyl sulfate], heated to 65°C for 15 min and measured by optical density at 260 nm (OD_{260}). Samples are stored at -20°C until assayed.

Because of its sensitivity, efficiency, and ability to quantify mRNA without densitometry, we chose to use solution hybridization to measure $mRNA^{PEPCK}$. The basic scheme of the method is to first hybridize specific $mRNA^{PEPCK}$ contained in a solution of tissue-derived nucleic acids with a ^{32}p-labeled, antisense riboprobe. The mixture is then exposed to RNase. Among the many messages in the tissue extract only the hybrid of $mRNA^{PEPCK}$ and ^{32}P-labeled riboprobe is protected from digestion by the RNase. It is then separated and quantified by scintillation counting. An 845-base pair *Eco*RI–*Ava*I fragment of the cDNA for PEPCK was kindly provided by S. McKnight, Ph.D., of the University of Washington Department of Pharmacology (Seattle). With standard protocols (48) this fragment is ligated into plasmid pGEM-4z (Promega, Madison, WI) prepared by digestion with *Eco*RI and *Ava*I (Boerhinger-Mannheim, Indianapolis, IN). Because of the SP6 and T7 promoters flanking the inserted cDNA, this plasmid allows transcription of either sense or antisense RNA by use of the appropriate RNA polymerase. [^{32}P]UTP-labeled, antisense riboprobe is transcribed according to Promega's directions for synthesis of high specific activity RNA probes and purified by passage over a G-50 Sephadex column. Unlabeled, "sense strand" RNA is transcribed for use as standards, according to Promega's instructions for transcribing large quantities of RNA. The DNA template is destroyed with DNase (Worthington, Freehold, NJ), and the RNA is quantified by OD_{260}. Four serial dilutions from 1 to 1000 ng/ml are made to serve as the standards. Total RNA is prepared by a quanidinium–thiocyanate–phenol–chloroform method (49) from the livers of a fed and a 2-day fasted rat. These RNA samples are included in every assay as "low"- and "high"-level $mRNA^{PEPCK}$ controls, respectively.

The TNA unknowns are diluted to 1 mg/ml in $0.1\times$ SET for the solution hybridization assay. The assay is set up with a 12-point standard curve (2–10,000 pg) according to McKnight *et al.* (47), except "sense" strand RNA is used for standards in place of single-stranded M13 DNA. Unknowns are assayed in triplicate with 5 μg of TNA per tube. Hybridization is carried out at 68°C overnight. RNase digestion and TCA precipitation are performed according to McKnight *et al.* (47). Filters are treated with Soluene-350 (Packard) and then counted in Ultima Gold (Beckman) scintillation cocktail for 5 min. Results are computed as follows. Counts per minute are converted to percentage hybridization by comparison to the zero and total count tubes.

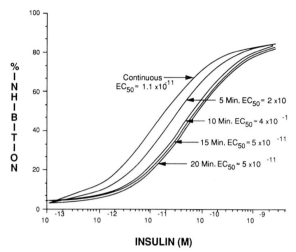

INSULIN (M)

FIG. 8   The effect of pulses of insulin delivered at four frequencies or continuously on expression of the gene for PEPCK. Cultured rat hepatoma (H-4-II E-C3) cells were perifused in three matched columns and exposed to a cAMP analog and insulin. All columns were stimulated with cAMP. One column received pulsed insulin, one received the same amount of insulin continuously, and one received no insulin. Pulses were delivered at intervals of 5, 10, 15, or 20 min for 3 hr. Cells were harvested and extracted for total nucleic acids and mRNA[PEPCK] was quantified with a solution hybridization RNase protection assay. The ability of insulin to inhibit cAMP-stimulated PEPCK expression was plotted as percentage inhibition versus the insulin concentration employed. The curves depicted are logistic functions fitted to the experimental data. The 50%-effective concentrations (EF_{50}) derived from these functions are listed on the graph. In marked contrast to the pulse enhancement seen with glucagon, insulin pulses were fourfold less effective than continuous insulin in this system. [Reproduced with permission from H. C. Harrison, Jr., C. J. Goodner, and M. A. Berrie (45).]

Using a curve-fitting program the most linear portion of the standard curve (usually from 2–500 pg) is fitted to a second-order polynomial equation and used to calculate the unknowns expressed as picograms mRNA[PEPCK] per microgram TNA. By knowing the molecular weight of the riboprobe, picograms mRNA[PEPCK] (numerator) can be converted to molecules of PEPCK. The DNA in each unknown sample is measured with a fluorometric method (39), percentage of DNA of each TNA sample is calculated, and all samples are averaged to give the mean percentage of DNA. With the published value for picograms of DNA per liver cell (9.3 pg DNA/liver cell) (50), micrograms of TNA (denominator) can be expressed as molecules per cell. By comparing results for the insulin-treated (inhibited) to the stimulated columns, percentage inhibition by insulin is calculated for continuous and pulsatile columns.

Experimental Results

Continuous insulin administration inhibited PEPCK expression in a dose-dependent fashion with an EC_{50} of 1×10^{-11} M. Equivalent time-averaged amounts of insulin delivered as pulses achieved significant inhibition but less effectively than continuous insulin. The apparent EC_{50} for pulsatile insulin increased from 2×10^{-11} to 5×10^{-11} M as the oscillatory period was raised from 5 to 20 min (Fig. 8). These data indicate that insulin-mediated inhibition of PEPCK transcription is diminished by pulsatile administration in marked contrast to the pulse-enhancement observed for glucagon-mediated hepatic glucose production. As illustrated by these studies, the use of solution hybridization in an RNase protection assay is a very powerful tool for studying hormonal regulation of gene expression. Not only because it is highly sensitive and reproducible, but also because the same total RNA extract from an experimental column may be analyzed for multiple specific mRNAs. In this way hormone interactions on expression and other complex characteristics of control may be investigated simultaneously.

References

1. C. J. Goodner, B. C. Walike, D. J. Koerker, J. W. Ensinck, A. C. Brown, E. W. Chideckel, J. Palmer, and L. Kalnasy, *Science* **195,** 177 (1977).
2. D. S. Weigle, *Diabetes* **36,** 764 (1987).
3. C. J. Goodner, F. G. Hom, and D. J. Koerker, *Science* **215,** 1257 (1982).
4. J. I. Stagner, E. Samols, and G. C. Weir, *J. Clin. Invest.* **65,** 939 (1980).
5. D. L. Cook, *Metabolism* **32,** 681 (1983).
6. E. A. Longo, K. Tornheim, J. T. Deeney, B. A. Varnum, D. Tillotson, M. Prentki, and B. E. Corkey, *J. Biol. Chem.* **266,** 9314 (1991).
7. C. Ammala, O. Larsson, P. O. Berggren, J. K. Bokvist, L. Berggren, H. Kindmark, and P. Rorsman, *Nature* (*London*) **353,** 849 (1991).
8. R. M. Santos, L. M. Rosario, A. Nadal, S. J. Garcia, B. Soria, and M. Valdeolmillos, *Pfluegers Arch.* **418,** 417 (1991).
9. H. F. Chou, N. Berman, and E. Ipp, *Am. J. Physiol.* **262,** E800 (1992).
10. J. I. Stagner and E. Samols, *Diabetes* **35,** 849 (1986).
11. C. J. Goodner, D. J. Koerker, J. I. Stagner, and E. Samols, *Am. J. Physiol.* **260,** E422 (1991).
12. J. I. Stagner, *in* "The Endocrine Pancreas" (E. Samols, ed.), p. 5. Raven Press, New York, 1990.

13. C. Simon, G. Brandenberger, and M. Follenius, *J. Clin. Endocrinol. Metab.* **64,** 669 (1987).
14. J. Sturis, C. E. Van, J. D. Blackman, and K. S. Polonsky, *J. Clin. Invest.* **87,** 439 (1991).
15. D. A. Lang, D. R. Matthews, M. Burnett, and R. C. Turner, *Diabetes* **30,** 435 (1981).
16. S. O'Rahilly, R. C. Turner, and D. R. Matthews, *N. Engl. J. Med.* **318,** 1225 (1988).
17. K. S. Polonsky, B. D. Given, L. J. Hirsch, H. Tillil, E. T. Shapiro, C. Beebe, B. H. Frank, J. A. Galloway, and E. Van Cautere, *N. Engl. J. Med.* **318,** 1231 (1988).
18. E. Samols, J. I. Stagner, R. B. Ewart, and V. Marks, *J. Clin. Invest.* **82,** 350 (1988).
19. E. Samols and J. I. Stagner, *Am. J. Med.* **85,** 31 (1988).
20. E. Samols and J. I. Stagner, *Metabolism* **39,** 55 (1990).
21. J. I. Stagner and E. Samols, *J. Clin. Invest.* **77,** 1034 (1986).
22. J. I. Stagner, E. Samols, and W. S. Bonner, *Diabetes* **37,** 1715 (1988).
23. D. K. Granner, *Kidney Int.* **32,** S82 (1987).
24. D. J. Koerker and C. J. Goodner, in "Textbook of Physiology" (Patton, Fuchs, Hille, Scher, and Steiner, eds.). Saunders, Philadelphia, 1989.
25. R. S. Sherwin, K. J. Kramer, J. D. Tobin, P. A. Insel, J. E. Liljenquist, M. Berman, and R. Andres, *J. Clin. Invest.* **53,** 1481 (1974).
26. Y. J. Yang, I. D. Hope, M. Ader, and R. N. Bergmann, *J. Clin. Invest.* **84,** 1620 (1989).
27. K. H. Norwich, "Molecular Dynamics in Biosystems." Pergamon Press, New York, 1977.
28. M. Komjati, M. P. Bratusch, and W. Waldhausl, *Endocrinology (Baltimore)* **118,** 312 (1986).
29. D. S. Weigle, D. J. Koerker, and C. J. Goodner, in "Isolation, Characterization and Use of Hepatocytes" (R. A. Harris and N. W. Cornell, eds.), p. 139. Elsevier Science, New York, 1983.
30. D. S. Weigle and C. J. Goodner, *Endocrinology (Baltimore)* **118,** 1606 (1986).
31. M. A. Smith and W. W. Vale, *Endocrinology (Baltimore)* **107,** 1425 (1980).
32. M. N. Berry and D. S. Friend, *J. Cell. Biol.* **43,** 506 (1969).
33. P. O. Seglen, *Methods Cell Biol.* **13,** 29 (1976).
34. N. M. Berry, R. L. Hamilton, E. M. Severinghaus, and M. C. Williams, in "Regulation of Hepatic Metabolism" (F. Lundquist and N. Tygstrup, eds.), p. 790. Munksgaard, Copenhagen, 1974.
35. D. M. Crisp, A. E. Sorman, J. M. Beirne, T. C. Orton, and A. P. Sturdee, *Eur. J. Biochem.* **123,** 377 (1982).
36. C. J. Goodner, I. R. Sweet, and H. C. J. Harrison, *Diabetes* **37,** 1316 (1988).
37. D. L. Eaton and C. D. Klaassen, *J. Pharmacol. Exp. Ther.* **205,** 480 (1978).
38. A. J. Leyva and W. N. Kelly, *Anal. Biochem.* **62,** 173 (1974).
39. C. Labarca and K. Paigen, *Anal. Biochem.* **102,** 344 (1980).
40. D. S. Weigle, I. R. Sweet, and C. J. Goodner, *Endocrinology (Baltimore)* **121,** 732 (1987).
41. D. S. Weigle, D. J. Koerker, and C. J. Goodner, *Am. J. Physiol.* **248,** E681 (1985).

42. D. J. Haisenleder, J. A. Katt, G. A. Ortolano, M. R. el-Gewely, J. A. Duncan, C. Dee, and J. C. Marshall, *Mol. Endocrinol.* **2,** 1033 (1988).

43. M. A. Cimbala, P. Van Lelyveld, and R. W. Hanson, *in* "Advances in Enzyme Regulation" (G. Weber, eds.), Vol. 19, p. 205. Pergamon Press, New York, 1980.

44. K. Sasaki and D. K. Granner, *Proc. Natl. Acad. Sci. U.S.A.* **85,** 2954 (1988).

45. H. C. Harrison, Jr., C. J. Goodner, and M. A. Berrie, *Diabetes* **40,** 990 (1991).

46. L. Agius, A. Battersby, and K. G. M. M. Alberti, *In Vitro Cell Dev. Biol.* **21,** 254 (1985).

47. G. S. McKnight, M. D. Uhler, C. H. Clegg, L. A. Correll, and G. G. Cadd, *in* "Methods in Enzymology" (J. D. Corbin and R. A. Johnson, eds.), Vol. 159, p. 299. Academic Press, San Diego, 1988.

48. F. M. Ausubel *et al.*, eds., "Current Protocols in Molecular Biology," Vol I. Wiley, New York, 1989.

49. P. Chomczynski and N. Sacchi, *Anal. Biochem.* **162,** 156 (1987).

50. R. Y. Thompson, F. C. Heagy, W. C. Hutchinson, and J. N. Davidson, *Biochem. J.* **53,** 460 (1953).

[12] Pulsatile Endocrine Secretion in the Ovine Fetus

Steven M. Yellon and Ede M. Apostolakis

Background

History of Chronic Fetal Sheep Model

In a seminal review by Donald Barron (1) the mammalian fetus is envisioned as developing within an environment where the availability of oxygen is limited by circumstances over which the fetus has no control. The fetus thus falls victim to its environment; as gestation advances growth occurs but conditions for continued maturation become less favorable. Sir Joseph Barcroft in 1947 concluded that "the alternatives [for the fetus] are escape through birth or death in utero" (cited in 1). Rather than a pessimistic view of fetal development, these classical assessments highlight the accomplishments that the fetus must make to survive in the world outside the womb. At some point the fetus enters into a race to establish the independent physiological functions required for life and to mature without depleting limited resources. Considerations related to the competing demands of this race are essential to understanding physiological function in the fetus.

The modern era of study in fetal physiology is relatively recent in the scope of biomedical sciences. In 1978, Reynolds (2) surmised that new and wide-ranging technological advancements in this century were, in a great part, responsible for scientific breakthroughs. The technologies referred to include new catheter materials, antibiotic therapies, and surgical expertise. In his review, Reynolds described the first time that blood was taken from the fetal circulation for chronic *in utero* studies without loss of amniotic fluid or opening of the amniotic sac. In 1953–1954, A. St. George Huggett, William Paul, Vittorio Danesino, and S. R. M. Reynolds catheterized an interplacental artery in the primate uterus to directly obtain fetal blood for analysis of transplacental carbohydrate metabolism. In 1959, Meschia *et al.* (3) obtained blood samples from the uterine vein via an indwelling catheter in the unanesthetized ewe. Following this initial study, fetal arterial blood was obtained from the uterine vein at intervals over a period of weeks without interfering with fetal development or natural birth at full term (4).

Methods in Neurosciences, Volume 20

The landmark series "Animal Models in Fetal Medicine," initiated in 1980 with Peter Nathanielsz as editor, established that the fetus had come of age as a reliable experimental model for research. Abraham Rudolph and Michael Heymann (5) contributed a pioneering review to that series and detailed the surgical methodology for instrumentation of the ovine fetus. The work summarized in the present chapter relies on the foundations described in their review.

The value of the fetal model for neuroscience research was also exemplified by another chapter in this publication series in which Gluckman and Parsons describe stereotaxic surgery on the brain of the ovine fetus (6). In their review, earlier studies by Comline *et al.* in 1970 and 1977 were indicated as the first to directly assess the neuroendocrine function of the pituitary in the ovine fetus; the technique of electrocoagulation was used to effect an *in vivo* hypophysectomy. Also noted was a study in the porcine fetus in 1983 in which electrical stimulation of the fetal brain increased gonadotropin secretion in the circulation. Yet it was not until 1990, that *in vivo* disconnection of the pituitary from the hypothalamus in the ovine fetus was accomplished (7). Thus, relatively recent studies demonstrate the capabilities of the fetal model for neuroendocrine research and highlight the limited literature on the topic.

Significance of the Fetal Model for Neuroendocrinology

For Growth and Development

Ontogenesis of neuroendocrine function and the physiological role of the hypothalamic-pituitary axis in the fetus are critical issues for understanding growth and development of the fetus *in utero*. Gluckman *et al.* (8) indicated that although differentiation of the hypothalamic–pituitary axis and its circulatory linkage occurs early in gestation in precocial mammals, functional maturation of the neuroendocrine axis and its regulation continues until well after birth. This conclusion as it applies to regulation of pulsatile hormone secretion was, in part, based on infrequently collected fetal blood samples or from blood samples obtained at 10- to 15-min intervals over a limited 1- to 2-hr period. These data provided the first evidence for the efficacy of thyrotropin-releasing factor, somatotropin release-inhibiting factor, β-endorphin, and neuropharmacological agents to regulate prolactin and growth hormone secretion in the fetal lamb. Current hypotheses consider these hormones as important for fetal growth, adrenal function, and glycogen metabolism.

For Parturition

Over the past 2 decades, the maturation and regulation of the hypothalamic–pituitary–adrenal axis in the ovine fetus have been extensively studied during late pregnancy (9). In part, this focus is due to the pivotal role that glucocorticoids play in the maturation of a number of organ systems that are necessary for extrauterine survival (10). Precocious activation of this axis is associated with premature delivery while fetal hypophysectomy or adrenalectomy or hypothalamic–pituitary disconnection prolongs gestation (reviewed in 7). Thus, regulation of ACTH secretion from the pituitary and cortisol from the adrenal gland is a critical focus of studies to test the hypothesis that the ovine fetus plays an important role in the mechanism initiating parturition. Our experience in the pursuit of this hypothesis is summarized by the procedures discussed in this chapter. However, as Liggins (11) has pointedly stated, "The expectation that a reasonably complete knowledge of parturitional physiology in one species would inevitably provide clues to an understanding of parturition in most other species is unfulfilled." This assessment is as true today as it was a decade ago. Efforts in other species are needed to develop a working hypothesis for the mechanism that initiates labor and parturition.

Methodology

Surgery and Instrumentation

Access to the fetus and its circulation requires technological expertise and extensive surgical skills to ensure the long-term viability of the experimental model. The review by Rudolph and Heymann (5) should be committed to memory as an initial step toward understanding the complex arrangements needed for a successful fetal surgery. A visit to an established fetal physiology laboratory is encouraged not only to observe the routine of a study but to gain an appreciation for the coordinated efforts that surround both surgical procedures and experiments. It is plain to see that chronic fetal research is expensive, labor intensive, and highly dependent upon teamwork.

The preparation for fetal surgery is critical to its success because the health and well-being of the fetus is an absolute prerequisite for experimentation. Proper training in the techniques of sterile surgery is essential for all involved with the project. Preceding surgery, four separate packages are sterilized. As listed in Table I, these packs have all the linens, instruments, and catheters for surgery. The *linen pack* consists of the gowns, towels, and drapes necessary for sterile surgery. The tools to perform surgery and catheterization are included in two *instrument packs*. The *catheter pack* contains catheters,

TABLE I Contents of Four Sterile Packs for Surgical Instrumentation of the Ovine Fetus

Linen pack	Instrument pack A (generic-fetal/surgery)
Gowns, three Hand towels, three absorbant Utility drapes with adhesive tape, eight 18 × 24 in., to isolate surgical field Half drapes, two 44 × 60 in., to cover upper and lower body Lap drape, 72 × 120 in., full cover except for 15 × 5-in. opening for surgical field Lap sponges, five 18 × 18 in., segregates uterus from other abdominal cavity organs	Small metal pan (filled during surgery with 10 U heparin/100 ml saline to flush catheters) Large metal pan, 30 × 15 × 5 cm (filled during surgery with saline for lavage) Knife holder (No. 4) and scalpel blade (No. 10), two Towel clamps, Roeder Gauze squares (10 × 10 cm, 5 × 5 cm), four Skewers with thin umbilical tape (to subcutaneously tunnel catheters), two Large needles, 3-in. curved cutting edge, two Forceps: two small Russian, one large Russian, two Allis tissue, three Hartman Mosquito, seven delicate Halsted-small Kelly, eight large Kelly, eight Babcock, eight Pennington, two Kocher, three Ochsner Retractors: one small Crile, one Goelet, one Richardson, two Army/Navy–USA Scissors: one large Metzenbaum, one small Metzenbaum, two Mayo (straight and curved, one ea), suture Needle holders: 6 and 8 in. Mayo Hegar, one Olsen Hegar

Catheter pack

Amniotic fluid catheter, 1 150-cm length of Tygon tubing, pretreated with TDMAC-heparin (i.d. 1.77 mm; o.d. 2.28 mm; wall 0.51 mm) and with 7.5 cm slotted 12 French tubing as end basket Fetal catheters, five 150-cm length (i.d. 1.02 mm; o.d. 1.78 mm; wall 0.38 mm) glued to a 20-mm extension (i.d. 0.51 mm; o.d. 1.53 mm; wall 0.5 mm) Maternal catheters, three 150-cm length (i.d. 1.27 mm; o.d. 2.28 mm; wall 0.51 mm) glued to a 25-mm extension (i.d. 1.02 mm; o.d. 1.78 mm; wall 0.38 mm) 15-gauge blunt needle hubs, four 18-gauge blunt needle hubs, five 3-way stopcocks, ten Suture, ten 20 cm each of No. 1, 2-0, 3-0 silk Cotton tip swabs, eight Thick umbilical tape, 80 cm (prevents catheter tangles in pouch) Nylon pouch (15 × 20 cm) with grommets, sewn to left flank for catheter storage	*(Instrument pack B (for catheterization))* Knife handle (No. 3) and scalpel blade (No. 15) Catheter introducers, two Bulldog, Johns Hopkins Forceps: two Graefe, two Dressing Scissors: two Vannas, one Iris Coated vicryl suture (4-0 Ethicon) with FS-1 curved cutting-edge needle

precut sutures, and other components that are needed to secure access to the venous and arterial circulation of the fetus and pregnant ewe. We follow the recommendations of Rudolph and Heymann (5) for catheter material and their preparation.

Before surgery, ewes need to be acclimated to the vivarium and visited frequently by personnel involved with the project to minimize the stressors surrounding a chronic study. The order of surgery can be segregated into six distinct stages: anesthesia, maternal catheters, approach to the fetus, fetal catheters, surgical closure, and postoperative care.

Anesthesia

Procedures that have been detailed previously (12) are briefly reviewed here. The pregnant ewe is first injected with the short-lived barbiturate Biotal by jugular venipuncture, then transferred to the surgery table and restrained in the supine position. The trachea is intubated with a cuffed tube and an adequate level of general anesthesia maintained with inspiration of 1–2% halothane in a 40% N_2O mixture (750 ml tidal volume). Periodic assessment of respiratory rate is an important indication of the depth of anesthesia; slow shallow breathing and hyperventilation should be avoided. The next step in preparation for surgery is for all surgical sites to be shaved of wool and the skin scrubbed clean with several washes using Betadine or Hibiclens. If abdominal bloating is detected during this time, it may indicate tracheal extubation; re-intubation or re-inflation of the tracheal tube cuff may be required.

Maternal Catheters

Catheters are placed first in the pregnant ewe to obtain an arterial blood-gas measurement and assess animal well-being. The approach to and catheterization of the fetal artery in the hind limb are the same as previously described (5). For the maternal venous line, a length of the jugular vein adjacent to the trachea is surgically exposed. A collateral vein flowing into the main jugular is identified and dissected free of all fatty, as well as connective, tissue. A catheter is inserted through this collateral vein and advanced approximately 10 cm toward the heart. Each catheter is anchored with a 2-0 silk suture, first to the vessel itself and then to nearby muscle tissue, separated by an intervening small loop of tubing. To expedite the next phase of surgery, the incision in the leg and neck are temporarily clamped and catheters stored in a sterile towel. The pregnant ewe is then draped for the next procedure.

Approach to the Fetus

An opening to expose the uterus is initially made with a superficial incision near midline and then into the abdominal cavity along the linea alba. Palpation within the peritoneal cavity is necessary to determine the number of fetuses and their orientation. The fetal forelimb is identified by its flexion and manipulated to an avascular portion of the uterine horn. A small incision is made with a scalpel in the thin-walled uterus. One fetal forelimb is withdrawn while a length of gauze is securely wrapped around the uterine opening to reduce the loss of amniotic fluid.

Fetal Catheters

An incision less than 2 cm in length is made along the medial aspect of the fetal humorus; blunt dissection readily exposes the deep brachial artery and more superficial but lateral cephalic vein. These vessels are fragile and easily induced to spasm. Instrumentation procedures follow those described previously (5) and the following is a brief review. Introduction of a slightly bevelled catheter is facilitated by the use of a catheter introducer and Dow–Corning silicone fluid. The length of catheter to be inserted into the vessel and advanced to the superior vena cava or dorsal aorta is an empirical estimate. Fetal catheters are anchored with 3-0 silk in a manner similar to that described for maternal catheters. Fetal skin incisions are closed with Ethicon 4-0 coated vicryl suture with an FS-1 curved cutting needle. Both fetal forelimbs are catheterized to provide a backup for lines that become occluded over the course of study. Finally, an amniotic fluid catheter is typically attached to the forelimb at this time. This catheter is used to monitor pressure, to obtain fluid samples, and for antibiotic administration. At this point during surgery, all catheters should be tested for patency. In our studies, we have not attempted to install a catheter in the cerebral sagittal sinus; however, a technique described by Tsoulos and colleagues indicates that cerebral venous blood may also be readily accessible (13).

Surgical Closure

After the second fetal forelimb is catheterized, it is pushed back into the amniotic cavity and catheters are brought out of the uterus. To compensate for tension created by fetal movement, about 10 cm of catheter length remains within the uterus. Membranes of the amnion and chorion are separated from the uterine muscle and double tied with No. 1 silk suture around the catheter bundle (each tie is twice wrapped). This creates a liquid-tight seal to prevent leakage of amniotic fluid into the peritoneal cavity. The uterus itself is then double-sutured (mattress stitch) using 2-0 chromic gut. The linea alba is closed with an individually tied 1-0 silk suture on a large curve needle. Catheters are individually clamped near the uterus with Pennington forceps, tunneled subcutaneously (catheters and hubs only) with a skewer, and exteriorized through a small incision on the right flank. A nylon pouch is sewn directly onto the left flank for storage of appropriately labeled catheters. Finally, the three skin incisions in the ewe, i.e., abdominal, leg, and neck, are conveniently closed with a subcuticular continuous stitch using 2-0 silk with a cutting edge needle.

Postoperative Care

Surgery should take less than 2 hr from anesthesia to closure. During the last 15 min of the procedure the ewe should be exclusively on N_2O anesthesia. Before the ewe is returned to an individual cage in the animal room, all indwelling catheters are flushed with saline and an antibiotic administered. For about 3 days, the ewe receives an intramuscular injection of combiotic (2.5 ml im; Pfizer, NY) and progesterone (100 mg, im; Rugby Laboratories, Rockville, NY). The fetus also receives antibiotics, gentamycin (40 mg daily; Elkins-Sinn, Cherry Hill, NJ) may be given for the duration of the study through the amniotic fluid catheter or intravenously (bolus or drip). Fetal intravenous administration has the advantage of dose specificity; however, the preparation must be adequately diluted and given over a 5- to 10-min interval to minimize deleterious effects on the vasculature. Several other antibiotics have proved useful to combat fetal infection, including Claforan (Hoechst-Roussel Pharmaceuticals, Somerville, NJ), Clindamycin (Upjohn, Kalamazoo, MI), Mezlin (Miles Pharmaceuticals, West Haven, CT), and Tobramycin (Lederle Labs, Wayne, NJ). The particular antibiotic used is empirically determined from cultures of fetal blood and amniotic fluid, as well as known contra-indicative side effects. Doses and treatment regimens are based on manufacturers recommendations for infants.

Fetal Health and Well-Being

The live birth of a lamb of normal weight may be considered to attest to the maintenance of fetal health during experimentation. Infection is the most common threat to the well-being of the chronically cannulated fetus. We have used a number of indices of fetal wellness, these include daily or more frequent assessment of fetal arterial pO_2, pCO_2, percentage oxyhemoglobin saturation (HbO_2), hemoglobin concentration (Hb), hematocrit, and pH. Serious signs of fetal distress are indicated by development of acidosis, a reduction in HbO_2 saturation, declining pO_2 or increasing pCO_2, and an acid-base imbalance. A normal range for fetal blood gases should be established within each laboratory using reliable and properly calibrated equipment (14, 16; Fig. 1). These parameters are also sensitive indices of fetal stress and, along with measurements of plasma of ACTH and cortisol concentrations, provide adequate information about the status of fetal health.

As a precaution, the best treatment for fetal infection is prevention. Preoperative care and strict adherence to sterile techniques during surgery have already been described to be essential. At the end of surgery and periodically thereafter, fetal blood and amniotic fluid samples are collected to culture bacterial flora and test antibiotic sensitivity. Preventive antibiotic treatment is routinely initiated in the ewe and fetus after surgery (described above). However, the antibiotic regimen may be modified in response to culture reports or perceived trends in fetal blood-gas data. Sodium bicarbonate (2 mEq/ml) has proved useful to acutely correct severe acidosis. Several days

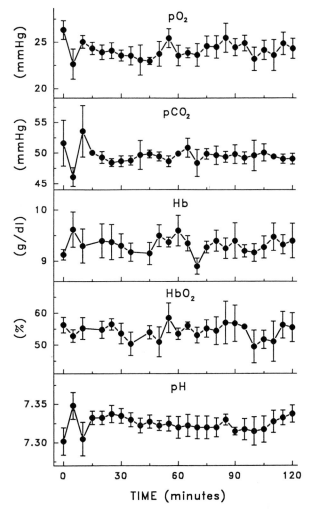

Fig. 1   Fetal blood-gas data (mean ± SE, $n = 4$) for the partial pressure of oxygen (pO_2) and carbon dioxide (pCO_2), hemoglobin concentration (Hb), percentage oxyhemoglobin saturation (HbO$_2$), and pH in blood samples withdrawn every 5 min for 2 hr. Differences over time for blood-gas data were not significant ($p > 0.05$, ANOVA with repeated measures).

of any new treatment may be required to stabilize and then restore fetal blood gases to normal; experiments should be delayed until the recovery of fetal health is sustained.

Catheter Patency and Maintenance

Regular catheter maintenance is critical to reliably access fetal circulation. After surgery and subsequently at least once each day, all catheters are flushed with 3 to 5 ml of heparinized saline. Within 24 hr of surgery, 10 U of heparin/ml of sterile saline has been used to reduce the risk of fetal hemorrhage, while at other times 100 U/ml of heparinized saline is the routine. A gentle and slow withdrawal of solutions or blood from the catheter with a sterile 3-ml syringe is recommended. The syringe is a lueger-locked type which helps prevent a blowout in the connection with the three-way plastic stopcock port. This stopcock is attached to the metal hub (15 or 18 ga) which is inserted into the tip of the catheter line. Stopcock hubs are covered with caps that are soaked in Omnicide (Baxter Hospital Supply, Irvine, CA). All connections and attachments to the catheter must be kept clean and, when not in use, carefully housed in the nylon storage pouch.

Generally, fetal arterial vessels are high flow conduits which rarely occlude compared to venous lines that often become closed with time or temporarily blocked with a rapid or high-pressure withdrawal. Venous catheters also more commonly occlude due to accumulated debris or clotting at the distal tip or position of the fetal limb at the time of blood withdrawal. An obstructed catheter may occasionally be cleared and free flow reestablished by filling the line with 5000 U heparin/ml saline for at least 6 hr or overnight.

Preparations for Frequent Blood Collection

In planning for a frequent blood collection study, protocol forms, supplies, equipment, and the facility itself must be prepared before the first sample is obtained. As part of the setup, a written protocol form should contain all information relating to the study, such as blood collection times and corresponding sample numbers, gestational age of fetus, and personnel involved, and space for notes during the bleed period. Tubes should be prelabeled for blood collection (12 × 75-mm borosilicate glass) and plasma storage (1.5 ml plastic microcentrifuge). Other relevant supplies need to be prepared, including sterile heparinized saline to clear catheters of blood, Ringers lactate solution to resuspend erythrocytes, pipettes to aliquot plasma for storage, extra tube racks, ice buckets, timers, and syringes (3 ml for sample and 10 ml to flush catheter). In a separate room near the ewe, a refrigerated desktop centrifuge was used to harvest plasma and perform blood-processing procedures. Finally, at least 12 hr before the study, 5 ml of fetal blood is collected in a sterile 10-ml syringe (preloaded with heparinized Ringers lactate) and stored at 4°C for the next day. This blood is returned to the fetus within the first 30 min of the frequent blood collection period to allow for the lag time in processing erythrocytes during the actual experiment.

On the day of the study, the ewe is tethered in a metabolic cage with full access to food and water. Next to, but out of reach from the ewe, was a small desk and chair which provided workspace for placement of the indwelling catheter lines, other supplies for blood sample collection, the actual location for blood withdrawal and a seat for the investigator. Primary and backup catheters are placed on a sterile towel or gauze (4 × 4 inches). A backup line helps maintain a rigid time regimen for frequent blood collections. We have found that catheter problems can be adequately addressed during the 2- to 3-minute interval between 5-min blood collections. By this time, the ewe has become acclimated to the presence of the investigator and activities related to the experiment. The less interested the ewe is in the experimental proceedings and the more the cud is chewed, the more prepared the animal is for the study to begin.

Frequent Sampling from Circulation and Fetal Blood Gases

In conducting the study, one person collects frequent blood samples from the ewe and fetus, as well as makes all decisions regarding catheter lines or the animal during the study. A second individual is needed to assist in the study and to process blood: harvest and aliquot plasma for storage, reconstitute erythrocytes, and periodically assess arterial samples for blood gases.

The frequency and duration of the blood-sampling protocol are critical issues to accurately discern the episodic pattern of hormone secretion in circulation. A number of considerations were factored into the decision to collect blood every 5 min for 2–4 hr in the fetal lamb. The episodic nature of secretion within pituitary–adrenal axis and the relatively short half-life for ACTH in fetal circulation of less than 10 min (14) suggested that blood samples needed to be collected as frequently as possible to resolve the relationship between the trophic stimulus and the endocrine response. In addition, the weight of the fetus, as estimated from the known gestational age at surgery, provides a good approximation of total fetal blood volume. Estimates of fetal blood volume were based on the observation that fetal blood volume appears to be a constant fraction of fetal body weight (15). In sheep and goats during the latter half of gestation, fetal blood volume has been reported to range from 106 to 116 ml/kg. We used the estimate of 110 ± 2 ml blood/kg body weight based on previous work in this breed of sheep by Lawrence D. Longo and Robert A. Brace in the Division of Perinatal Biology.

Hormones that exert profound effects on fetal circulation are released in response to hemorrhage, e.g., plasma ACTH, cortisol, and arginine vasopressin. Withdrawal of more than 10% of fetal–placental blood volume can induce significant secretion of these hormones of interest. Even so, a minimum number of secretory episodes over a period of time is required to accurately assess hormone pulse frequency. Thus we decided to withdraw as little blood as possible over a 2- to 4-hr period, immediately replace with saline the volume withdrawn, and, after plasma was harvested for assays, return to the fetus reconstituted erythrocytes to reduce the hazards inherent in the methodology. To minimize blood withdrawal, less than 3 ml of fetal whole blood was obtained for any one sample. Over the course of a 2-hr experiment, typically less than 80 ml of blood is withdrawn and up to 125 ml of saline or Ringers lactate reinfused to the fetus.

Another consideration was whether endocrine pulse patterns are associated with fluctuations in certain indices of fetal well-being such as moment-to-moment changes in fetal pO_2. Therefore, to test the hypothesis that episodic hormone secretion was not related to specific hemodynamic characteristics, frequent blood-gas measurements were made at 5-min intervals and in sequence with withdrawal of blood for hormone determinations. Over the course of the 2-hr blood sampling period, fetal blood-gas data for pO_2, pCO_2, percentage HbO_2 saturation, Hb, and pH in blood remain relatively constant within a narrow range (Fig. 1). Even when the frequent blood withdrawal protocol was repeated at intervals ranging from 22 hr to 7 days, there was little change in blood-gas parameters (data from animals in reference 16). Although not indicated in Fig. 1, fetal erythrocytes were reconstituted in a volume of 2–5 ml of Ringers lactate and were reinfused into fetal circulation at 10- to 15-minute intervals beginning about 30 min after the onset of the frequent blood collection protocol. Any effect of returning fetal erythrocytes or infusate solutions on these blood-gas measurements were not apparent.

Hormone Assays

ACTH and cortisol in fetal plasma were measured by radioimmunoassay. Parallelism, quantitative accuracy, and repeatability were verified using plasma pools from pregnant and fetal sheep. The ACTH radioimmunoassay, purchased from Incstar Corp. (Stillwater, MN), had an average assay sensitivity of 1 pg/ml; intra- and interassay coefficients of variation were less than 11%. Antiserum for the cortisol radioimmunoassay was provided by John Challis and used at a dilution of 1 : 3500/0.1 ml assay buffer. Assay sensitivity averaged 0.2 ng/ml; coefficients of variations within and between assays average better than 13%. To reduce variability and enhance reliability, all plasma samples collected during a 2- to 4-hr study period were processed in a single assay. Whenever possible, plasma samples from a single animal at different gestational ages were processed in the same assay.

The plasma concentrations of the catecholamines, norepinephrine (NE), and epinephrine (E), were quantified by high-pressure liquid chromatography with electrochemical detection (17). Assay sensitivity averaged 1 pg/ml.

Pulse Analysis and Statistics

For the study of fetal ACTH and cortisol secretion (16), a pulse was characterized by peak concentrations that exceeded the 95% confidence interval of both the preceding and the subsequent nadirs, with an amplitude (peak minus preceding nadir) that exceeded assay sensitivity. This criterion has demonstrated good agreement with the Cluster analysis algorithm for pulse detection (18). The coincidence of pulsatile ACTH and cortisol secretion was empirically defined by a peak ACTH episode that was coincident with or followed within 10 min by a pulse peak in plasma cortisol.

Application Examples

ACTH and Cortisol in Fetal Circulation

Episodic variations in ACTH and cortisol in fetal circulation lead to the conclusion that these hormones are secreted as discrete pulses (Fig. 2). ACTH and cortisol pulses were identified in all fetuses (16). Approximately one-third of all ACTH pulses were coincident with cortisol pulses in circulation; the number of coincident pulses did not exceed random association. Moreover, as gestation progressed, increases in mean cortisol concentrations in circulation, as well as pulse frequency and amplitude, were not associated with any change in pulsatile ACTH secretion. The pattern of pulsatile ACTH, as well as cortisol, in the fetus was found to be independent of that observed in maternal circulation. These data suggest that a trophic drive other than the pulsatile secretion of ACTH may be the principal stimulus for cortisol pulses in the ovine fetus during the latter days of gestation near paturition. The data further suggest that pulses of ACTH or cortisol in the fetus are

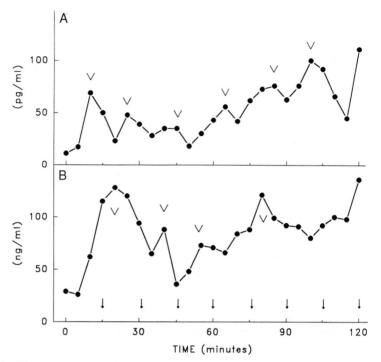

FIG. 2   Plasma concentrations of ACTH (A) and cortisol (B) in the circulation of fetus No. 257 at 137 days gestation (morning). This lamb was born alive on Day 145 of pregnancy and weighed 3.64 kg. Inverted arrowheads indicate episodes that meet pulse criteria. Inverted arrows indicate reinfusion into fetal circulation of fetal erythrocytes reconstituted with Ringers lactate.

not dependent on the pulsatile pattern of either of these hormones in the pregnant ewe.

The technology to study pulsatile hormone secretion has also been applied to questions of neuroendocrine regulation of constitutive ACTH secretion. The principal hypothalamic releasing factor for ACTH in the ovine fetus appears to be arginine vasopressin. To determine whether arginine vasopressin is involved in the regulation of pulsatile ACTH secretion, a specific arginine vasopressin pituitary receptor antagonist was administered to the fetus during late gestation (14). Although arginine vasopressin-induced ACTH release was effectively blocked by the arginine vasopressin antagonist treatment, basal pulsatile ACTH and cortisol secretion were unaffected during the weeks preceding parturition. Moreover, basal cortisol secretion is maintained in the fetus late in gestation even when the hypothalamus has

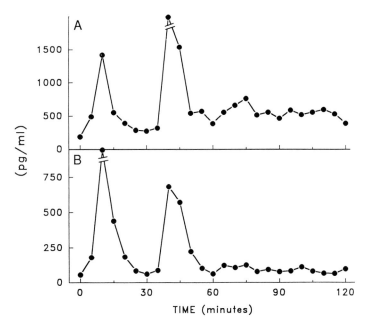

FIG. 3   Plasma norepinephrine (NE) in (A) and epinephrine (E) in (B) concentrations in the circulation of fetus No. 257 on the morning of 137 days gestation (17). Two data points were above scale: for NE at 40 min, 1702 pg/ml, and for E at 10 min, 2003 pg/ml. See Fig. 2 legend for further details.

been disconnected from the pituitary (7). These data raise the hypothesis that near-term increased pulsatile cortisol secretion in the fetal lamb is driven by a mechanism that is independent of the neuroendocrine regulation by arginine vasopressin or pulsatile ACTH secretion.

Catecholamines in Fetal Circulation

In fetal sheep, catecholamines are involved in the cardiovascular response to stress and increased secretion of cortisol from the adrenal. Episodes of pulsatile secretion of the catecholamines, norepinephrine and epinephrine, in fetal circulation are present throughout the last 2 weeks of gestation (Fig. 3). The temporal coincidence of plasma norepinephrine and epinephrine pulses was nearly 80% (17). As gestation progressed, there was little evidence to suggest any change in the pulsatile characteristics of catecholamine secretion. Exogenous treatment with cortisol, however, was found to selectively enhance the amplitude but not frequency of norepinephrine and epinephrine pulses. These data lead to the hypothesis that rather than precede the endogenous increase in cortisol in circulation during late gestation, enhanced catecholamine secretion appears to follow the changes in the hypothalamic pituitary axis that are associated with the process of parturition.

Other Endocrine Patterns in Fetal Circulation

Considerable data are available on the ontogeny of pituitary hormone secretion in the ovine fetus. By the last third of gestation, the mean concentrations of prolactin and growth hormone but not luteinizing hormone are on the rise in fetal circulation (8, 19). The secretion of each of these hormones has been characterized as pulsatile based on a 15-min blood sampling frequency. Even so, the physiological importance of the pulsatile nature of secretion for these hormones and, as Gluckman *et al.* (8) have remarked, their function in the fetus have yet to be defined.

In contrast to the ultradian patterns of secretion for these hormones, a circadian variation has also been reported in the ovine fetus for melatonin, prolactin, and growth hormone (12, 20). Although the significance of 24-hr prolactin and growth hormone rhythms is not known, the circadian melatonin rhythm is thought to convey information about environmental photoperiod to temporally regulate physiological function. Thus neuroendocrine studies of pulsatile or circadian hormone secretion may lead to important insights about physiological mechanisms if linked with such processes as growth and development in the fetus.

Summary Considerations

Catheterization of the fetus for the chronic study of its physiology *in utero* has become a routine research model in laboratories with surgical expertise and broad-based resources. A success rate of better than 80% survival to term is, in our experience, attainable with careful attention to the details surrounding fetal health. The invasive procedures themselves, i.e., surgery and frequency or duration of blood withdrawal, may affect the end points of research interest and must be addressed with objective criteria. To this end our studies have used the pituitary–adrenal axis not just as an index of fetal maturation but also as an indicator of stress to the fetus. The absence of chronically elevated concentrations of ACTH and cortisol, along with a normal range of blood-gas parameters and catecholamines in circulation, suggests that physiological processes in the fetus are not masked by the experimental intervention.

The resolution of a true endogenous physiological signal from either background noise or a periodic stimulus-induced response is critical for any analysis of pulsatile endocrine secretion. This goal is especially true of studies in the fetus where interpretation of results may be complicated by issues related to placental or maternal influences on fetal physiology. Simultaneous collection of blood from the ewe and fetus may be necessary to study placental metabolism or distinguish any maternal contribution to the pulsatile hormone pattern that is present in the fetus.

At the foundation of understanding pulsatile endocrine secretion in the fetus is the adequacy of the blood collection protocol. As with other systems, both the frequency and the duration of blood sampling are important to define the pulsatile characteristics of hormone secretion. Technical limitations related to the amount of blood withdrawn from the fetus over a period of time appear to be surmountable by volume replacement and reinfusing erythrocytes. Certainly, the most relevant assessment that these precautions are effective is the apparent absence of long-term effects on fetal growth and development. Moreover, lambs are typically born alive and at normal term. Thus, the ovine fetus presents a strong model for neuroendocrine studies of pulsatile hormone secretion.

Acknowledgments

The authors thank Dr. Lawrence D. Longo for instruction in fetal surgery, participation in the experiments, and his commitment to excellence. Ms. Lela Spears, Ms. Larkin Buyak, and Mr. Christian P. Haase provided technical assistance for these studies. Support for the work described in this chapter came from the Department of Pediatrics at Loma Linda University School of Medicine, NIH Grant HD 03817, NIH Center for Nursing Research NRSA 06042, and the Graduate School of Loma Linda University.

References

1. D. H. Barron, in ''Perinatal Life'' (H. Mack, ed.), p. 109. Wayne State Univ. Press, Detroit, 1970.
2. S. R. M. Reynolds, in ''Fetal and Newborn Cardiovascular Physiology'' (L. D. Longo and D. D. Reneau, eds.), p. 33. Garland STPM Press, New York, 1978.
3. G. Meschia, A. S. Wolkoff, and D. H. Barron, Q. J. Exp. Physiol. 44, 333 (1959).
4. G. Meschia, J. R. Cotter, C. S. Breathnach, and D. H. Barron, Q. J. Exp. Physiol. 50, 185 (1965).

5. A. M. Rudolph and M. A. Heymann, *in* "Animal Models in Fetal Medicine" (P. W. Nathanielsz, ed.), p. 1. Elsevier-North Holland Biomedical Press, Amsterdam, 1980.

6. P. D. Gluckman and Y. Parsons, *in* "Animal Models in Fetal Medicine" (P. W. Nathanielsz, ed.), p. 69. Perinatology Press, Ithaca, NY, 1984.

7. I. Z. Ozolins, I. R. Young, and I. C. McMillen, *Endocrinology (Baltimore)* **127,** 1833 (1990).

8. P. D. Gluckman, M. M. Grumbach, and S. L. Kaplan, *Endocrine Rev.* **2,** 363 (1981).

9. J. R. G. Challis, A. N. Brooks, L. J. Fraher, L. J. Norman, A. D. Bocking, S. A. Jones, and L. Power, *in* "The Endocrine Control of the Fetus" (W. Künzel and A. Jensen, eds.), p. 374. Springer-Verlag, Berlin/Heidelberg, 1988.

10. P. L. Ballard, *in* "Glucocorticoid Hormone Action" (J. D. Baxter and G. G. Rousseau, eds.), p. 493. Springer-Verlag, New York, 1979.

11. G. C. Liggins, *in* "Fetal Endocrinology," p. 211. Academic Press, San Diego, 1981.

12. S. M. Yellon and L. D. Longo, *Am. J. Physiol.* **252,** E799 (1987).

13. N. G. Tsoulos, J. M. Schneider, J. Colwell, G. Meschia, E. L. Makowski, and F. C. Battaglia, *Pediatr. Res.* **6,** 182 (1972).

14. E. M. Apostolakis, L. D. Longo, and S. M. Yellon, *Endocrinology (Baltimore)* **129,** 295 (1991).

15. R. A. Brace, *in* "Animal Models in Fetal Medicine" (P. W. Nathanielsz, ed.), p. 19. Perinatology Press, Ithaca, NY, 1984.

16. E. M. Apostolakis, L. D. Longo, J. D. Veldhuis, and S. M. Yellon, *Endocrinology (Baltimore)* **130,** 2571 (1992).

17. E. A. Apostolakis, T. Matsumoto, L. D. Longo, and C. A. Ducsay, *Biol. Reprod.* **44** (Suppl.), 167 (1991).

18. J. D. Veldhuis, J. Moorman, and M. L. Johnson, Chapter 15, this volume.

19. N. Albers, M. Bettendorf, H. Herrmann, S. L. Kaplan, and M. M. Grumbach, *Endocrinology (Baltimore)* **132,** 701 (1993).

20. I. C. McMillen, G. D. Thorburn, and D. W. Walker, *J. Endocrinol.* **114,** 65 (1987).

[13] Pulsatile Corticosterone Secretion as Measured by Intraadrenal Microdialysis

Michael S. Jasper, Jill T. Walworth, and William C. Engeland

Introduction

The hypothalamic–pituitary–adrenal axis is characterized by its rhythmic secretion under nonstress conditions. In addition to a circadian rhythm in plasma corticosteroids that is driven by parallel rhythms in plasma ACTH and in adrenal sensitivity to ACTH (1), pulsatile changes in corticosteroids have been described. There is some controversy as to whether episodes of secretion are random events (2) or occur at regular intervals producing an ultradian rhythm (3, 4). In addition, the mechanisms responsible for producing and controlling secretory episodes have not been delineated. Since plasma ACTH concentration changes in a pulsatile fashion (5), adrenal responses most likely are driven in part by ACTH. It is probable that neural and humoral mechanisms in addition to ACTH contribute to the control of corticosterone pulsatility.

Our interest has been directed toward understanding the role of extra-ACTH factors in modulating adrenocortical responsiveness to ACTH. To examine the influence of ACTH and non-ACTH factors on control of ultradian adrenal rhythmicity in rats, a preparation was required that enabled direct measurement of adrenal secretion. By measuring secretion directly rather than inferring it from plasma steroid concentration, one could be assured that measurements reflected changes in adrenal output and not changes in steroid distribution, binding, or metabolism. *In situ*-perfused adrenals, in which the normal relationship between cells and neural input is preserved, have been used successfully to assess adrenal responses to putative secretagogues (6); however, this approach does not permit studies of adrenal secretion under physiological conditions in behaving animals. Since collection of adrenal venous output in rats can only be accomplished in anesthetized, acutely prepared animals, an intraadrenal microdialysis technique, adapted from previous work by Jarry and co-workers (7), was developed. This preparation enabled the collection of adrenal extracellular corticosterone in awake, behaving rats and the monitoring of adrenal secretory rhythms.

In this review we discuss methods used to apply adrenal microdialysis to study pulsatile secretion of corticosterone in rats. An attempt has been made

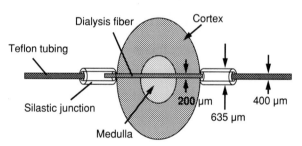

FIG. 1   Schematic drawing of microdialysis probe placed in the rat adrenal gland. The probe is secured to the adrenal by adhering the Silastic tubing to the adrenal capsule using cyanoacrylate adhesive.

to strike a balance between presenting a guide for validating the microdialysis technique for monitoring adrenal dialysate corticosterone in behaving rats and providing the basis and the techniques for statistical analysis of pulsatile changes in adrenal corticosterone secretion. In addition, examples are presented of the use of adrenal microdialysis to study changes in pulsatile secretion of corticosterone under differing physiological conditions.

Construction of the Microdialysis Probe

Microdialysis probes are constructed as described previously (8) with some modifications (Fig. 1). Probes are made from single dialysis fibers obtained from manufacturers of hemodialysis or bioreactor units. An 8-mm piece of dialysis fiber (200–250 μm O.D.) is inserted between two 23-mm sections of Silastic tubing (I.D. = 0.012 in.) and fastened using silicon adhesive (Corning Medical, Corning, NY); a 2-mm section of dialysis fiber is exposed using care to avoid covering dialysis pores with cement. The Silastic junctions are connected to lengths of Teflon tubing (Zeus Industrial Products, Inc., Raritan, NJ; O.D. = 0.016 in., I.D. = 0.004 in.) by threading the Teflon tubing into the Silastic tubing until it abuts the dialysis fiber; no adhesive is required to maintain these connections. In a modification, a 15-mm piece of tungsten wire (O.D. = 0.003 in., World Precision Instruments, FL) is threaded through the dialysis fiber prior to attaching the Silastic tubing. This addition appears to increase the mechanical stability of the probe preventing it from twisting or collapsing during insertion into the adrenal.

In Vitro Validation of Microdialysis Probes

The recovery and dynamic response of microdialysis probes is characterized *in vitro* by immersing probes sequentially in a 37°C saline solution and a solution of epinephrine (2.58 μM), corticosterone (14.5 μM), and ascorbic

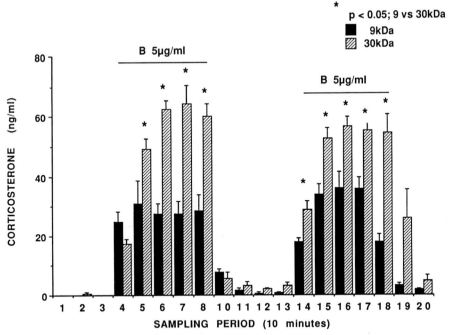

FIG. 2   *In vitro* corticosterone recovery of 9- and 30-kDa microdialysis probes. Horizontal lines indicate periods during which probes were immersed in a 5 μg/ml solution (14.5 μM) of corticosterone (compound B); probes were immersed in Ringers lactate solution in between corticosterone pulses. Vertical bars represent the mean $\pm$ SEM of four probes. Corticosterone recovery was greater using the 30-kDa microdialysis probe relative to the 9-kDa probe ($p < 0.05$ by ANOVA), but there were no differences in recovery for either probe during repeated exposure to corticosterone.

acid (600 μM) to simulate the hormonal milieu within the adrenal; this sequence is repeated to assess the reproducibility of the response. Probes are perfused with Ringers solution at a flow rate of 10 μl/min and the corticosterone concentration in the collected dialysate is assayed by radioimmunoassay using a commercially available kit (ICN Biomedical, Costa Mesa, CA). *In vitro* comparisons are made between a cellulose dialysis membrane (Marco HF) with a molecular weight (MW) cutoff of 9000 and a cellulose acetate dialysis membrane (Unisyn Fibertec Corp., San Diego, CA) with a MW cutoff of 30,000. Probes respond rapidly to acute changes in corticosterone concentration and give quantitatively similar responses when exposure to corticosterone is repeated (Fig. 2). Fibers with a MW cutoff of 9000 show a lower recovery of corticosterone compared to fibers with a MW cutoff of 30,000 (0.6–0.7 vs 0.9–1.2%), suggesting that increasing the MW cutoff may

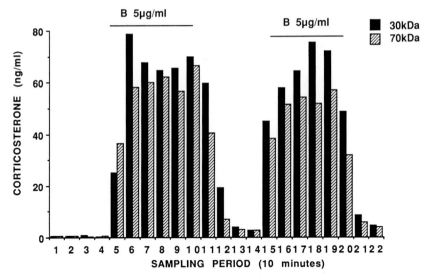

FIG. 3   *In vitro* corticosterone recovery of 30- and 70-kDa microdialysis probes. Applying the same procedure described in Fig. 2, there were no consistent differences in recovery. Average recoveries for the 30- and 70-dKa probes were 1.35 and 1.14%, respectively.

be advantageous for recovering corticosterone. However, using a probe made with a cellulose acetate membrane with a 70,000 MW cutoff (Unisyn Fibertec Corp., San Diego, CA) did not result in further augmentation of corticosterone recovery (Fig. 3).

Although *in vitro* tests of corticosterone recovery should be done to select a membrane through which corticosterone will diffuse, diffusion characteristics of dialysis probes *in vitro* may not reflect quantitatively those occurring *in vivo*. Diffusion of steroids *in vivo* most likely is affected by components of the interstitium including extracellular matrix that cannot easily be simulated during *in vitro* testing. To quantitate adrenal extracellular concentration of corticosterone, knowledge of *in vivo* recovery of corticosterone would be required. Although it is possible to perform *in vivo* calibration of microdialysis probes as done previously for estimating glucose recovery in subcutaneous tissue (9), the estimate of recovery requires that steady-state concentrations of analyte are maintained during the collection period. This requirement cannot be met by estimating recovery of corticosterone in adrenal extracellular fluid, since pulsatile changes in corticosterone concentration occur (see Fig. 5). *In vivo* recovery after long-term placement also may be affected by changes in the probe's diffusion efficiency. For example, fibrosis would decrease diffusion by reducing the number of pores available for transport. To control for *in vivo* differences in recovery, adrenal corticosterone secretion in each experiment is normalized to the secretory maximum defined by the response to a supraphysiological bolus of ACTH (described below).

Surgical Implantation of Microdialysis Probe

Male Sprague–Dawley rats (250–500 g body weight, Charles River Laboratories) are housed two to a cage in a light-controlled facility, lights on from 0700 to 1900 hr. Food and water are provided *ad libitum* and animals are allowed to acclimate to the housing facility and light cycle for at least 1 week before experiments. Rats are anesthetized with sodium pentabarbital (60–70 mg/kg) and the adrenal gland is exposed through a subcostal abdominal skin and muscle incision. Probes are flushed with saline, 10% ethanol, and saline again prior to insertion. The probe is inserted by attaching a 26-ga needle to the Teflon tube and threading the needle, tube, and probe through the center of the adrenal gland until the two Silastic junctions are located at the edge of the gland (see Fig. 1). The Silastic junctions are cemented to the outside of the adrenal gland using cyanoacrylate. Prior to applying adhesive, the patency of the probe and its connectors is determined by attaching the Teflon tubing to a Harvard syringe pump and perfusing the system with saline. If flow is absent or reduced, it is probable that the dialysis fiber has been twisted during insertion into the adrenal; manipulation of the tubing usually increases flow which is continuously monitored while the Silastic junctions are glued to the adrenal. The abdominal musculature is closed with suture and the Teflon tubing is secured to the abdominal musculature, tunneled subcutaneously, and exteriorized between the scapulae. The abdominal skin is sutured and the exteriorized Teflon tubing is either coiled and placed in a subcutaneous pocket on the dorsum of the neck or threaded through a stainless steel spring that is tethered to a swivel above the animal's cage. Prior to placement of the adrenal probe, an indwelling Silastic catheter (I.D. = 0.020 in., O.D. = 0.037 in.) is inserted in the right jugular vein via a ventral incision and, in experiments requiring the infusion of ACTH or saline, a PE10 polyethylene catheter is also inserted into the right jugular vein. The incision is closed with wound clips and the catheters are tunneled subcutaneously and exteriorized between the scapulae. Antibiotics (Ancef, 10 mg/kg im) are given and the animal is kept warm until fully ambulatory. Animals are studied 1–5 days after surgical preparation.

Calculation of *In Vivo* Secretion Rate

Corticosterone concentrations in dialysate are multiplied by dialysate flow rate and divided by sample period (10 min) to express secretion as average picograms per minute. Because corticosterone concentrations in dialysate are relatively low, samples are diluted 10-fold less than the plasma samples, in order to keep measured values on the linear portion of the standard curve. Thus, plasma samples are diluted 1 : 200 [standard for this radioimmunoassay (RIA) kit], whereas dialysate samples are diluted 1 : 20. Samples from experiments involving dexamethasone administration without ACTH replacement are diluted 1 : 2 due to the very low levels of corticosterone. The sensitivity of the assay, as defined by the ED_{95}, was 6.25 ng/ml. This corresponds to a secretion rate of 6.25 pg/min in the data reported here. The intraassay coefficient of variation (CV) was 7.6% and the interassay CV was 13.3%, on a pool value of 78 ng/ml.

Variation in absolute secretion between similarly treated animals is observed. Interanimal differences in corticosterone secretion could result from variations between dialysis probes in diffusion efficiency. In addition, the intraadrenal position of dialysis probes will vary; it is likely that probes in contact primarily with cortical cells will be exposed to higher corticosterone concentrations compared to those in contact with both cortical and medullary cells. In order to control for interanimal differences in absolute corticosterone secretion, secretion rates are normalized by dividing by the maximal secretory rate elicited by the injection of a 50 ng bolus of ACTH [hACTH 1-39 or ACTH 1-24 (Cortrosyn)].

Methods for Analysis of Pulsatile Corticosterone Secretion

Pulse-Detection Method

Peaks in the data series can be identified by one of several pulse-detection methods. We have used an IBM-AT computer and PC-Pulsar, a version of the Pulsar pulse-analysis program of Merriam and Wachter (10), as modified by Gitzin and Ramirez (11). Pulsar first calculates a baseline trend in the data using a weighted moving average smoothing algorithm. Residuals are then calculated between individual data points and the baseline, and these residuals are expressed in units of assay standard deviation at the appropriate dose level. Thus, residuals are expressed in "signal/noise" units. Program parameters are chosen to produce a theoretical maximum false-positive rate of approximately 5% (i.e., a 5% likelihood of detecting a pulse in pure noise). The following values are used: $G(1) = 3.98$, $G(2) = 2.4$, $G(3) = 1.68$, $G(4) = 1.24$, $G(5) = 0.93$, smoothing time = 225 min (i.e., half the experimental duration).

Pulsar is used to determine the pulse duration, pulse amplitude, and interpulse interval (IPI). Preliminary data analysis revealed nongaussian distributions in all three parameters. Therefore, in each experiment, the median value and maximum value for each parameter are determined, and a group mean and standard error is determined to compare treatment effects. Median IPI is an indicator of the overall frequency of pulses and thus corresponds to the primary frequency in a spectral analysis. Maximum IPI is useful as an index of the longest period without significant active secretion. This has been referred to as the quiescent period and may be altered in pathological conditions (12). Maximum pulse amplitude is used to test for the presence of unusually large pulses under different conditions. Median and maximum IPI, duration, and amplitude are compared between groups using ANOVA.

Time-Domain versus Frequency-Domain Analysis

Analyses of episodic variations frequently use time-domain methods (13) such as Pulsar (10) or CLUSTER (14). These algorithms differ primarily in the manner in which they decide if a transient increase represents a significant pulse. Discrete pulse-detection methods are very sensitive to sampling frequency. Since all pulse-detection methods yield an average pulse frequency, multiple underlying periodicities in the data cannot be separated. Different control mechanisms may impinge on episodic systems driving rhythms with different frequencies; thus, the method of analysis must be capable of distinguishing multiple component periodicities in a complex waveform. In contrast to time-domain methods, frequency-domain analysis (power spectrum analysis, Fourier analysis) partitions overall variability into variations at different frequencies, decomposing an arbitrary signal into a sum of sine waves and thus allowing detection of multiple periodicities. Providing that the sampling rate is at least twice as high as the highest frequency of interest (Nyquist sampling rate), power spectrum analysis will be comparatively insensitive to sampling frequency. Frequency domain methods are preferable for the detection of underlying periodicities in episodic secretory data. On the other hand, pulse-detection methods facilitate quantitative comparisons of waveform features such as pulse amplitude or duration, which are less easily extracted from spectral analyses. In experimental situations, where the ideal conditions for either approach are usually not present, time- and frequency-domain analysis complement each other and provide more information in sum than either technique alone.

Power Spectral Analysis and Permutation Rank Test

It is usually helpful to condition the data before applying spectral analysis techniques to maximize the likelihood of detection of the information of interest. Signal conditioning prior to application of the FFT consists of DC bias removal, trend removal, adjustment of statistical outliers, time-domain windowing, and zero padding. DC bias removal is equivalent to subtracting the baseline or zero-frequency component from the data. In measuring adrenal corticosterone by microdialysis, baseline differences might be caused by differing efficiencies from probe to probe. Similarly, trend removal subtracts very slowly varying signals from the data. Slow trends may be introduced by assay drift if many samples are analyzed sequentially. If trend removal is not done, a large zero- or low-frequency component may obscure a small, but significant higher-frequency oscillation. We removed slow trends in the data using the algorithm contained in PC-Pulsar. Any residual linear trend was subtracted using a routine from Mathpak 87 (Precision Plus Software, Oakville, Ontario). Statistical outliers are also adjusted to avoid their having disproportional effects on the frequency spectrum (15). Distortion also may be introduced into frequency spectra by the process of analyzing short series of data which are presumed to represent infinitely long series in the ideal case. The process of abruptly starting and stopping the data series has the effect of causing ''leakage'' in the frequency spectrum, resulting in signal power displacement into incorrect frequency bins. To reduce this leakage, it is desirable to multiply the data series by a ''window'' which smoothly tapers the data to zero at the ends of the series, eliminating the discontinuity caused by the implicit rectangular window. A discussion of the characteristics of the different functions available for this purpose is beyond the scope of this paper, but detailed information is available (e.g., 16, 17). We empirically tested five window types using random series and combinations of sine waves with and without noise. The 20% cosine taper was chosen as the best compromise between detection of known signal components and discrimination against spurious signals in random series. Finally, in order to maximize the resolution of distinct periodic components in the frequency spectrum, ''zero padding'' is employed. This procedure involves the addition of zero values to the data series to increase its total length. Because the frequency resolution produced by Fourier analysis is proportional to the number of data points analyzed, this produces more bins in the power spectrum. The FFT was computed by the split radix algorithm using an assembly language routine included in Mathpak. Other software was developed for these experiments using Turbo Pascal (Borland, Scotts Valley, CA). Power spectrum magnitudes are expressed as the fraction of total power contributed by each frequency bin, allowing comparison between animals with different absolute secretion rates. Individual spectra in each group should be averaged to produce an ensemble average spectrum. If periodicities are spurious and occur at random frequencies, the ensemble average will approach a flat spectrum.

It is important to realize that power spectrum analysis is not a decision-making technique, but rather a transformation of the data into a form which makes the presence of periodicity more apparent. Thus, a statistical test is needed to determine if any given peak in the spectrum is indicative of a rhythmic process. It is possible to evaluate spectra using analysis of variance. However, a more sensitive test has been described, which relies on nonparametric rank testing. The permutation rank test (PRT) of Odell *et al.* (18) involves constructing 100 random permutations of the original data series. Because these permuted series involve random rearrangements of the same data, each of these comparison data sets has the same amplitude distribution as the original data. Only the temporal information has been altered. Each of these series is subjected to the same analysis as the original series, and power spectrum magnitudes at each frequency are compared. If no more than two of the permuted series produce greater power at a given frequency than the original series, that value is considered significant. In addition, when consecutive frequency bins are judged to be significant, only the maximum value in the group is considered to be an independent periodicity. Detection of multiple independent periodicities requires separation by at least three frequency bins, with at least one nonsignificant value in between.

When assessing rhythmicity in data series, the analysis should only consider periodicities for which two complete cycles can be observed. However, large low-frequency peaks may be present and may obscure relatively low-amplitude spectral components in the region of interest, preventing their detection by the PRT. To remove low-frequency variations from the data, a digital high-pass filter was developed and incorporated into the program which performed the FFT and PRT. The filter was designed with a seventh-order Butterworth characteristic and a cutoff at 213 min.

A deficiency of the PRT is that it does not explicitly consider the impact of assay variance on the detection of rhythmicity. However, it is possible to derive an index of replication from intrasample replicate variability (19). From this quantity, a lower bound can be set on the amplitude of a periodic signal which can be detected with 95% confidence. The index of replication is calculated for each experiment, and the amplitude of any periodic signal detected is estimated by fitting a sinusoid to the data series at the frequency determined by the PRT, using a curve-fitting algorithm (Sigmaplot, Jandel Scientific, Corte Madera, CA). If the signal amplitude is too small in relation to the replicate variability, the periodicity is rejected. Of 12 animals studied 1 or 2 days after surgery, all but 1 passed this test.

An alternative means of detecting rhythmicity in time series is the use of autocorrelation analysis. Like Fourier analysis, this technique represents a transformation of the data. Indeed, the autocorrelation function and the power spectrum form a Fourier transform pair and are thus interconvertible. Although power spectrum analysis is more appropriate for the extraction of dominant periodicities (20, 21), we initially used both techniques to facilitate comparison to previous studies (e.g., 22). A periodic signal would be expected to produce an autocorrelogram with a significant correlation at a lag corresponding to the periodicity. The 95% confidence intervals on autocorrelograms can be approximated as $r \pm 2/\sqrt{N}$, where r is the correlation coefficient and N is the number of data points. Observed values of r which fall outside these limits are significantly different from zero ($p < 0.05$) (20). However, the autocorrelation technique is best used with large data series and may not be very sensitive for short series.

Validation of the Methods Using Control Data Sets

Time series methods of analysis may sometimes introduce spurious rhythmicities into otherwise nonrhythmic data. Therefore, it is important to demonstrate that the technique of choice can distinguish truly random data. For this purpose, we used two different types of control data sets. The first set consisted of corticosterone concentrations determined by running 50 samples from one plasma pool (concentration 8 μg/dl) in our standard corticosterone assay. This data series was subsequently analyzed with both Pulsar and power spectral analysis to test the analysis techniques on data in which no physiological signal was present. Pulsar detected no peaks in the series of plasma pools. Using power spectral analysis and the PRT, a significant periodicity was found in this series. This rhythm was of very low amplitude and was rejected based on the index of replication. Thus, the index of replication is an important indicator of the limits imposed by the inherent variance of the assay used and provides a statistical basis for the rejection of signals that are too small to be detected reliably. To test whether apparent rhythmicity might be introduced into a signal consisting of pure noise, 10-min sampling experiments were simulated with random time series. Seven sets of random numbers were generated with amplitude distributions similar to seven experiments in which dialysate corticosterone was measured. When these series were individually tested by the PRT, four of seven produced significant rhythmicity. However, the periods of these rhythms were not consistent, varying from the equivalent of 45 min to 213 min. When the spectra of the seven series were averaged, a flat spectrum resulted, as would be expected for a random or "white noise" process. Thus, although some individual random series appeared to contain significant rhythmicities, the ensemble average did not support a conclusion of rhythmicity. The index of replication test was not applied to these controls, since the data were not collected using an assay with defined variance.

In Vivo Experiments Using Adrenal Microdialysis

Experimental Protocol

Animals have been studied 1, 2, or 5 days after surgery. For experiments performed more than 1 day after surgery, animals are placed in the experimental chamber for several hours on the day before the experiment to familiarize them with the apparatus. On the day of experiment, animals are brought to the laboratory at 0730 hr, and the tubes are removed from the subcutaneous pocket under local anesthesia. Animals are then placed singly in the experimental chamber and the tubes are connected to a syringe pump (Harvard No. 933). From 0800 to 1000 hr, animals are allowed to stabilize and the dialysis system is flushed with saline or Ringers solution at 10 μl/min. This rate of flow is used continuously throughout all experiments. Dialysate is sampled continuously at 10-min intervals throughout all experiments. At the conclusion of all experiments, 50 ng of ACTH1-24 (Cortrosyn) or ACTH1-39 is administered intravenously to determine the maximal corticosterone secretion rate. Peripheral venous blood is sampled 10 and 30 min after this stimulus. The experiments reported here were performed in complete accordance with the NIH Guidelines for humane use of experimental animals and all protocols were approved by the RI Hospital Animal Care Committee.

Since *in vivo* calibration of the probes was not possible, we sought to demonstrate that changes in dialysate corticosterone were indicative of changes in plasma corticosterone. A linear regression of plasma corticosterone concentration on dialysate corticosterone concentration was performed, using plasma and dialysate samples obtained simultaneously under a variety of conditions (Fig. 4). Regression of plasma corticosterone on dialysate corticosterone was significant ($r = 0.74$, $p < 0.001$), suggesting that dialysate concentration of corticosterone is a good predictor of plasma concentrations of corticosterone. It may seem surprising that a higher correlation is not observed; however, plasma concentration of corticosterone is affected by plasma protein buffering and may not reflect transient changes in the secretion rate of adrenal corticosterone.

In Vivo Application of Adrenal Microdialysis for Monitoring Pulsatile Secretion

The calculated corticosterone secretion rate for a representative animal 1 day postsurgery is shown in Fig. 5A. Pulsatile secretion of corticosterone is clearly evident. A maximal adrenocortical response was elicited after sample

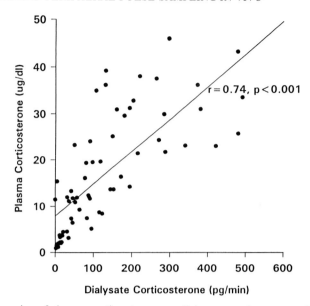

FIG. 4   Regression of plasma corticosterone on dialysate corticosterone. The correlation coefficient was significant, suggesting that dialysate corticosterone is a good predictor of plasma corticosterone.

No. 46 by iv injection of 50 ng of ACTH. The median pulse amplitude was 102 pg/min, the median pulse duration was 20 min, and the median IPI was 35 min. Note that the median pulse amplitude is about 25% of the maximal secretory rate and that corticosterone secretion frequently falls to zero in between pulses. The result of power spectral analysis is shown in Fig. 5B. The first eight data points were discarded from the power spectrum calculation because the rapidly falling baseline suggested a nonstationary signal. Two significant rhythmicities were detected with periods equal to 91 and 64 min (black bars). These periods are about twice as long as the IPI determined by Pulsar. The reason for this apparent discrepancy can be seen by examining the pulse profile in Fig. 5A. Pulsar is equally influenced by the small frequent pulses and larger, more infrequent pulses. In contrast, spectral analysis shows that only the lower frequency periodicity is significant, although a small, nonsignificant peak can be seen in the spectrum corresponding to a periodicity of 35 min (cross-hatching). Autocorrelation analysis suggested that periodicities of 70 and 120 min might be present; however, these peaks were not statistically significant. These results reflect data published previously (8) showing an ultradian rhythm in adrenal secretion of corticosterone at 24 and 48 hr after placement of an adrenal microdialysis probe. Animals

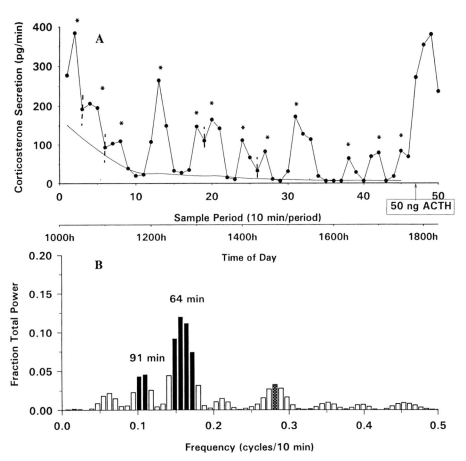

FIG. 5   (A) Corticosterone secretion rate in an animal studied 1 day after surgery. Asterisks indicate significant pulses as determined by Pulsar. Broken vertical lines indicate peaks split by Pulsar algorithm. The smooth curve shows the baseline determined by Pulsar. Arrow indicates time of injection of 50 ng bolus of ACTH to elicit maximal adrenocortical response. (B) Power spectrum of secretion rate data shown in A. Black bars indicate significant periodicities as determined by PRT. Crosshatching indicates period corresponding to IPI determined by Pulsar.

were studied 5 days after surgery to determine if additional recovery time influenced the secretory pattern. Figure 6 shows the results of time-domain and frequency-domain analysis of a representative animal in this group. Unlike the animals studied 1 and 2 days after surgery, very little pulsatile activity is present during the morning and early afternoon hours. No signifi-

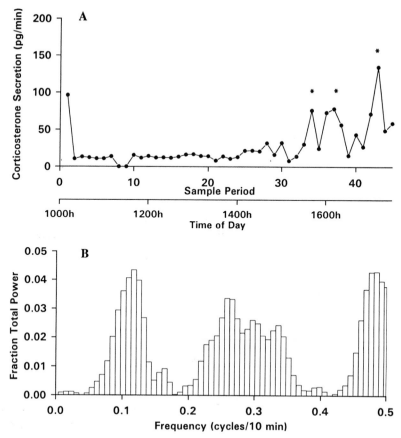

FIG. 6   (A) Corticosterone secretion rate in an animal studied 5 days after surgery. Symbols as in Fig. 5. Note the long quiescent period during which no pulses are observed. (B) Power spectrum of data shown in A. Power is present throughout the spectrum indicating a noise process. No significant periodicities were detected by the PRT.

cant pulses were detected by Pulsar until 1430 hr (sample No. 34). The spectral profile (Fig. 6B) contains no significant periodicities and resembles a noise process. These findings suggest that after prolonged recovery from surgery the ultradian rhythm in corticosterone secretion observed at 1 and 2 days is lost; it is probable that the reduced pulsatility observed in the morning at 5 days reflects the normal quiescence in adrenal corticosterone secretion observed during the nadir of the circadian rhythm (1).

To investigate the role of ACTH in controlling pulsatile corticosterone

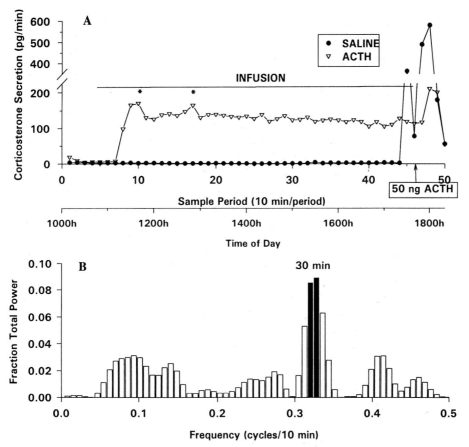

FIG. 7 (A) Corticosterone secretion rate in dexamethasone-treated animals with and without ACTH replacement. Horizontal bar indicates the period of saline or ACTH infusion. Other symbols as in previous figures. (B) Power spectrum of secretion rate in ACTH-infused animal. Although a significant periodicity was detected (black bar), the amplitude of this rhythm was very close to the sensitivity limits of the assay.

secretion, animals were administered a synthetic steroid, dexamethasone (25 μg/100 g body weight), 2 hr before experiments to block endogenous ACTH secretion. Figure 7A shows corticosterone secretion in animals receiving iv infusions of saline or of ACTH (75 pg/min/100 g body weight in 5 μl saline/min). As expected, no corticosterone secretion was detected in the animal receiving saline alone (i.e., no ACTH replacement). However, there was a robust corticosterone secretory response to the iv ACTH bolus at the end of the experiment. A large corticosterone pulse is seen just before the bolus was administered. The reason for this could not be determined, but may indicate a nonanterior pituitary stimulatory factor. Infusion of ACTH increased the secretory rate rapidly, producing a near-maximal initial response followed by a gradually falling plateau at about half the maximal secretory rate. Pulsar detected two pulses soon after the onset of the ACTH infusion. Spectral analysis indicated the presence of a significant rhythmicity with a period equal to 31 min. However, since the amplitude of this rhythmicity exceeded the index of replication by less than the standard error determined by the curve-fitting algorithm, the reliability of this result may be marginal. Although a low-amplitude rhythm may still be present under conditions of constant ACTH replacement, it is clear that the normal expression of pulsatile corticosterone secretion has been abolished. A more physiological pattern of ACTH secretion was presented in the experiment depicted in Fig. 8, in which ACTH was administered in pulses of 30 min duration (65 pg/min/100 g), separated by 40-min periods of baseline ACTH infusion (7.5 pg/min/100 g). The stimulation produced a pulsatile corticosterone secretory response which follows the stimulus faithfully. This rate of infusion produced a response which was approximately 30% of the maximal response elicited by the bolus injection of ACTH. These experiments suggest that the normal pulsatility in adrenal corticosterone observed at 1 and 2 days after surgery requires pulsatile exposure to ACTH.

Additional Applications of Adrenal Microdialysis for Study of Adrenal Function

Use of microdialysis to sample adrenal extracellular fluid is ideally suited for the study of pulsatile corticosterone secretion, since it permits chronic and continuous collection of adrenal dialysate in awake, behaving rats. By monitoring adrenal secretion after long-term recovery from the stress of surgical preparation (e.g., 5–7 days), circadian rhythms in corticosterone as well as ultradian rhythms can be evaluated in nonstressed rats. Following reestablishment of normal rhythmicity, rats can be exposed to stressors and adrenal secretory responses can be examined in relationship to basal secretion. In addition, experiments can be performed to determine how altered light/dark cycles, activity rhythms, or feeding schedules affect ultradian rhythms in corticosterone secretion.

There is evidence that factors in addition to ACTH affect adrenocortical secretion, including neurotransmitters localized in nerve terminals in the adrenal cortex and in the adrenal medulla (23). In addition to collection of adrenal extracellular fluid, dialysis presentation of pharmacological agents

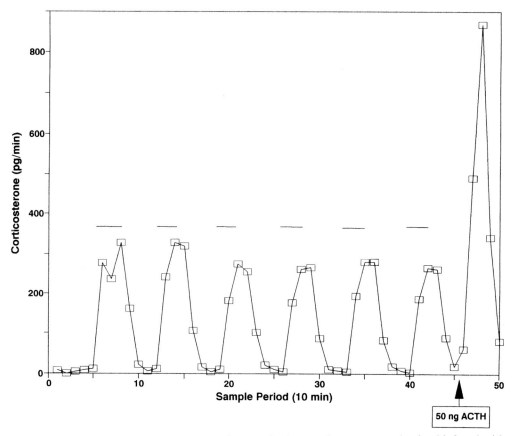

FIG. 8 Corticosterone secretion rate in dexamethasone-treated animal infused with pulses of ACTH. Pulses were 30 min long and separated by 40-min periods of low infusion rate. Note that adrenocortical response follows the stimulus faithfully with no indication of desensitization or priming.

can be done to assess the effect of direct activation or blockade of putative neurotransmitters on adrenocortical rhythms and responses to stress. This approach has proved successful in determining the role of neuropeptides in control of adrenomedullary secretion in rats (24). Since the microdialysis probe spans the cortex and the medulla, it would be possible to design experiments to compare adrenocortical and adrenal medullary secretion by measuring corticosterone and catecholamines in adrenal dialysate. In addition to comparing responses to stress, studies could be designed to compare rhythmicity. Although both plasma catecholamines and corticosterone vary diurnally (25), it would be of interest to assess whether pulsatile catecholamine secretion is associated with pulsatile corticosterone secretion.

Acknowledgments

This work was supported in part by NIH Grant DK38951 and funds from RI Hospital and the Department of Surgery at the University of Minnesota.

References

1. M. F. Dallman, W. C. Engeland, J. C. Rose, C. W. Wilkinson, J. Shinsako, and F. Siedenburg, *Am. J. Physiol.* **235,** R210 (1978).
2. J. D. Veldhuis, A. Iranmanesh, G. Lizarralde, and M. L. Johnson, *Am. J. Physiol.* **257,** E6 (1989).
3. L. A. Benton and F. E. Yates, *Am. J. Physiol.* **258,** R578 (1990).
4. J. W. Holaday, H. M. Martinez, and B. H. Natelson, *Science* **198,** 56 (1987).
5. M. Carnes, S. Lent, J. Fenyzi, and D. Hazel, *Neuroendocrinology* **50,** 17 (1989).
6. J. P. Hinson, G. P. Vinson, and B. J. Whitehouse, *J. Endocrinol.* **111,** 391 (1986).
7. H. Jarry, E. M. Duker, and W. Wuttke, *Neurosci. Lett.* **60,** 273 (1985).
8. M. S. Jasper and W. C. Engeland, *Am. J. Physiol.* **261,** 30, R1257 (1991).
9. P. Lonnroth, P.-A. Jansson, and U. Smith, *Am. J. Physiol.* **253,** E228 (1987).
10. G. R. Merriam and K. W. Wachter, *Am. J. Physiol.* **243,** E310 (1982).
11. J. F. Gitzen and V. D. Ramirez, *Psychoneuroendocrinology* **12,** 3 (1987).
12. P. Linkowski, J. Mendlewicz, R. Leclercq, M. Brasseur, P. Hubain, J. Golstein, G. Copinschi, and E. Van Cauter, *J. Clin. Endocrinol. Metab.* **61,** 429 (1985).
13. R. J. Urban, W. S. Evans, A. D. Rogol, D. L. Kaiser, M. L. Johnson, and J. D. Veldhuis, *Endocr. Rev.* **9,** 3 (1988).
14. J. D. Veldhuis and M. L. Johnson, *Am. J. Physiol.* **250,** E486 (1986).
15. W. N. Tapp, J. W. Holaday, and B. H. Natelson, *Am. J. Physiol.* **247,** R866 (1984).
16. R. W. Ramirez, "The FFT, Fundamentals and Concepts." Tektronix, Inc., Englewood Cliffs, NJ, 1985.
17. F. J. Harris, *Proc. IEEE* **66,** 51 (1978).
18. R. H. Odell, Jr., S. W. Smith, and F. E. Yates, *Ann. Biomed. Eng.* **3,** 160 (1975).
19. S. W. Smith and R. H. Odell, Jr., *Ann. Biomed. Eng.* **4,** 68 (1976).
20. C. Chatfield, "The Analysis of Time Series: Theory and Practice" Chapman & Hall, London, 1975.
21. J. S. Bendat and A. G. Piersol, "Random Data: Analysis and Measurement Procedures," 2nd Ed. Wiley, New York, 1986.
22. A. Iranmesh, G. Lizarralde, M. L. Johnson, and J. D. Veldhuis, *J. Clin. Endocrinol. Metab.* **68,** 1019 (1989).
23. M. A. Holzwarth, L. A. Cunningham, and N. Kleitman, *Ann. N. Y. Acad. Sci.* **512,** 449 (1987).
24. H. Jarry, M. Dietrich, A. Barthel, A. Giesler, and W. Wuttke, *Endocrinology (Baltimore)* **125,** 624 (1989).
25. S. F. DeBoer and J. Van Der Gugten, *Physiol. Behav.* **40,** 323 (1987).

Section IV

Mathematical Procedures for Pulse Analysis

[14] Comparative Analysis and Procedures for Validation of Pulse-Detection Algorithms

Randall J. Urban

Introduction

The episodic release of hormones into the peripheral circulation is a naturally occurring biologic phenomenon that is important in regulating physiologic function in many species. Studies indicate that this episodic release of hormones is an important physiologic component of endocrine systems, and altered episodic release of hormones may constitute pathophysiologic conditions in living organisms.

As such, over the past several decades with the advancing technology of computer science and immunochemistry, computer-based algorithms have been developed to identify and characterize episodic or pulsatile release of hormones as measured by immunoassays that are reproducible, sensitive, and specific. Multiple pulse-detection algorithms have been published based on various mathematical functions and subsequently used to assess endocrine time series for pulsatile release of hormones. This diversity of methods has led to a lack of standardization in analyzing endocrine time series and has often raised the question of validity in published reports. For example, a published study by one group of investigators analyzing the pulsatile release of a particular hormone in a certain species by using a pulse-detection algorithm may differ considerably from that of another group studying the same hormone in the same species but using a different pulse-detection algorithm. This diversity is further demonstrated by Fig. 1, which shows the number of luteinizing hormone (LH) peaks detected from LH time series (edited by successive deletions to vary sampling intensity) in eight men analyzed by eight different pulse-detection algorithms. The greater the sampling frequency, the greater the diversity in pulse detection among the different algorithms.

In lieu of the diversity in pulse detection shown in Fig. 1, this chapter outlines the steps necessary to validate pulse-detection algorithms for an endocrine time series. Although it is impossible to determine absolutely the ability of a pulse-detection algorithm to identify the true signal in an endocrine time series, the method described below establishes constraints to greatly improve the validity of pulse detection. This chapter defines relevant valida-

Methods in Neurosciences, Volume 20

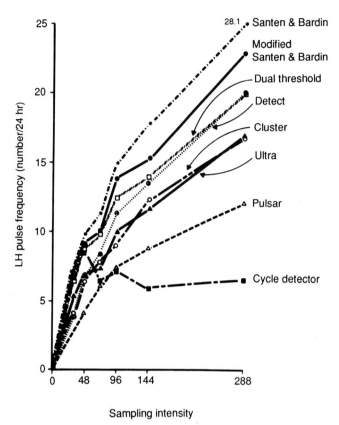

FIG. 1 Variability in pulse detection by eight different algorithms. Influences of sampling intensity (horizontal axis) and discrete pulse-detection algorithm type (individual curves) on mean luteinizing hormone (LH) pulse frequency estimates (vertical axis). Pulse detection programs were constrained to a 1% false-positive error rate on signal-free noise whenever possible. Mean LH pulse-frequency estimates were derived by analyzing LH time series in eight healthy men, each of whom underwent blood sampling at 5-min intervals for 24 hr. [Adapted with permission from Urban *et al.* (11).]

tion terminology, discusses information about endocrine time series necessary for proper validation studies, and describes validation methods.

Definitions

False-Positive Peak

A pulse-detection algorithm finds a peak that is not a true peak. False-positive errors in pulse detection increase when algorithm constraints are lowered.

False-Negative Peak

A pulse-detection algorithm fails to identify a true peak. False-negative errors in pulse detection increase when algorithm constraints are increased.

Sensitivity

One minus the number of false-negative peaks divided by the total number of detected true peaks plus the number of false-negative peaks. The sensitivity value denotes the fractional probability of detecting true peaks in the data (1).

Positive Accuracy

One minus the number of false-positive peaks divided by the total number of true peaks detected plus the number of false-positive peaks. Positive accuracy denotes the fractional probability that any identified peak is a true peak (1).

Pulse-detection algorithms when used on endocrine time series with stringent constraints for pulse detection show increased positive accuracy (i.e., every peak the program finds has a greater probability of being a true peak), but diminished sensitivity (i.e., many true peaks in the time series will not be detected). This inverse relationship between positive accuracy and sensitivity is shown in Fig. 2. The constraints for pulse detection that give both the highest sensitivity and positive accuracy (where the lines cross in Fig. 2) is the ultimate goal when validating pulse-detection algorithms.

Assessment of Endocrine Time Series

Hormone

Knowledge of the hormone from which the time series is generated has important implications in pulse-detection validation. Under the system to be tested, the concentration of the hormone is very important. For example, when assessing the pulsatile release of LH in hypogonadotropic young women with hypothalamic amenorrhea, the LH concentration is low, the LH pulse amplitude is low, and the pulse-detection algorithm should be adjusted to detect pulses in a setting of a low signal/noise ratio. On the other hand, the pulse-detection algorithm settings would be much different when

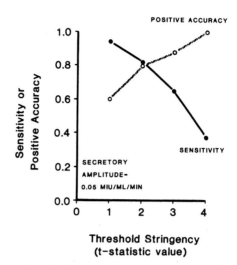

FIG. 2   Reciprocal relationship between pulse-detection sensitivity and positive accuracy for varying threshold stringency. Synthetic LH time series were created to conform to a mean interpulse interval of 90 min (±30%), a mean subphysiological secretory pulse amplitude of 0.05 mIU·ml⁻¹·min⁻¹ (±30%), and superimposed random variance of ±8% (noise). Cluster parameters of one point in test nadirs and one point in test peaks were used, with indicated *t* statistics to identify significant increases and decreases in data (upstrokes and downstrokes constituting peaks). [Adapted with permission from Urban *et al.* (1).]

assessing the pulsatile release of LH in young women in the luteal phase of the menstrual cycle when the LH concentration is high, the LH pulse amplitude is large, and there is a high signal/noise ratio.

Another important characteristic of the hormone is its metabolic clearance. Pulse-detection algorithms must be adjusted to account for fast or slow hormone clearances. It has been shown previously that increasing half-times of hormone clearance diminish hormone pulse detection sensitivity and positive accuracy (2). Therefore, if a hormone time series is being evaluated for a hormone that has a long half-life [e.g., follicle-stimulating hormone (FSH)], then the investigator must realize that pulse detection by any algorithm known at this time is not as accurate as that for a hormone with a shorter clearance (e.g., LH).

Assay

The hormone assay used to generate the endocrine time series also influences pulse-detection validation. One important consideration is the amount of serum required to perform the assay with respect to the amount of serum the species can safely tolerate having removed by phlebotomy. For example, assessing LH time series in prepubertal children has many more restrictions on the amount of blood that can be withdrawn over 24 hr compared with assessing LH time series in adults. Moreover, an assay that requires 200 μl of serum per sample compared with an assay that requires 20 μl of serum per sample also limits the number of samples that can be withdrawn over a certain time period. As shown in Fig. 1 and discussed below, sampling intensity influences the constraints of pulse-detection algorithms.

The reproducibility and precision of the assay also directly influences the amount of noise present in the endocrine time series. An assay shown to have a low coefficient of variation (CV) for both interassay and intraassay measurements produces an endocrine time series with a higher signal/noise ratio than an assay with higher CVs. An estimate of the CV of an assay is an essential component for validation of a pulse-detection algorithm using computer modeling as described below.

Finally, the number of replicates that can be measured on each time point in the endocrine time series is also important. Any endocrine time series to be analyzed by a statistically based pulse-detection algorithm must be measured at least in duplicate. Additional replicates improve the precision of the assay and should lower the noise, which could in turn influence the pulse-detection validation parameters. Due to serum constraints, most endocrine time series are done in duplicate or at most triplicate.

Sampling

The frequency with which the endocrine time series is generated over a certain period of time is another important consideration in pulse-detection validation. As has been stated, many times the constraints of the amount of serum that can be taken from a species or the amount of serum used for assay present set limitations on sampling intensity. In addition, the clearance of the hormone generating the endocrine time series may influence the desired sampling intensity. For example, an endocrine time series determined for a hormone with a very fast clearance requires more intense sampling to capture all possible true hormone peaks. If a hormone is cleared from the serum in 10 min, a sampling paradigm of every 20 min would fail to identify many true peaks. Analysis of LH time series has shown an increased detection of LH pulses with an increase in sampling intensity (3). Moreover, computer simulations have shown that sampling more often not only increases the sensitivity of pulse detection but also lowers the positive accuracy (1), implying that with greater sampling intensity of a hormone time series, more stringent detection criteria for pulse detection would be needed to maintain acceptable estimates of positive accuracy.

The pulsatile release of a hormone may also vary over a 24-hr period. For example, release of hormones might be increased during the night, with the onset of sleep, or after meals. If there is knowledge of such variability in an endocrine time series, breaking the series into parts and analyzing each separately may be the best method to analyze the data accurately. Regardless, any known estimates of the pulsatile release of a hormone greatly facilitate pulse-detection validation.

Validation of Pulse-Detection Algorithms

Selection of Pulse-Detection Algorithm

Before beginning validation procedures, it is necessary to select a pulse-detection algorithm. The mathematical formulations for eight pulse-detection algorithms have been reviewed previously (4). Cluster analysis (5), Detect (6), and Ultra (7) are three such programs that have been used extensively to analyze pulsatile hormone time series and have undergone validation studies. Multiple-parameter deconvolution of endocrine time series has also been extensively used to assess pulsatile hormone release (8, 9). Ease of attainment, adaptability to computer hardware, and simplicity in use are all factors to consider when selecting an algorithm.

Another consideration for selection is the variety of variance models that can be used by the pulse-detection algorithm. All pulse-detection algorithms must use some variance model to apply statistical methods to pulse detection. Using a linear, quadratic, or power function variance can be related to dose from actual sample replicates or from the standard curve and quality control replicates. Some programs may use a stable estimate of assay precision such as a constant CV or constant standard deviation (SD). Finally, variance may be estimated from a pooled t test of actual data replicates (4). Depending on the assay of the hormone in question, one variance model may more accurately encompass assay variability and determine pulse-detection algorithm selection.

If possible, selection of two separate pulse-detection algorithms to validate and analyze a pulsatile hormone time series will substantiate study results if findings from the two algorithms are similar. However, most published studies assessing pulsatile secretion in endocrine time series have used only one pulse-detection algorithm.

Computer-Simulated Time Series

Signal-Free Noise

Generation of signal-free time series and subsequent analysis by a pulse-detection algorithm allow an estimate of positive accuracy based on the

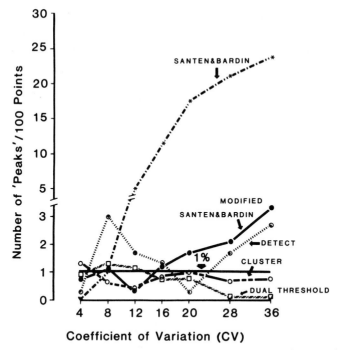

FIG. 3 Influence of the intraseries coefficient of variation on false-positive error rate for five different pulse-detection algorithms. Signal-free random (Gaussian) noise was generated to form synthetic hormone series with indicated intraseries coefficients of variation (*x*-axis). A presumptive target ("ideal") false-positive rate of 1% was used whenever allowed by program. [Adapted with permission from Urban *et al.* (11).]

number of false-positive peaks detected in the signal-free noise. However, there must be some estimate of intraassay CV for the hormone in the assay in which the experimental samples are to be analyzed. Moreover, this CV should be determined at a concentration of hormone present in the hormone time series to be tested (10). This CV should then be used to generate the signal-free time series and the pulse detection algorithm adjusted to yield a predetermined false-positive error rate (positive accuracy). Figure 3 shows the number of peaks detected in signal-free noise by using a 1% false-positive error rate when possible for five different pulse-detection algorithms across a range of CVs (11).

Biophysical Modeling

Although the establishment of false-positive error rates for pulse-detection algorithms on signal-free noise was an important first step in standardization of pulse-detection validation, it could not assess the interaction of signal and noise on pulse detection in endocrine time series. As such, additional computer modeling has allowed generation of computer-based endocrine time series with the ability to mix signal and noise. These computer-based endocrine time series permit identification of true signals from which sensitivity and positive accuracy can be exactly determined at various constraints of a pulse-detection algorithm. Several different biophysical modeling paradigms have been developed and when analyzed by Ultra (12), Detect (13), and Cluster (1, 14) the paradigms showed that the presence of signal lowers false-positive rates that have been determined on signal-free noise. Therefore, pulse-detection algorithms that have been constrained to a false-positive error rate based on signal-free noise may actually function at a much lower false-positive error rate when used on the actual hormone time series with true signal present. As such, these stringent constraints, while having an excellent positive accuracy, would have diminished sensitivity.

The parameters that can be used for each biophysical modeling paradigm vary between algorithms. The ability to vary peak amplitude, frequency, and CV noise is important. These parameters should be adjustable to carefully assess sensitivity and positive accuracy for an endocrine time series. Information as outlined above for assessing the endocrine time series can now be used to generate hormone time series which resemble the actual experimental data. Various settings of the pulse-detection algorithm to be used on the experimental data can be tested to find the setting that has the highest positive accuracy and sensitivity. Figure 4 shows various computer-based synthetic time series generated by a biophysical model that uses a multiple-parameter convolution integral to generate time series (14).

In Vivo Biologic Modeling

Although biophysical modeling is an improvement over signal-free noise, it still cannot include additional variance that may occur with performance of the actual study, i.e., withdrawal of samples from subjects or processing samples. Moreover, a computer-generated signal may mimic but never exactly replicate an experimental signal. For these reasons, additional pulse-detection validation can be attempted through an appropriate biologic model. This biologic model is a unique situation in which an actual endocrine time series has been measured on a subject and the exact location of the true signal is known. Figure 5 shows an example of a biologic model for detection of LH peaks. In this model, the timing of the episodic release of gonadotropin-releasing hormone (GnRH) has been identified electrically and can be compared with the concomitant LH time series (15). Thus, the true signal for

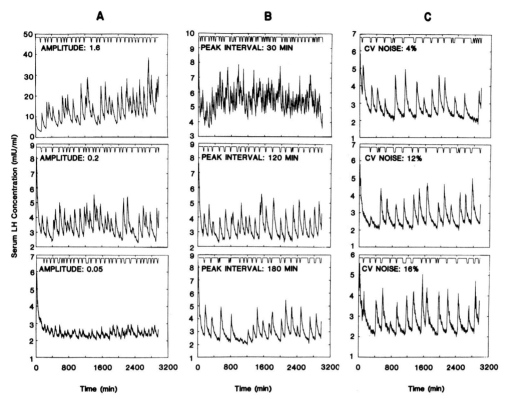

FIG. 4 Synthetic LH time series generated by computer-based biophysical model using a multiple-parameter convolution integral. (A) Variable LH secretory pulse amplitudes (0.05, 0.2, and 1.6 mIU·ml^{-1}·min^{-1}). (B) Variable LH interpulse intervals (30, 120, and 180 min). (C) Indicated ranges of random variance (noise). Peak secretory amplitudes (maximal rate of secretion attained in secretory burst) and interpulse intervals (time elapsed between successive secretory bursts centers) were varied randomly around their indicated mean values by ±30% coefficient of variation (CV). Data were computer synthesized in duplicate at an apparent sampling interval of 10 min over 50 hr. [Adapted with permission from Urban *et al.* (1).]

LH can be identified and estimates of pulse detection determined on actual experimental data.

However, a biologic model also has limitations that must be considered in pulse-detection validation. Usually the biologic model is in another species of animal which for some reason allows for the attainment of the true endocrine signal. In another species, the hormone clearance, pulsatile release,

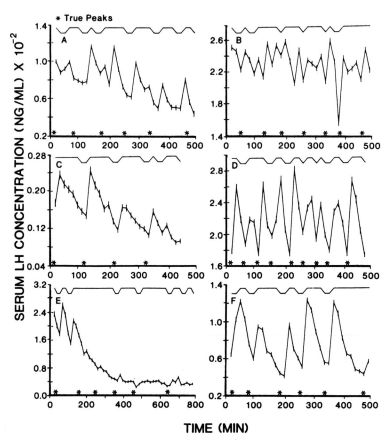

FIG. 5   LH time series from electrophysiologically monitored rhesus monkeys as an *in vivo* biologic model. These biologic time series were analyzed to define false-negative and false-positive errors on *in vivo* data. Deflections on the *top* of each panel denote Cluster-identified peaks (settings as follows: test cluster nadir and peak size of 2 × 1 with a *t* statistic of 2.0 for both the up- and downstroke thresholds). The *asterisks* on the abscissa represent true peaks, as documented by multiunit electrical discharge in the medial basal hypothalamus. Note the wide range of values for the vertical scales in the different subpanels that reflect measurements in intact (C) or castrate (all other panels) animals. [Adapted with permission from Urban *et al.* (15).]

and assay are different. As such, a biologic model is also not without its limitations but, when used in conjunction with computer-based biophysical modeling, it may yield the most accurate assessment of sensitivity and positive accuracy for the endocrine time series to be studied.

Conclusion

Investigators planning to analyze an endocrine time series with a pulse-detection algorithm can use the information in this chapter to guide the framework of their study. They must first understand conventional definitions used in pulse-detection validation. With this understanding, they must then collect information about the hormone they are planning to study. The assay to measure the hormone, the clearance of the hormone, the amount of blood required to measure the hormone, etc., are all important information for pulse-detection validation. Next, the investigator must select a pulse-detection algorithm and validate its performance in the endocrine time series to be studied. This can be done by one of three methods, (a) signal-free noise, (b) biophysical modeling, or (c) an *in vivo* biologic model. Although no method is without its limitations, assessment of signal-free noise for false-positive errors is the least desirable because it cannot assess the interaction of signal and noise. Use of both biophysical modeling and an *in vivo* biologic model will yield pulse-detection algorithm constraints that have the highest estimate of sensitivity and positive accuracy.

References

1. R. J. Urban, M. L. Johnson, and J. D. Veldhuis, *Am. J. Physiol.* **257,** E88 (1989).
2. R. J. Urban, M. L. Johnson, and J. D. Veldhuis, *Endocrinology* (*Baltimore*) **128,** 2008 (1991).
3. J. D. Veldhuis, W. S. Evans, A. D. Rogol, C. R. Drake, M. O. Thorner, G. R. Merriam, and M. L. Johnson, *Am. J. Physiol.* **247,** E554 (1984).
4. R. J. Urban, W. S. Evans, A. D. Rogol, D. L. Kaiser, M. L. Johnson, and J. D. Veldhuis, *Endocrinol. Rev.* **9,** 3 (1988).
5. J. D. Veldhuis and M. L. Johnson, *Am. J. Physiol.* **250,** E488 (1986).
6. K. E. Oerter, V. Guardabasso, and D. Rodbard, *Comput. Biomed. Res.* **19,** 170 (1986).
7. E. Van Cauter, M. L'Hermite, G. Copinischi, S. Refetoff, D. Desir, and D. Robyn, *Am. J. Physiol.* **241,** E355 (1981).
8. J. D. Veldhuis, M. L. Carlson, and M. L. Johnson, *Proc. Natl. Acad. Sci. U.S.A.* **84,** 7686 (1987).
9. J. D. Veldhuis and M. L. Johnson, *in* "Methods in Enzymology" (L. Brand and M. L. Johnson, eds.), Vol. 210, p. 539. Academic Press, San Diego, 1992.
10. J. D. Veldhuis, A. D. Rogol, and M. L. Johnson, *Am. J. Physiol.* **248,** E475 (1985).
11. R. J. Urban, D. L. Kaiser, E. Van Cauter, M. L. Johnson, and J. D. Veldhuis, *Am. J. Physiol.* **254,** E113 (1988).
12. E. Van Cauter, *Am. J. Physiol.* **254,** E786 (1988).

13. A. D. Genazzani and D. Rodbard, *Acta Endocrinol. (Copenhagen)* **124,** 295 (1991).
14. J. D. Veldhuis and M. L. Johnson, *Am. J. Physiol.* **255,** E749 (1988).
15. R. J. Urban, M. L. Johnson, and J. D. Veldhuis, *Endocrinology (Baltimore)* **124,** 2541 (1989).

[15] Deconvolution* Analysis of Neuroendocrine Data: Waveform-Specific and Waveform-Independent Methods and Applications

Johannes D. Veldhuis, John Moorman, and
Michael L. Johnson

I. Introduction

Rapid changes in the secretion of neuroendocrine effectors over time provide a cogent signaling method by which neuroendocrine glands communicate with their remote as well as proximal target tissues. The analysis of neuroendocrine signaling can entail investigation of regulated neurohormone secretion and metabolic clearance (deconvolution analysis) or an examination of physiologically controlled variations over time in plasma hormone concentrations bathing the target tissue (e.g., Cluster analysis). We present our two general forms of deconvolution analysis and illustrate their applications to the analysis of neuroendocrine data. The two categories of deconvolution techniques include first a *waveform-specific model* in which the experimenter assumes some general a priori form for the underlying secretion episodes, and seeks to estimate their number, mass, duration, and amplitude as well as simultaneously compute the apparent hormone half-life (1, 2). The second category of our deconvolution methodologies is *waveform independent* in which individual sample hormone secretion rates are calculated for all the observed hormone concentration data, but the investigator requires a priori knowledge of appropriate two-compartment elimination kinetics. Some important applications of deconvolution analysis are given in Table I. Of considerable importance, the waveform-specific convolution integral permits one to create mathematically explicit pulse trains, which very closely emulate physiological pulse patterns. These "synthetic pulsatile series" are then suitable for validation of discrete peak-detection methods, including, for

---

* The term deconvolution, as used here, refers to a numerical and analytical procedure designed to calculate hormone secretory rates from hormone concentrations measured as a function of time and/or to estimate simultaneously the elimination half-life (2). As described in the text, observed neurohormone concentrations over time can be expressed as a *convolution integral* of relevant secretory and clearance functions. Accordingly, the *inverse* process of calculating secretion and elimination rates from the neurohormone concentration data is referred to as *deconvolution*.

TABLE I   Applications of Deconvolution Analysis in Neuroendocrinology[a]

1. Evaluate the temporal behavior of a secretory ensemble.
2. Estimate endogenous hormone half-lives without hormone injections.
3. Estimate sensitivity of peak detection (e.g., discern otherwise summated peaks).
4. Improve specificity of pulse identification.
5. Assess concordance of secretory events after removing the effects of different half-lives, baselines, etc.
6. Delineate circadian and ultradian rhythms in secretion.
7. Carry out simultaneous analysis of two or more pulse generators.
8. Model physiological events (e.g., proestrous LH surge).

[a] Adapted with permission from J. D. Veldhuis and M. L. Johnson, *Fron. Neuroendocrinol.* **11**, 365, 1991.

example, Cluster analysis, Cycle Detector, Pulsar, Detect, Ultra (3), etc. We illustrate the use of the convolution integral in (i) the construction of synthetic pulsatile neurohormone series as analyzed by the Cluster methodology; (ii) the assessment of nonlinear dynamics of secreted free, bound, and total neurohormone concentrations in the presence of a circulating binding protein; and (iii) the evaluation of concordant neuroendocrine secretory activity.

II. Waveform-Specific Deconvolution

As intimated above, our laboratory has developed specific techniques within two broad classes of computer-assisted deconvolution methods that are applicable to neurohormonal data. First, we present a waveform-specific methodology in which a variety of putative secretory waveforms can be postulated or observed by an investigator and used as a basis for estimating underlying secretory event amplitude, frequency, duration, and mass (1, 2). Given a particular assumed or documented relevant secretory burst waveform that can be defined by a specific algebraic expression, one can estimate neurohormone secretion rates and neurohormone disposal rates simultaneously (1, 2, 4). We refer to this procedure generally as a *waveform-specific deconvolution* method because the secretion function is assumed to be described by a specific mathematical expression. For example, we have postulated that neurohormone secretory bursts can be approximated by one of several algebraic forms, e.g., a Gaussian distribution of instantaneous secretory rates; a square-wave secretory burst, a very rapid delta impulse function; or a skewed distribution of secretion velocities, among many considerations (see

Fig. 1). In evaluating anterior pituitary hormone secretion *in vivo*, we have inferred that a Gaussian or minimally skewed model of individual secretory events approximates many neuroendocrine bursts quite reasonably and provides nominal half-life estimates that conform to independently published values in the literature (1, 5–13).

The general form of the waveform-specific deconvolution model is given by Eq. (1), which is designated as a convolution integral.

$$C(t) = \int_0^t S(z)E(t - z)dz \tag{1}$$

where $S(z)$ and $E(t - z)$ denote, respectively, relevant secretory and elimination functions. The integral of the convolution (dot product) of these two functions provides a description of their combined contributions to the neurohormone concentrations over time.

As summarized in Fig. 1, any of a variety of specific algebraic functions can be considered for $S(z)$, the secretion function. Indeed, independent experimental evaluation of the secretory time course is important in selecting among possible functions. For example, to evaluate hypophyseal secretory bursts, studies have placed catheters in proximity to pituitary venous effluent blood as illustrated in Fig. 2. Specifically, blood was sampled at very frequent intervals (viz., every 30 sec) in the conscious male horse, and plasma luteinizing hormone (LH) and follicle-stimulating hormone (FSH) concentrations were measured (14). Note the generally symmetric form of the LH and FSH secretory bursts with relatively minimal interburst secretion, as appraised centrally in close apposition to the pituitary gland. Other studies in the mare suggest that a more complex waveform of pituitary LH secretion can also exist (data provided by Susan Alexander and Clifford Irvine, Christchurch, New Zealand). In the mare's estrous cycle, large secretory cascades of LH can be captured in pituitary effluent blood and represented mathematically as volleys of partially overlapping nearly symmetric release episodes (or summated Gaussian-like distributions).

Although the secretory event can be estimated by direct measurements in blood leaving the neuroendocrine gland or ensemble, we would note that the original secretory waveform is subject to significant admixture, streaming, convection, and other distorting influences as it enters the general circulation and is transferred throughout the sampling compartment. Indeed, arguments from fluid mechanics can be advanced to support the notion that even a delta function or square-wave secretory burst emanating from a remote central source would resemble a Gaussian or somewhat skewed distribution of secretory rates in the periphery if it could be reconstructed at a distal point of blood sampling. Accordingly, we have found that for many applications,

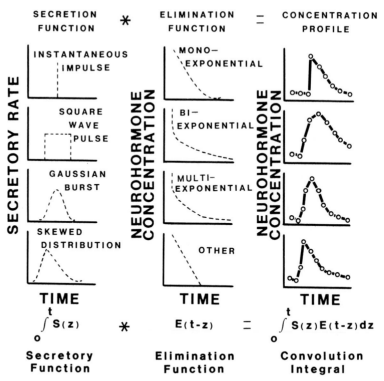

FIG. 1 Concept of convolution integral. A convolution integral is used to express the combined ("convolved or intertwined") effects of two functions that contribute jointly to an observed process. For example, a convolution integral containing a secretion and elimination function can define expected changes in hormone concentrations over time. As illustrated, the secretion function in principle could assume any one of several theoretical forms; e.g., an instantaneous impulse (zero duration secretory burst), a square-wave time course of secretion, a Gaussian waveform, or a skewed distribution of secretion rates. The elimination function most often is represented as a mono- or biexponential decay curve, but could in certain physiological circumstances exhibit different properties (e.g., log–linear concentration-dependent decay). Because several algebraic functions might provide good descriptions of neuroendocrine data, independent experimental knowledge of the system's secretory behavior aids in choosing the most appropriate convolution form. Note that the indicated combination of functions is purely hypothetical. Biologically relevant secretions and elimination terms must be defined by physiological experiments. [Adapted with permission from J. D. Veldhuis and M. L. Johnson (4).]

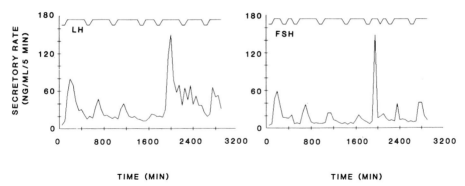

FIG. 2 Simultaneous monitoring of blood concentrations of LH and FSH in pituitary venous effluent of a conscious male horse catheterized via a midfacial vein. Valid deconvolution of the peripheral blood profiles of LH and FSH should yield LH and FSH secretion events that correspond reasonably with independently monitored pituitary secretory pulses at least as modified by propagation throughout the circulation. Secretory rates are in units of ng gonadotropin/ml blood/5 min. [Adapted with permission from J. D. Veldhuis and M. L. Johnson (4). Data were provided by Drs. S. Alexander and C. Irvine, Christchurch, New Zealand.] Schematized deflections above the data denote cluster-identified peaks (3).

an approximately Gaussian or slightly skewed distribution provides a good description of neuroendocrine data in a variety of physiological and experimental contexts (2, 15).

The detailed mathematical presentation of our waveform-specific deconvolution method has been given (2, 16). The reader is referred to this detailed summary. Accordingly, we direct the investigator to a particular application of the waveform-specific deconvolution methodology, namely, the mathematical simulation of explicitly pulsatile neurohormone series using the convolution integral (Eq. 1 above) (15, 17–20).

The development of simulation models for pulsatile neuroendocrine data is of great importance and constitutes a major application of the convolution integral (15, 17, 21). Indeed, a variety of mathematically explicit secretory waveforms have been considered, ranging from a simple sawtooth concentration peak (22) to a simple triangular secretion burst (23), an instantaneous secretion episode (21), and our representation of a Gaussian burst or a skewed distribution of secretion rates with a particular amplitude, half-duration (duration of secretion at half-maximal event amplitude), mass, and frequency (2, 15, 17). In each circumstance, convolution of the assumed secretion function with relevant kinetics of neurohormone elimination offers a suitable means of constructing mathematically explicit synthetic neurohormone data, which can then be submitted to traditional or novel discrete peak-detection methods (13, 15, 17–19, 24). Since the investigator has explicit knowledge of the number, amplitude, duration, mass, and location in time of all synthetic secretory bursts contained in the data and is aware of the simultaneously convolved half-life appropriate for the kinetics of hormone elimination, true-positive, true-negative, false-positive, and false-negative errors in pulse detection following the application of discrete peak detector procedures, such as Cluster analysis (15, 17–20), can be evaluated. We illustrate this important application below (see Section IV, A).

III.   Waveform-Independent Deconvolution Analysis

A. Statement of Problem

Pulsatile hormone release is believed to represent a fundamental physiological feature of most neuroendocrine ensembles (25–27). The evidently episodic nature of hormone secretion resuls in abrupt variations in circulating hormone concentrations termed pulses, whose regulated frequency and/or amplitude often convey important biological information to target tissues (28–31). In addition, in principle, appropriate analysis of pulsatile hormone concentrations should yield significant insights into the essential mechanisms that control endocrine glandular secretion (3). Unfortunately, many studies of the putatively pulsatile mode of hormone secretion *in vivo* have failed to apply objective methodologies or, when using objective techniques, have neglected to provide statistically bounded estimates of computed secretion rates. Specifically, most available deconvolution procedures designed to calculate hormone secretion do not estimate the experimental uncertainty inherent in the secretion estimate. Such uncertainty is contributed to by random variations in the experimental preparation, sample collection and processing, and the hormone assay sytem [e.g., radioimmunoassay (RIA), immunoradiometric assay (IRMA), and bioassay], as well as by variance in the measured hormone half-life (2).

Relevant error estimates in the secretion calculations are essential, because without them one cannot determine adequately whether secretion rates fall to values that are statistically indistinguishable from zero during intervals that separate successive secretory events (i.e., whether there is basal secretion) and whether peak secretory rates achieved within presumptive release episodes are themselves significantly nonzero (i.e., whether there are discrete pulses). Moreover, available procedures designed to calculate hormone secretion rates on a sample-by-sample basis are built on algebraic formulations that express the time differential (*dt*) in one or more denominator terms resulting in an *ill-posed problem*. The ill-posed nature of these numerical formulations arises because variations in calculated secretion rates increase

inversely as the value of *dt* (the sampling interval between successive observations) decreases. Consequently, at high data densities when an experimenter would like a secretory signal to be more highly resolved, there is an
amplification of "noise" as well as a tendency of the secretion estimate to
oscillate or "ring" (3). Additionally, many available deconvolution procedures yield estimates of hormone secretion that are either zero or negative
real numbers, even though negative secretion rates cannot be physically realized.

We have addressed in some measure the preceding problems by formulating and implementing a new deconvolution methodology designed to accomplish the following: (i) Calculate *in vivo* endocrine glandular secretory rates
from hormone concentration time series using nonlinear least-squares techniques with well-defined methods of joint-parameter error propagation. This
yields *statistically bounded estimates of hormone secretion rates* that incor-
porate the combined variances contributed by dose-dependent experimental
uncertainty in the measurement system and errors in the estimate of hormone
half-life. (ii) Provide an algebraic formulation of the deconvolution problem
that does not require (ill-posed) point-by-point derivatives of the data so that
model performance is more stable at high sampling or data densities. (iii)
Use two simple numerical procedures to *eliminate the occurrence of negative
hormone secretion rates* and thereby constrain secretion estimates to the
domain of positive real nonzero numbers. The results of this new deconvolution technique are illustrated for typical hormone time series of the anterior
pituitary gland [deconvolution-resolved secretion profiles of LH, FSH,
growth hormone (GH), ACTH], the adrenal gland zona fasciculata (cortisol
secretion), and the pancreatic β-cell (posthepatic insulin delivery).

B. Deconvolution Technique (Waveform-Independent)

The above concept of deconvolution analysis is illustrated schematically
in Fig. 3 in which secretion rates (and their variances) are estimated
simultaneously for all sample observations, given a relevant two-component
hormone half-life and associated variance. The deconvolution algorithm
involves two principal steps. The first step is a nonlinear least-squares
iterative deconvolution of concentration as a function of time to yield
sample secretory rates as a function of time. This first step makes no
assumptions about the shape of the secretion events, other than to require
zero or positive values. Thus, the first step can yield any admixture of
pulses and a constant secretory rate with no pulsatile activity. Second,
the sample secretory rates are examined and probable pulsatile secretory
events identified statistically.

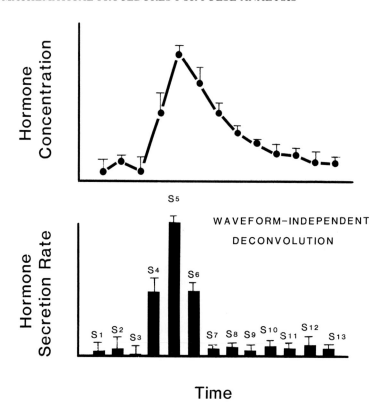

FIG. 3   Schematized depiction of our waveform-independent deconvolution technique, which is designed to quantitate the sample-by-sample secretory contribution to the hormone concentration profile over time. Each measured hormone concentration with its corresponding intrasample variance (dose-dependent standard deviation of the measured replicates) is considered to arise from the combined effects of sample secretion (S_1, S_2, ...), hormone-specific elimination kinetics, and experimental uncertainty. Secretion rates associated with each n measured serial hormone concentrations are calculated from a family of n simultaneous equations containing n secretion rates using an independently estimated one- or two-compartment hormone half-life ($t_{1/2} \pm$ SD). Nonlinear least-squares steepest descent methods of parameter estimation and error propagation are used to specify the maximum-likelihood secretory rates and their joint variances endowed by experimental uncertainties in the measured hormone concentrations and presumptive half-lives (see Section IV, A). Note that the sample secretory rates also manifest individual statistical confidence intervals, which can be denoted by their corresponding asymmetric SDs.

In our waveform-independent deconvolution method, the concentration of a hormone at any particular time is defined as the sum of the amount of hormone secreted at each previous time corrected for the amount of hormone eliminated between the time at which it was secreted and the time at which its concentration is observed. The amount of hormone secreted per unit distribution volume at some time T is given by $sec_i T$ where sec_i is the sample hormone secretory rate (mass/unit distribution volume/unit time) associated with the ith data point and T is the time interval between successive data points. The elimination function for a monoexponential model, which describes the concentration of a hormone remaining at some given time t, assuming a starting concentration of A, is given by Eq. (2).

$$\begin{aligned} \mathrm{elim}(t) &= A \exp(-0.693t/\mathrm{HL}) \quad &\text{for } t > 0 \\ &= 0 &\text{for } t \leq 0 \end{aligned} \quad (2)$$

where HL is the elimination half-life of the hormone and t is time. The form of the corresponding biexponential function is analogous and contains two half-lives and a fraction denoting their relative contributions (2). By combining the secretion and elimination terms, we can describe each measured concentration of a hormone at time t in relation to all n samples observed before and at time t as shown in Eq. (3).

$$\mathrm{conc}(t) = \sum_{i=1}^{n} sec_i \Delta \mathrm{T}\, \mathrm{elim}\,(t - T_i) \quad (3)$$

The initial estimates for the n secretory rates are found using Gold's ratio deconvolution method (32), assuming given elimination rate constants or corresponding half-lives (the rate constant corresponds to ln 2/HL). Gold's proportional method results in only positive secretion estimates. Using the secretory rates obtained by Gold's convergent method as initial guesses, the sample secretory rates are refined further using a weighted, constrained, steepest descent least-squares procedure for parameter estimation (33, 34). Each data point is weighted by the inverse of its observed standard deviation. The least-squares nonlinear convergence algorithm actually estimates the logarithm of the secretory rate at each data point. The logarithm of the secretory rate is used to guarantee positive secretory estimates in each sample (2, 33).

The confidence intervals of the derived secretory rates and their first derivatives are evaluated as the root-mean-square sum of the deviations that are introduced (i) by varying the assumed elimination half-life and repeating the deconvolution process and (ii) by point-by-point perturbation of the data set and repeating the deconvolution process (33, 34). Assuming Gaussian-distributed random experimental uncertainty that is restricted largely to the dependent variable, the above weighted least-squares procedure yields the maximum-likelihood secretory rates and their standard deviations corresponding to each data point.

There are a multitude of ways to evaluate the occurrence of distinct secretory pulses or peaks in the calculated sample secretion profiles. For example, we can fit the serial secretory rates to a series of discrete polynomials that define 3, 5, or 7 or more successive data points and estimate first derivatives of the secretory rates at all sampling points. We can then define a possible *nadir* as a region in which a significantly negative first derivative, as calculated from these polynomials, precedes a significantly positive first derivative. We test the regions between these identified nadirs for statistically significant (nonzero) secretory rates at some given probability value or corresponding z-score based on the secretory rate confidence intervals and designate a secretory peak as significant consecutive nonzero sample secretory rates located between successive nadirs. In this strategy, a significant secretory event must pass two tests applied to the sample secretory rates and their corresponding statistical confidence limits: (i) a significant first derivative; and (ii) a significant (nonzero) absolute secretory rate. The bounds of the originally defined nadirs are then extended to include all regions (sample secretory rate values) between significant secretory peaks.

This deconvolution methodology requires that one independently know, estimate, or assume values for the elimination rate constants or half-lives in order to evaluate the sample secretory rates. In our experience, the process is successful so long as the assumed values for the half-lives are less than or equal to the actual values contributing to the observed data. However, an inappropriately short half-life will alter the absolute values and calculated shapes of secretory events, and increase false-positive errors, whereas an erroneously prolonged half-life estimate will underfit the observed data and increase false-negative errors.

In our methodology, in order to identify peaks at various levels of stringency, values must be specified for three variables: (1) number of data points (e.g., 3, 5, or 7 or more) to use in calculating the fitted polynomials and their derivatives; (ii) z-score for a significant derivative; and (iii) z-score for a significant secretion value. A nominal value for the number of data points used to calculate the derivatives is three, and a typical value for both z-scores is 1.645. The latter corresponds to a 95% probability level in a one-tailed test of the null hypothesis of zero secretion, or a zero change in the sample secretion rate (first derivative).

C. Behavior of Our Waveform-Independent Deconvolution Methodology on Neurohormonal Data

Waveform-independent deconvolution analyses applied to human GH, FSH, LH, and cortisol time series are illustrated in Fig. 4. The conditions of blood sampling and assumed hormone half-lives (and their standard deviations) are given in the legend. For illustrative purposes, we employed the same z-score value in the first-derivative test for a significant nadir and peak and in the statistical test for significant nonzero secretion rate(s) within a putative peak; a three-point polynomial first-derivative calculation; and a Gaussian smoothing function with an SD equal to one-half the sampling interval. For each hormone, we show (i) the relationship between the observed serial serum hormone concentrations and the predicted hormone concentrations calcu-

--→

FIG. 4   Waveform-independent deconvolution analysis of *in vivo* hormone secretion. Deconvolution analysis can be applied to physiological profiles of plasma GH (A), FSH (B), LH (C), and cortisol (D) in individual normal men. Concentrations of pituitary hormones were measured by IRMA (immunoradiometric assay) and cortisol by RIA (radioimmunoassay) in sera derived from blood that was sampled at 10-min intervals for 24 hr. For each hormone depicted, the upper subpanel gives the observed serial hormone concentrations over time with their dose-dependent intrasample standard deviations and the deconvolution-predicted (fitted) curve. The middle subpanel gives the calculated sample secretion rates ($\pm$SD), and the lower subpanel the secretion-rate first derivatives ($\pm$SD). Above each time series, the upward and downward deflections denote significant secretory events identified by z-scores for the first derivative and the calculated sample secretion rate, which both exceed 1.0 (LH and FSH) or 1.645 (GH and cortisol). The nominal half-life values (min $\pm$SD) used here (and in Fig. 5) correspond to the following mono- or biexponential models of hormone disappearance commonly cited, (e.g., Refs. 1, 50):

Hormone	First $t_{1/2}$	Second $t_{1/2}$	Fraction[a] Second $t_{1/2}$
LH	18 ± 5	90 ± 21	0.37
FSH	102 ± 10	498 ± 45	0.48
GH	3.5 ± 0.7	21 ± 0.7	0.63
ACTH	3.0 ± 1.0	14 ± 2.0	0.33
Cortisol	3.5 ± 1.0	65 ± 5.0	0.75
Insulin	3.8 ± 0.7	—	—

[a] Fraction of total amplitude contributed by the second component (longer) half-life.

A

SERUM
GH
CONCENTRATION
(NG/ML)

GH
SECRETION
RATE
(NG/ML/MIN)

DERIVATIVE

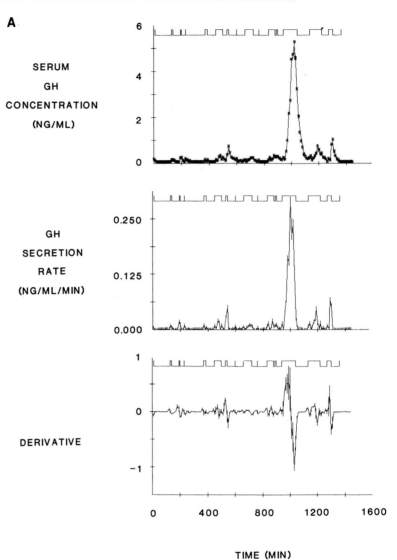

TIME (MIN)

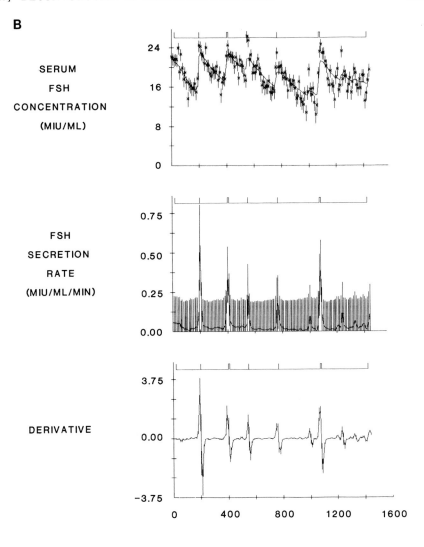

B

SERUM FSH CONCENTRATION (MIU/ML)

FSH SECRETION RATE (MIU/ML/MIN)

DERIVATIVE

TIME (MIN)

FIG. 4 (*continued*)

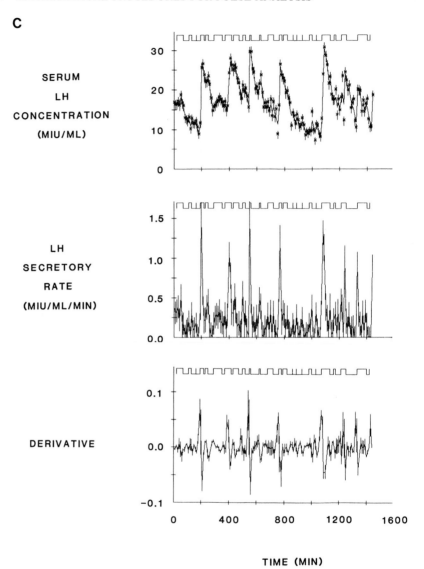

FIG. 4 (*continued*)

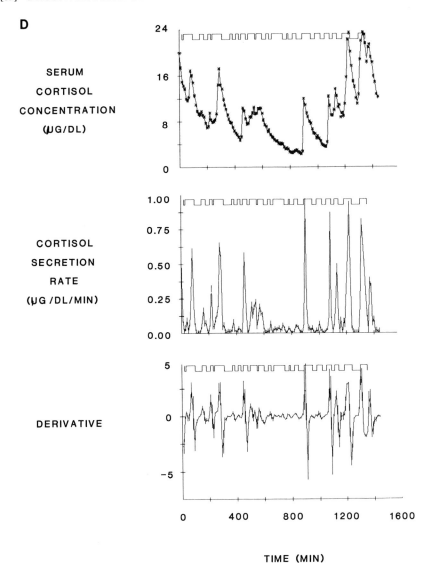

FIG. 4   (*continued*)

lated from the secretory rates; (ii) the calculated sample hormone secretory rates and their standard deviations over time; (iii) the corresponding first-derivative values and their standard deviations; and (iv) the individually identified peaks. The resulting estimates of sample secretion rates for the illustrated hormones (LH, FSH, GH, and cortisol) all fall within published physiological estimates.

To illustrate the behavior of the deconvolution technique on highly intensively sampled data, analyses of sample observations for ACTH (sampled every 2 min), insulin (sampled every 1 min), and GH (sampled every 30 sec) are given in Fig. 5.

Although available deconvolution models in the physiological sciences have yielded important and experimentally useful information regarding the operating characteristics of many endocrine systems (1, 3, 35–45), several significant limitations exist in their application. For instance, first, many deconvolution formulations utilized in endocrine physiology are *ill conditioned*, inasmuch as high observation intensities or data densities can result in deterioration of the resolving ability of the technique; e.g., at high blood sampling intensities, estimated hormone secretion rates tend to approach and/or oscillate about zero with large variations (2, 42). Second, certain physiological questions of interest, such as do endocrine glands secrete in an exclusively burst-like or pulsatile mode without any significant degree of interpulse tonic (basal or constitutive) secretion, cannot be answered without knowledge of the experimental uncertainty in each sample secretion estimate. We believe that the magnitude of this experimental uncertainty should be estimated from at least two sources; viz., the error in the calculation of

---

→

FIG. 5   Behavior of our waveform-independent deconvolution technique on intensively sampled GH (A), insulin (B), and ACTH (C) concentration time series. GH concentrations were measured by IRMA in heparinized blood withdrawn at 30-sec intervals over the entire night (hours of sleep) in a young healthy man. Insulin and ACTH were assayed in plasma and serum samples withdrawn at, respectively, 1- and 2-min intervals. Data were analyzed by waveform-independent deconvolution using threshold z-scores of 1.645. Results are presented as described in the legend of Fig. 4, except that in the case of GH a 2-min SD was used for the smoothing Gaussian, critical z-scores were 0.5, derivative values were computed over five points (SDs not shown), and the dose-dependent intrasample variance in the GH assay was estimated from a large panel of external standards. In the insulin profile, glucagon (1.0 mg intravenously) was administered at 120 min. [GH data are from R. Holl, M. Hartman, M. L. Vance, J. D. Veldhuis, and M. O. Thorner; insulin data are from C. Asplin, J. D. Veldhuis, W. S. Evans; and ACTH data are from A. Iranmanesh, G. Lizzaralde, and J. D. Veldhuis.]

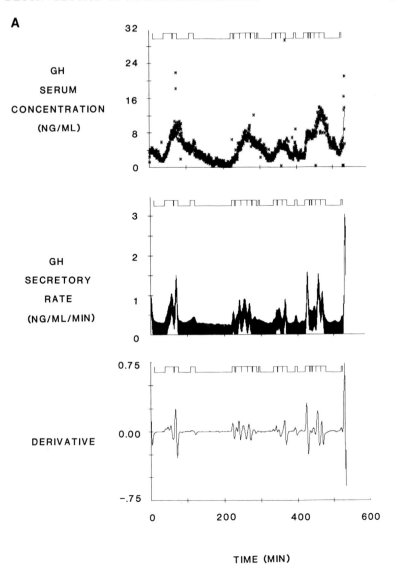

TIME (MIN)

B

PLASMA
INSULIN
CONCENTRATION
(UU/ML)

INSULIN
SECRETORY
RATE
(UU/ML/MIN)

DERIVATIVE

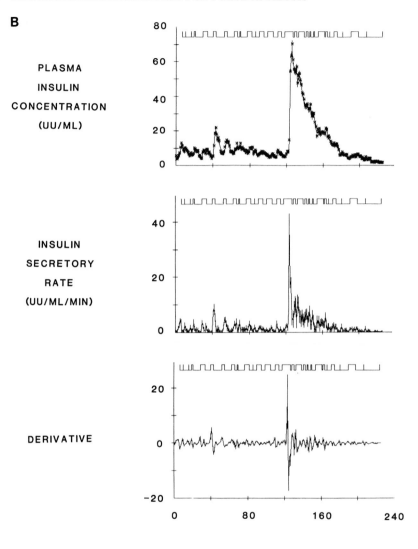

TIME (MIN)

FIG. 5   (*continued*)

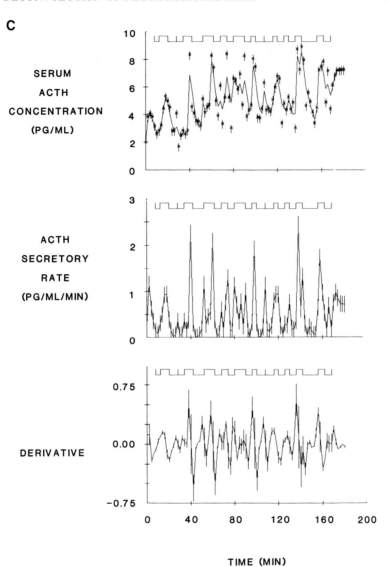

FIG. 5   (*continued*)

hormone half-life and the error in the sample withdrawal, processing, and measurement systems. And, third, although a waveform-specific model of hormone secretion and clearance can overcome the preceding two limitations (ill conditioning and lack of propagation of experimental error) (1, 2), some physiological experiments would benefit from a method of deconvolution, in which no a priori known or assumed waveform for the secretion event is required. Our proposed deconvolution technique favors well-behaved estimates of sample hormone secretion rates, specifies statistical confidence limits for each sample secretory estimate, and is secretion waveform independent in its assumptions. Error propagation is accomplished via established procedures used in nonlinear, least-squares curve fitting and is subject to the same assumptions (33). Under these conditions, any given sample secretion estimate represents a maximum-likelihood value that can be distinguished from zero at some statistical probability level. This important aspect of our deconvolution method permits one to address various questions of experimental interest in endocrine physiology (below).

An important physiological issue is the extent to which fluctuating plasma hormone concentration profiles can be accounted for exclusively (i) by distinct, *burst-like* episodes of hormone secretion without intervening tonic or basal hormone release, or (ii) by secretion events superimposed on a significantly nonzero *baseline* of tonic hormone release. Our waveform-independent deconvolution technique can provide a versatile instrument for examining this query in a quantitative and statistically based manner. Particularly, one can estimate whether hormone secretion rates within and between successive release episodes approach zero or are statistically distinguishable from zero at some a priori probability level. Therefore, the extent to which a secretion time course is composed of discrete secretory bursts and/or sample secretion rates having individually significant nonzero positive real values can be inferred at some desired probability level. For example, an investigator may require that significant hormone secretory bursts contain at least one sample secretion rate whose value differs from zero at some desired p value. The exact suitability of any stipulated p value (e.g., 0.05 or 0.01) will depend on various factors that typically guide experimental and statistical design. Finally, since the model is secretion-waveform independent, the temporal characteristics of the secretion event (e.g., whether it conforms to a Gaussian distribution of release rates or some particular consistently skewed distribution) can be inferred objectively.

Some deconvolution techniques exhibit "ringing" or erratic oscillations (e.g., about zero) when used to calculate hormone secretory rates from high observation density neuroendocrine data (2, 3). This difficulty can be obviated in part by numerical smoothing procedures, although the latter can introduce autocorrelations in the serial secretory estimates. Such serial correlations challenge the assumption of statistical independence often required in available secretory peak-detection methods. Therefore, deconvolution algorithms that employ correct error propagation (above) and are well behaved at high data densities (large numbers of sample observations per unit time) are useful. The present deconvolution formulation yields minimally nonoscillating estimates of sample hormone secretion rates even at high data densities, e.g., samples collected every 0.5, 1, or 2 min (see illustrative GH, insulin, and ACTH profiles in Fig. 4).

Analyses using this waveform-independent methodology predict a predominantly burst-like mode of hormone secretion, in which sample hormone secretion rates tend to fall to values statistically indistinguishable from zero between successive episodes of hormone release. This inference agrees with an earlier waveform-specific model of hormone secretion and clearance in which delimited hormone release episodes can be defined algebraically as symmetric (Gaussian) distributions of instantaneous molecular secretion rates without detectable interpulse (basal) hormone secretion (5, 6, 17, 24, 46). Moreover, hormone secretion assessed by our waveform-independent deconvolution procedure occurs as distinct events having finite and nonzero duration, rather than as instantaneous release impulses. Although the assumption of (nearly) instantaneous impulses to denote the hormone secretion function has been useful mathematically (36, 37), our waveform-independent deconvolution technique indicates that zero-duration impulses are not a physiological characteristic of endogenous hormone secretory patterns, at least for illustrative profiles of LH, FSH, GH, ACTH, cortisol, and insulin in normal men subjected to relatively intensive and extended blood sampling. A similar inference regarding GH secretion was made by McIntosh and McIntosh, who suggested that physiological GH secretory bursts unlike those initially surmised for LH (36; Chapter 20, this volume) are significantly nonzero in duration (43). Other reports based on model-specific deconvolution analysis (1, 46) also support a prolonged *in vivo* GH secretory event.

Another application of waveform-independent methods is to determine the mechanisms by which ultradian rhythms give rise to circadian plasma neurohormone concentration changes (47). To this end, we have shown that 24-hr modulation of hormone secretory burst amplitude alone, or amplitude and frequency (but not frequency alone) (47), generates normal nyctohemeral serum hormone concentration rhythms.

An interesting application of our proposed secretion waveform-independent, statistically based deconvolution procedure is the *elucidation of a particular presumptive secretory waveform* for a given endocrine gland under specified physiological conditions. If a homogeneous secretory waveform is identified, this waveform can then be used in a model-specific method of deconvolution analysis, e.g., to estimate both secretory behavior and hormone clearance rates simultaneously (1–3, 42). In addition, since the secretory waveform may be altered in pathologically and/or pharmacologically distinct states, we suggest that a waveform-independent deconvolution algorithm be used first to estimate underlying secretory properties in all novel contexts. This suggested approach is reasonable so long as the hormone half-life is known (and/or shown to be unchanged) in the specific condition being evaluated. In general, we recommend that physiological state-specific estimates of hormone half-life be obtained independently by equilibrium infusion, bolus injection, and/or other methods (44, 45, 48–51) under experimental conditions that are similar or identical to those associated with collecting the data of interest. Faulty half-life estimates can be expected to yield erroneous inferences regarding secretory rates and waveforms.

In summary, we present a secretion waveform-independent, statistically based, quantitative deconvolution technique that is relatively well behaved at high sampling rates. Application of this deconvolution method to physiological endocrine data suggests that a predominantly burst-like mode of noninstantaneous hormone release characterizes the operating behavior of endocrine glands such as the pituitary, adrenal, and pancreatic islet cells *in vivo*. We also emphasize that an array of possible discrete peak-evaluation methods can be applied to the calculated sample secretory rates to identify and quantitate pulsatile and/or basal secretion; e.g., Cluster, Pulsar, Ultra, Cycle Detector, and Detect (3, 17, 22, 52–54).

IV. Applications of Deconvolution Methodology

A. *Validating GH Peak Detection by Cluster Analysis Using Deconvolution Modeling*

1. Introduction

The somatotropic axis utilizes an episodic mode of GH secretion rather than tonic release to signal end-organ receptor systems (55–65). The opportunity to modulate both the frequency and the amplitude characteristics of such intermittent GH signals can allow for precision and flexibility in regulating ligand–receptor interactions and subsequent intracellular events. However, the reliable and valid detection of episodic GH release is made difficult by the apparently random dispersion of GH secretory bursts over time, the frequent occurrence of minimally detectable plasma GH concentrations in some species, the relatively rapid disappearance of endogenous GH from plasma, and the large number of metabolic and environmental cues that alter GH secretory dynamics (43, 46, 57, 59, 66–68). Thus, a significant limiting factor in the physiological investigation of GH signaling patterns has been the accurate identification and characterization of GH secretory pulses in a statistically defined and independently validated manner. In fact, to our knowledge the detection of GH peaks has not been validated formally in any species. Hence, we illustrate this application of the convolution integral here.

To quantitate the amplitude and frequency of GH signals in a valid manner, investigators require an independent knowledge of the GH secretory pulse configuration, its true frequency, and its true amplitude. As discussed in Section II, the formulation of an algebraically explicit convolution model of episodic hormone secretion convolved with relevant clearance kinetics allows objective and specific simulations of hormone secretory and clearance dynamics to be quantified (1, 2, 17, 42). This simulation model comprises a multiple-parameter convolution integral, which defines simultaneously the number, amplitude, mass, duration, and temporal locations of randomly occurring hormone secretory bursts and a pertinent half-life of hormone disappearance. The resultant *synthetic* pulsatile hormone concentration time series can be perturbed by desired amounts (and types) of random experimental variance (noise). Such explicitly defined, computer-synthesized hormone series can then be used to test the false-positive and false-negative errors associated with endocrine peak detection (see Fig. 6A).

We apply the convolution model to assess the ability of an objective pulse-detection algorithm, Cluster (69), to identify GH peaks in an accurate and valid manner in relation to (i) a physiological range of underlying GH pulse frequencies; (ii) various GH secretory burst amplitudes; (iii) distinct GH secretory burst durations; (iv) several half-lives of GH disappearance; (v) multiple expected sampling intensities (numbers of samples examined per unit time); and (vi) a spectrum of threshold stringencies for the peak-detection algorithm. This approach delineates specific determinants of false-positive and false-negative errors inherent in GH peak detection and thereby offers guidelines for GH peak detection in physiological data.

2. Computer Simulations

The mathematical construct used to produce simulated pulsatile neuroendocrine time series is a convolution integral, as described above (15, 17, 18). This algebraic formulation defines the fluctuating profile of plasma hormone concentrations as the output or consequence of a family of distinct secretion and metabolic clearance parameters. Specifically, the investigator stipulates the following individual relevant parameters of hormone secretory and clearance dynamics quantitatively: (i) secretory burst amplitude, frequency, mass, and duration; (ii) hormone half-life (min); (iii) sample number and spacing (min); and (iv) experimental variance (''noise'') given as a coefficient of variation and a minimal intrasample standard deviation. The structure of

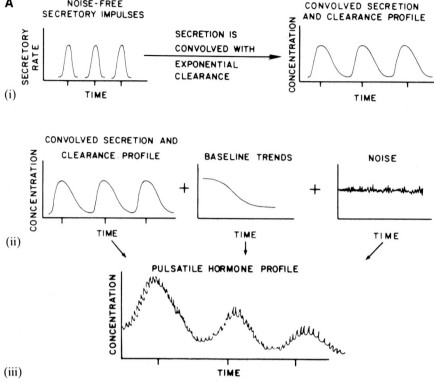

FIG. 6   (A) Schematic illustration of proposed multiple-parameter convolution modeling of pulsatile hormone time series. Scheme indicates in summary form sequential process for building a simulated pulsatile hormone time series using a convolution of random secretory bursts with specific clearance (i). The combined secretion and clearance profile is superimposed on systematic baseline trends, if any, and perturbed by random experimental noise (ii). The final synthetic hormone time series (iii) results from algebraic summation of these constituent contributions. [Adapted with permission from J. D. Veldhuis and M. L. Johnson (17).] (B) Use of convolution modeling to test the performance accuracy of discrete peak-detector algorithms. This figure illustrates the impact of random experimental variance (bottom) on false-positive (FP) and false-negative (FN) errors exhibited by a particular discrete peak-detection algorithm, Cluster (69) applied to simulated plasma LH concentration profiles. Deflections above the top profile denotes Cluster-identified peaks. Synthetic ("observed") profiles (top and middle) were created by convolving LH secretory and clearance functions, which were further perturbed with random biological and/or procedural noise. [Adapted with permission from J. D. Veldhuis and M. L. Johnson (4).]

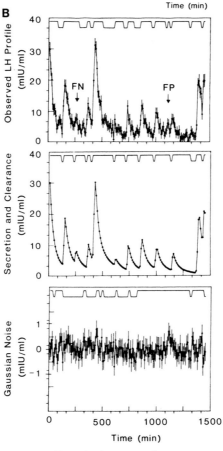

FIG. 6   (*continued*)

this model conforms to physiological expectations (i.e., random bursts of hormone secretion are acted on by endogenous exponential clearance kinetics); the parameter response characteristics are known [i.e., how changes in secretion and/or clearance parameters influence hormone concentrations (model output)]; and the model will correctly predict endogenous hormone production rates and half-lives and reconstruct 24-hr pulsatile serum hormone concentration series obtained under physiological conditions (1, 2, 15, 17, 18). We can use this general model to generate synthetic GH time series containing randomly dispersed GH secretory bursts that occur at desired mean pulse frequencies, amplitudes, and durations, with metabolic clearance rates corresponding to endogenous GH disappearance rate constants as recently measured in man (50). We can vary the half-lives of GH disappearance used in the convolution model by one or two standard deviations from the mean to recapitulate the variability in clearance rates recognized among different individuals. Nominal GH secretory burst amplitudes (maximal rate of secretion/burst, ng/ml/min) and secretory burst half-durations (duration in minutes of the secretion pulse at half-maximal amplitude) are based on results obtained from deconvolution of spontaneous GH time series observed by sampling blood every 5 min for 24 hr in normal men (10).

Synthetic GH time series shown here each consist of 300 "samples" generated in duplicate. Profiles are created to correspond to sampling intervals of 5, 10, 15, 20, 30, and 45 min. An intrasample experimental coefficient of variation of 10% (random Gaussian noise) with a minimum intrasample standard duration of 0.1 ng/ml is imposed on the time series, assuming an intraassay coefficient of variation of 4–6% for GH and additional preassay variance of 4–6% attributable to experimental variation and sample withdrawal, storage, and/or processing.

The simulated GH time series are then subjected to peak analysis by the Cluster program using cluster sizes (numbers of samples in the *test* nadirs and peaks, respectively) of 1×1, 2×1, 2×2, and 3×3 (69). Each of these different test cluster sizes can be evaluated over a range of pooled t statistics for both upstroke and downstroke thresholds; viz., t values of 1.0, 2.0, 3.0, 4.0, and 5.0. A power function model of intrasample variance versus dose is used by the Cluster algorithm to estimate dose-dependent within-sample standard deviations from all sample replicates in any given time series (3). Thus, for each synthetic series, at least 20 Cluster parameter permutations are studied here.

True-positive identification of a peak requires that Cluster correctly identify points in the synthetic data containing the true peak maximum (Fig. 6B). Peak maxima found by Cluster are then compared to the known synthetically generated peak maxima to yield estimates of *false-negative* (a true peak maximum is missed) and *false-positive* (an erroneous peak maximum is found) errors in peak detection. *Sensitivity* is defined as one minus the number of false-negative peaks divided by the total number of peaks actually synthesized. This expression is algebraically equivalent to the formal statistical definition of test sensitivity (70, 71). *Positive accuracy* is defined as one minus the number of false-positive peaks divided by the total number of peaks synthesized. The sensitivity value denotes the fractional probability of detecting any given true peak in the data. Positive accuracy denotes the fractional probability that any identified peak is a true peak. In order to calculate *negative accuracy and specificity*, a "true-negative" result must be defined. A true-negative result in our system would be any "valley" identified by Cluster which included no true peak maxima. However, the

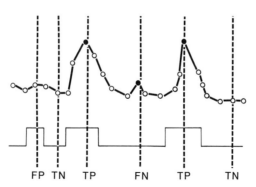

FIG. 7 Schematized depiction of definitions of *false-positive* and *false-negative* errors inherent in analyzing episodic hormone peaks. A false-positive (FP) error occurs when the peak-detection algorithm identifies a presumptive peak when no true peak is present. A false-negative (FN) error occurs when the peak detection algorithm fails to enumerate a peak present in the data. Based on the numbers of false-positive and false-negative errors, the sensitivity and positive accuracy of the peak-detection procedure can be calculated. *Sensitivity* denotes the probability of detecting a true peak present in the data. *Positive accuracy* designates the probability that any given algorithm-identified "peak" is a true peak. True-positive (TP) and true-negative (TN) events are also marked.

presence of false-positive peaks would falsely elevate the number of apparently true-negative events by creating additional flanking valleys. Since we are primarily concerned with positive peak detection, we have not used a modified true-negative term here, which would take the preceding into account. These statistical concepts are schematized in Fig. 7.

3. Sensitivity and Positive Accuracy of Peak Detection

As illustrated in Figs. 8A and 8B, the biophysical model of pulsatile GH release yields GH time series qualitatively and quantitatively similar to physiological data. Series can be created with varying mean GH pulse frequencies (Fig. 8A); viz., mean GH interpulse intervals of 45 min ($\pm 30\%$ coefficient of variation), 90 min ($\pm 30\%$), and 180 min ($\pm 30\%$). In addition, profiles of GH-simulated pulsatility can be created for several different secretory amplitudes (maximal rate of GH secretion attained within an underlying GH secretory burst); viz., secretory amplitudes of 0.6 ($\pm 33\%$), 0.9 ($\pm 33\%$), and 1.2 ($\pm 33\%$) ng/ml/min. In these examples, we use an experimentally imposed intrasample coefficient of variation of $\pm 10\%$, a GH half-life of 20 min (50), and GH secretory burst half-duration of 33 min (10).

The impact of sampling intensity on the number of apparently superim-

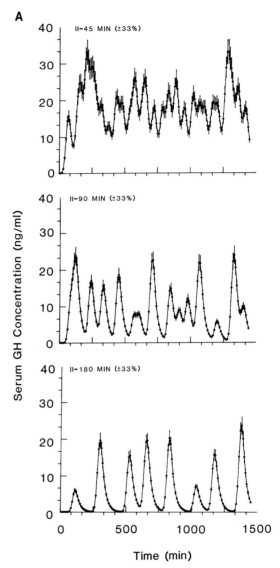

A

FIG. 8   Illustrative pulsatile serum GH concentration profiles of simulated GH secretion and clearance using our multiple-parameter convolution integral. (A) Pulsatile GH profiles are simulated to correspond to mean interpulse intervals (II) of 45 min (±33%), 90 min (±33%), and 180 min (±33%) at a mean GH secretory burst amplitude of 0.9 ng/ml/min (±33%) and half-duration of 33 min, associated with an apparent half-life of GH disappearance from plasma of 20 min. Experimental variance is superimposed at an intrasample coefficient variation of ±10%. (B) Physiological GH pulse profiles obtained from three normal men sampled at 10-min intervals for 24 hr. Data are sample means ± SD of the replicates.

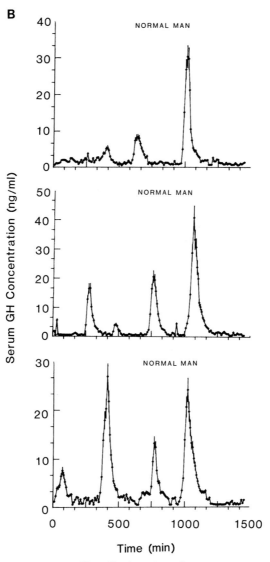

FIG. 8   (*continued*)

posed GH peaks was assessed first. As summarized in Fig. 9, both sampling intensity (number of samples collected and assayed per unit/time) and GH pulse frequency (inversely proportional to GH interpulse interval) control the percentage of GH peaks apparently superimposed. The latter are defined as peaks not separated by any intervening GH concentration lower than the flanking peak maxima (i.e., no intervening nadir). At high GH pulse frequencies, the number of apparently superimposed GH peaks increases substantially; the effect of this increase is magnified at less-frequent sampling intervals. Accordingly, rapidly pulsating GH time series, if sampled with insufficient intensity, pose a considerable risk of *obligatory false-negative* errors for peak-detection algorithms that require a decline in GH concentrations between consecutive peak maxima in order to detect the consecutive peaks. Consequently, in the remaining analyses, we calculate corrected sensitivity values using the number of nonsuperimposed peaks (total minus number superimposed).

The influences of threshold stringency and sampling intensity on false-negative and false-positive errors in GH peak detection are illustrated in Fig. 10. For any particular test cluster size used in the peak-detection algorithm, increasing t statistics (thresholds) results in enhanced positive accuracy over a wide range of sampling intensities (Fig. 10A). Increasing t statistics affects sensitivity in a reciprocal manner (Fig. 10B). At low sampling frequency (blood samples drawn every 20, 30, or 45 min), there is a marked decrease in (GH) peak-detection sensitivity. These analyses were performed at one particular cluster configuration (two points in the test nadir and two points in the test peak). Thus, further studies were conducted to assess the impact of a range of cluster configurations on positive accuracy and sensitivity.

As summarized in Fig. 11A, more stringent cluster configurations (larger numbers of points in the test nadirs and peaks) enhance GH peak-detection positive accuracy. The effect of cluster stringency is observed across a range of sampling intensities from simulated sampling at 5-, 10-, 15-, 20-, 30-, and 45-min intervals. Conversely, increased cluster sizes negatively affect GH peak-detection sensitivity, especially at low sampling intensities (Fig. 11B). Thus, sampling intensity and peak-detection stringency (defined in relation to either the threshold t statistic or the cluster size) jointly control positive accuracy as well as sensitivity. The impact of sampling intensity and threshold stringency on positive accuracy and sensitivity are related reciprocally.

The impact of the GH interpulse interval on sensitivity and positive accuracy is shown next (Fig. 12). There are significant interactions between GH pulse frequency and detector stringency (t statistic threshold and cluster size). In general, positive accuracy declines with lower GH pulse frequency at any given peak detector t statistic threshold and/or cluster size (left).

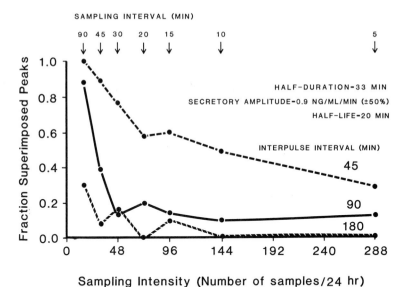

FIG. 9 Influence of blood sampling intensity (number of blood samples examined per unit time) and GH pulse frequency on the number of apparently superimposed GH peaks. Sampling intensity is shown on the horizontal axis as the number of samples collected per 24 hr (e.g., 289 samples correspond to 5-min sampling interval, 145 samples to a 10-min sampling interval). The fraction of peaks that are apparently superimposed is given on the vertical axis. Two peaks are considered to be apparently superimposed if there is no intervening sample valley. The three individual curves shown correspond to simulated GH pulse series having mean interpulse intervals of 45, 90, and 180 min (±33%). Each data point is estimated from a series of 300 simulated samples.

Conversely, GH peak-detection sensitivity improves at lower GH pulse frequencies and lower peak-detection stringencies (right).

The effects of varying secretory burst half-duration (duration of the synthetic GH secretory event at half-maximal amplitude) on positive accuracy and sensitivity are less marked than those of interpulse interval. Doubling GH secretory burst duration only slightly decreases positive accuracy at any given threshold; higher thresholds overcome this detrimental effect. Sensitivity is minimally (but reciprocally) affected by severalfold changes in GH secretory pulse duration (not shown).

We find a reciprocal relationship between positive accuracy and sensitivity over a twofold range of GH half-lives. Varying GH half-lives over an approximately physiological range of 15–27 min (50) for normal men does not greatly

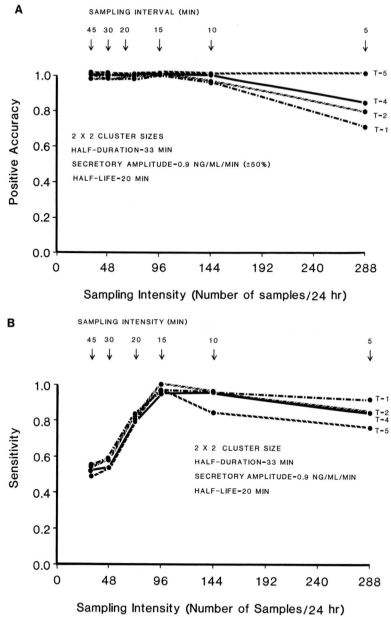

FIG. 10   Impact of blood sampling intensity on the positive accuracy (A) and sensitivity (B) of GH peak detection. Sampling intensity is defined as given in the legend of Fig. 9. The effects of varying threshold *t* statistics (*t* = 1, 2, 4, 5) and varying the sampling interval (from 5 to 10, 15, 20, 30, or 45 min) on the positive accuracy

influence peak detection (not shown). Rather, threshold (t statistic) and peak-detection stringency (number of points in the test nadirs and test peaks) more significantly control the positive accuracy and sensitivity at any given half-life of GH at high sampling densities.

Increasing GH secretory burst amplitude (maximal rate of GH secretion attained within a release episode) improves both the positive accuracy and the sensitivity of GH peak detection across a range of detector thresholds and degrees of stringency. However, even at reduced GH secretory burst amplitudes, appropriate selection of the threshold (e.g., t statistic of 3.0 to 4.0) and cluster stringency (e.g., three points in the test nadirs and three points in the test peaks) results in greater than 90% positive accuracy and sensitivity.

Based on the simulation studies described above, we can identify *optimal Cluster detector parameters* for maintaining both a high positive accuracy and sensitivity of GH peak detection. As summarized in Table II, we suggest the sum of the sensitivity and positive accuracy as an index of peak detection performance. Ideally, the positive accuracy (probability that any particular detected peak is a true peak) as well as the sensitivity (probability of detecting true peaks in the data) would each equal 1, so that the sum of the sensitivity and positive accuracy would be 2. Thus, optimal peak-detection parameters are those that maximize the sum of the sensitivity and positive accuracy and yield a summed value that approaches 2.

After identifying the optimal peak-detection parameters as a function of sampling intensity from Table II, we can apply these sampling rate-adjusted parameters to the identification of GH pulses in time series from nine normal men who underwent blood sampling at 5-min intervals for 24 hr (72). The parent 5-min GH time series can be edited to yield their constituent 10-, 15-, 20-, 30-, and 45-min subsets. Using the optimal parameters of Table II, we demonstrate a highly significant effect of sampling intensity on the estimate of GH pulse frequency ($p < 0.001$). The increase in estimated GH pulse frequency at higher sampling intensities yields maximal and stable estimates of GH pulse frequency in the 10- and 5-min series but not in 20-min or less frequently collected data (see Fig. 13).

---

and sensitivity of GH peak detection are presented. Simulated GH pulse series are composed of a mean secretory burst amplitude of 0.9 ng/ml/min ($\pm$50%), a secretory burst half-duration of 33 min, and a mean interpulse interval of 90 min ($\pm$33%) with 10% superimposed noise (intrasample coefficient of variation). A fixed Cluster (69) stringency of two points in the test peak and two points in the test nadir is used for illustrative purposes.

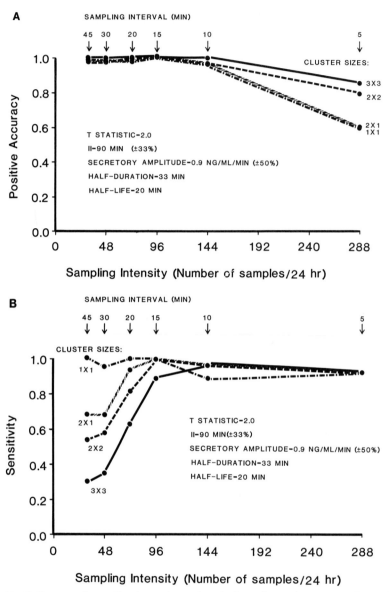

FIG. 11 Influence of sampling intensity and peak-detection stringency on the positive accuracy (A) and sensitivity (B) of GH pulse detection. Data are presented as described in the legend of Fig. 9, except that a fixed *t* statistic value of 2.0 is used, and the Cluster stringency is allowed to vary (test nadirs and peaks consisting of one point, two points, or three points, as indicated). Other features of simulated GH secretion and clearance are the same as those given in Fig. 10.

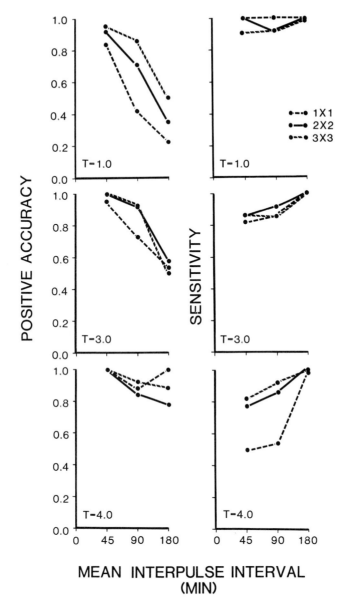

FIG. 12 Combined influences of GH interpulse interval and peak-detection threshold (*t* statistic) and stringency (Cluster size) on the positive accuracy (left) and sensitivity (right) of GH peak detection. Pulsatile GH time series are created here as described in the legend of Fig. 9, except that the mean GH interpulse interval is 45, 90, or 180 min (±33%). A range of threshold *t* statistics (*t* = 1.0, 3.0, and 4.0) is shown as well as a range of peak-detection stringencies (one, two, or three points in the test nadirs and peaks). A sampling interval of 5 min is simulated.

TABLE II   Optimizing GH Pulse-Detection Parameters in Relation to Sampling Intensity Using Summed Sensitivity and Positive Accuracy[a]

Sampling interval	Threshold t statistic				
	$t = 1.0$	$t = 2.0$	$t = 3.0$	$t = 4.0$	$t = 5.0$
5 min					
1 × 1[b]	1.42[a]	1.52	1.58	1.42	1.23
2 × 1	1.59	1.52	1.58	1.70	1.59
2 × 2	1.63	1.72	1.84	1.70	1.77
3 × 3	1.78	1.78	<u>1.84</u>	1.84	1.85
10 min					
1 × 1	1.93	1.85	1.85	1.81	1.78
2 × 1	1.96	1.92	1.89	1.85	1.89
2 × 2	<u>1.96</u>	1.92	1.92	1.96	1.85
3 × 3	1.96	1.96	1.89	1.85	1.85
15 min					
1 × 1	1.98	2.00	1.97	1.97	1.92
2 × 1	<u>2.00</u>	2.00	1.97	1.95	1.97
2 × 2	1.97	2.00	1.95	1.95	1.97
3 × 3	1.89	1.89	1.89	1.89	1.89
20 min					
1 × 1	<u>1.98</u>	1.98	1.96	1.94	1.92
2 × 1	1.92	1.92	1.92	1.90	1.88
2 × 2	1.82	1.82	1.80	1.80	1.82
3 × 3	1.65	1.63	1.59	1.61	1.59
30 min					
1 × 1	<u>1.97</u>	1.94	1.92	1.86	1.86
2 × 1	1.69	1.66	1.67	1.69	1.70
2 × 2	1.58	1.56	1.54	1.54	1.54
3 × 3	1.32	1.35	1.32	1.32	1.31
45 min					
1 × 1	<u>1.99</u>	1.99	1.98	1.97	1.93
2 × 1	1.68	1.66	1.66	1.64	1.65
2 × 2	1.55	1.52	1.55	1.52	1.49
3 × 3	1.30	1.30	1.31	1.32	1.31

[a] Data are summed sensitivity and positive accuracy for the indicated Cluster parameters (69). Underscored values denote optimized peak-detector parameters. Synthetic GH pulse series were created as defined in the legends of Figs. 6 and 8.

[b] Number of points in the test Cluster peak and nadir for any given threshold t statistic.

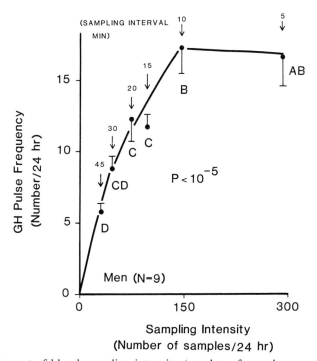

FIG. 13   Impact of blood sampling intensity (number of samples examined per 24 hr) on estimated GH pulse frequency (number of GH pulses detected per 24 hr) in nine normal men. Subjects underwent blood collection at 5-min intervals for 24 hr. The parent 5-min GH time series containing 289 samples were edited to yield their constituent 10-, 15-, 20-, 30-, and 45-min subsets. Cluster analysis was used at optimized threshold stringency adjusted to sampling rate (Table II), so as to maintain at least 90% positive accuracy and sensitivity barring peak superimposition. Significantly different mean GH pulse frequencies ($\pm$SEM, $N = 8$ men) at the different sampling intensities were assessed by analysis of variance and Duncan's multiple-range test and are denoted by different alphabetic superscripts. The plateau values at 10- and 5-min sampling were 18 ± 1.9 and 17 ± 2.3 GH pulses/24 hr.

4. Summary of Optimizing Cluster Parameters for GH Peak Detection

Type I statistical errors in hormone pulse detection occur whenever "false-positive" peaks are identified, i.e., denoting an apparent pulse when no true signal is present. Conversely, a *type II* (false-negative) *statistical error* occurs when a true pulse is overlooked (Figs. 6B and 7). In other available analyses to date, neither type I nor type II error rates have been defined for published GH pulse profiles.

To test Cluster's validity in GH peak detection, we selected a strategy that includes the following important features of convolution model adequacy: (i) *model validity:* physiological GH (and other hormone) pulse profiles can be recovered by our convolution formulation quantitatively with statistically demonstrated goodness of fit (1, 15, 17, 18). In addition, recent studies of the LH and FSH axes using independent *in vivo* electrophysiological monitoring of mediobasal hypothalamic multiunit electrical activity in rhesus monkeys have documented excellent correspondence between predictions by the *in vivo* and mathematical models (19, 20); (ii) *model relevance:* the present mathematical model correctly estimates endogenous hormone secretion and metabolic clearance rates (1, 2, 15, 17); (iii) *model operating characteristics:* the quantitative interactions among input parameters (e.g., secretory pulse amplitude, frequency, mass, and duration, as well as half-life of hormone disappearance) and their impact on model output (the pulsatile hormone concentration profile) have been reported (15, 17); and (iv) *explicit model structure:* our algebraic formulation is specified by a specific closed-form, multiple-parameter convolution integral (15).

Using the above convolution model (Section II), we are able to demonstrate that the valid detection and accurate identification of discrete GH peaks are jointly influenced by underlying GH pulse frequency and investigator-stipulated sampling intensity (number of samples observed per unit time). In particular, if few blood samples are withdrawn per unit time and high GH pulse frequencies are present, a substantial fraction of superimposed GH peaks will occur on an obligatory basis; i.e., peaks with maxima in the same or consecutive samples without any intervening valleys. This problem of apparent peak superimposition cannot be overcome readily by discrete peak detection algorithms. Rather, peak superimposition requires the use of a more frequent sampling paradigm experimentally (see Veldhuis et al., Chapter 17, this volume). This objectively delineated inference corroborates earlier suggestions from physiological observations that an adequately high sampling intensity is required to capture the majority of GH peaks present in the circulation (64). However, the latter report made inferences about GH peak frequency without independent statistical validation of GH pulse-detection sensitivity and specificity (see below).

Increasing peak-detector thresholds (higher *t* statistics) and/or peak-detector stringency (numbers of points in the test nadirs and test peaks) resulted in enhanced positive accuracy of GH peak detection; i.e., a higher probability that any particular algorithm-identified GH peak was actually a true peak. However, as detector threshold and stringency increased, there was a reciprocal decline in GH peak-detection sensitivity; i.e., the probability of finding all true peaks present in the data decreased. This reciprocal relationship between positive accuracy and sensitivity was hypothesized previously (3, 46). Two important implications of these findings to neuroendocrine physiologists are (i) peak-detection threshold and stringency must be selected judiciously, so that both positive accuracy and sensitivity are maintained at experimentally acceptable levels; and (ii) valid peak-detection parameters can vary among different specific hormones studied.

The duration of the GH secretory burst, as well as the half-life of GH disappearance from plasma, both influence sensitivity and positive accuracy but to a lesser degree than do GH pulse frequency, sampling intensity, and peak-detector threshold and stringency. In addition, we can demonstrate that the impact of GH secretory burst amplitude conforms to expectations, inasmuch as GH secretory bursts of larger amplitudes can be detected with greater sensitivity and positive accuracy.

Based on the optimized peak-detector thresholds identified in the mathematical simulations (above), we could reevaluate GH pulsatility in nine normal men, who had previously undergone blood sampling at 5-min intervals for 24 hr (64). Estimates of GH pulse frequency were carried out using Cluster detector thresholds specifically adjusted to sampling intensity, so as to maintain at least a 90% sensitivity and positive accuracy at different sampling rates. Under these conditions, our estimates of mean GH pulse frequency in normal men approach a stable asymptotic value when the sampling interval is decreased to every 10 or 5 min. This new observation differs from our earlier inference that GH pulse frequency continues to increase as the sampling interval is progressively reduced (64), but agrees with independent deconvolution estimates (10). On the basis of the present analyses, we can infer that our earlier conclusion using peak-detection parameters not constrained to a known sensitivity and positive accuracy across different sampling intensities (64) yielded underestimates of GH pulse frequency at a 10-min sampling rate and overestimates of GH pulse frequency at a 5-min sampling rate. Accordingly, we emphasize that the use of objectively validated peak-detection thresholds that are sampling intensity adjusted can materially alter the interpretation of physiological neuroendocrine pulsatility data.

B. Influence of One or More High-Affinity Plasma Neurohormone-Binding Proteins on the Nonlinear Dynamics of Hormone Secretion and Removal

The discovery of a specific high-affinity GH-binding protein (GH-BP) in plasma adds complexity to the dynamics of GH secretion and clearance. Intuitive predictions are that such a protein would damp sharp oscillations in blood GH concentrations otherwise caused by abrupt bursts of GH secre-

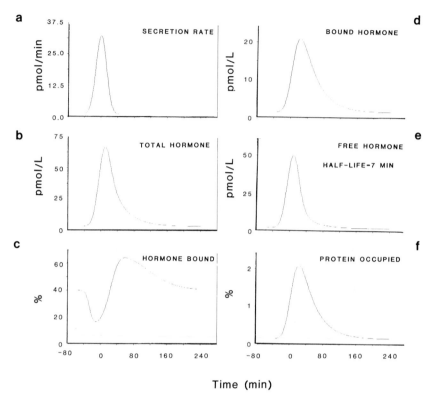

Time (min)

FIG. 14   Impact of a high-affinity GH-binding protein on the dynamic properties of a single burst of GH secretion. Panels show time courses of calculated GH secretory rates, as well as total, bound, and free plasma GH concentrations, and percentages of GH bound and protein occupied assuming (a) a single high-affinity plasma GH-BP (k_d = 1.5 nmol/liter, capacity = 1.0 nmol/liter); (b) a GH distribution volume of 4.9 liter; (c) a total GH $t_{1/2}$ of 18 min and a free GH $t_{1/2}$ of 3 min; (d) a molecular weight of GH of 22,000; (e) a k_{off} of 0.037 min^{-1}; and (f) a symmetric (Gaussian) GH secretory burst with a half-duration (duration at half-maximal amplitude) of 30 min centered about zero and a mass of 1 nmol (22 μg). For ease of visualization, the inset pulses have been elevated to reflect a low rate of constant basal secretion (1 pmol/min). [Adapted with permission from J. D. Veldhuis *et al.* (66).]

tion into the blood volume, prolong the apparent pulse duration and half-life of circulating GH, and contribute a reservoir function. To test these implicit considerations, we can formulate an explicit mathematical model of pulsatile GH secretion and clearance in the presence or absence of a specific high-affinity GH-BP (66). Simulation experiments reveal that the pulsatile mode of physiological GH secretion creates a highly dynamic (nonequilibrium) system in which the half-life of free GH, its instantaneous secretion rate, the distribution volume, and the GH-BP affinity and capacity all contribute to defining momentary levels of free, bound, and total GH; the percentage of GH bound to protein; and the percentage occupancy of GH-BP. In contrast, the amount of free GH at equilibrium is specified only by the GH distribution volume and secretion rate, and the half-life of free hormone. Thus, the *in vivo* dynamics of GH secretion, trapping, and clearance from the circulation offer a variety of regulatory loci at which the time structure of free, bound, and total GH delivery to target tissues can be controlled physiologically.

This application of convolution modeling in the presence of a single high-affinity binding protein for GH is illustrated in Fig. 14. Our formulation by pertinent differential equations is described in detail elsewhere, in which a predominant high-affinity binding protein in plasma creates a trapping mechanism that markedly modifies the time course of free, bound, and total GH concentrations following the pulsed secretion of GH into the sampling compartment (66). We emphasize that this general model can be expanded to two, three, or more ligands and binding proteins, as are appropriate in the case of sex-steroid hormones such as testosterone and estradiol. which bind to prealbumin, albumin, and sex-steroid binding globulin. Indeed, we have expanded the foregoing model to include two ligands (testosterone and estradiol) and three binding proteins in a system of either constant steroid hormone delivery or pulsatile steroid hormone secretion into the sampling compartment. This model is also pertinent to triiodothyronine and thyroxine and their corresponding plasma transport proteins, namely albumin, prealbumin, and thyroid-binding globulin.

C. Use of the Convolution Integral to Simulate Pulsatile Hormone Series Coincidences

As discussed in Chapter 17 in this volume, a straightforward modeling of *pulse-train coincidence* entails discretizing or quantizing the locations of pulses in the two or more neurohormone time series to be compared (15, 24, 73). In this coincidence modeling method, one assigns peak locations (e.g., defined by peak maxima or the initial or midpoint of significant upstroke) to individual samples, thus creating in essence a *binary train* rather than a more complex pattern of nonuniform pulse widths, amplitudes, baselines, and apparently random locations. However, a fully realistic description of spontaneous neurohormone pulse series can also be modeled, simply at the expense of somewhat greater computational time. The latter we have

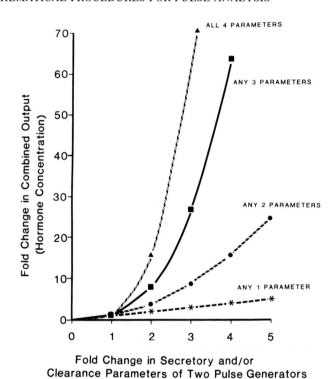

FIG. 15 Impact of changing one to four secretory and/or clearance parameters simultaneously in both of two pulse generators on their combined output (resultant steady-state hormone concentrations in plasma). Equal fold changes in any one, two, three, or all four secretory and/or clearance parameters (e.g., secretory burst frequency, duration, amplitude, and/or hormone half-life) were carried out for two independent pulse generators, and the combined output was analyzed. Fold changes in input and output are given. [Adapted with permission from J. D. Veldhuis *et al.* (15).]

carried out by creating a pulse simulator consisting of one to three independent pulse generators (2, 15, 24). As illustrated in Fig. 15, two pulse generators firing independently exhibit strong joint effects, as assessed by the expected mean plasma neurohormone concentrations resulting from their combined effects. Importantly, multiple altering of the frequency, amplitude, or duration of two or more independent pulse generators simultaneously evokes a multiplicative change in the measured plasma neurohormone concentration. Moreover, the half-life is also a linear operator, so that combined changes in secretory burst characteristics and half-life result in multiplicative changes in neurohormone output (assessed by predicted plasma effector concentrations) (2, 15).

In addition to evaluating the effects of regulating multiple neuroendocrine pulse generators on the overall plasma hormone concentration, convolution modeling is suitable for generating statistically independent pulse trains of defined frequency and distributions, which can be used to assess expected random coincident behavior anticipated solely on the basis of chance peak associations. Indeed, we can estimate the expected mean number of coincident events between two, or among three, four, or more neuroendocrine pulse trains resulting from chance associations alone, as well as calculate the corresponding variance and cumulative probability distribution (24, 73). From this information, one can then determine the probability that any given or observed number of coincidences in a particular pair (or triplet or quadruplet) of biological pulse trains can be attributed to chance associations (random assortment) alone. Moreover, as discussed elsewhere, we can estimate the statistical power ($1-\beta$, where β is the type II error, or probability of falsely accepting the null hypothesis of no significant peak associations) of an analysis. The statistical power of a co-pulsatility analysis is an estimate of the probability that the investigator's declaration of no significant copulsatility has not been flawed by overlooking significant co-pulsatility actually present. Thus, a statistical power of 80% (0.8) denotes an 80% probability of identifying significant copulsatility at some particular α (or p value, e.g., 0.05) given particular preliminary or pilot observations, e.g., number of neurohormone pairs and pulse frequencies in the various pairs. Such information is of particular importance in planning experiments and determining when to terminate a study after suitable statistical power has been achieved.

V. Summary

We present two of our waveform-specific and waveform-independent deconvolution methodologies and illustrate their application in three domains: (i) validating discrete hormone peak-detection methods, such as Cluster analysis; (ii) estimating the influence of one or more high-affinity plasma-binding proteins on the time course of free, bound, and total hormone, when a neurohormone is secreted into the bloodstream in the form of a nonlinear pulse; and (iii) evaluating the coincident behavior of multiple neuroendocrine pulse trains, given nonuniformity of peak frequency over time, unequal peak amplitudes and durations, and varying baselines of hormone secretion. In short, the development, refinement, and extension of deconvolution technologies in the arena of neuroscience investigation now offer a substantial and informative foundation for reliable statistical quantitation of neuroendocrine data.

Acknowledgments

We thank Patsy Craig for her skillful preparation of the manuscript; Paula P. Azimi for the artwork; and Sandra Jackson and the nursing staff at the University of Virginia Clinical Research Center for conduct of the research protocols. This work was supported in part by NIH Grant No. RR 00847 to the Clinical Research Center of the University of Virginia; RCDA 1 K04 HD00634 (J.D.V.); GM-28928 (M.L.J.); Diabetes and Endocrinology Research Center Grant DK-38942; NIH-supported Clinfo Data Reduction Systems; and Baxter Healthcare Corp (Round Lake, IL), the Pratt Foundation, the University of Virginia Academic Enhancement Fund, the National Science Foundation Center for Biological Timing (J.D.V., M.L.J.).

References

1. J. D. Veldhuis, M. L. Carlson, and M. L. Johnson, *Proc. Natl. Acad. Sci. U.S.A.* **84,** 7686 (1987).
2. J. D. Veldhuis and M. L. Johnson, *in* "Methods in Enzymology" (L. Brand and M. L. Johnson, eds.), Vol. 210, p. 539. Academic Press, San Diego, 1992.
3. R. J. Urban, W. S. Evans, A. D. Rogol, D. L. Kaiser, M. L. Johnson, and J. D. Veldhuis, *Endocr. Rev.* **9,** 3 (1988).
4. J. D. Veldhuis and M. L. Johnson, *J. Neuroendocrinol.* **2**(6), 755 (1991).
5. J. D. Veldhuis, A. Iranmanesh, G. Lizarralde, and M. L. Johnson, *Am. J. Physiol.* **257,** E6 (1989).
6. J. D. Veldhuis, M. L. Johnson, and M. L. Dufau, *Am. J. Physiol.* **256,** E199 (1989).
7. J. D. Veldhuis and M. L. Johnson, "Frontiers in Neuroendocrinology," Vol. 11, p. 363. Raven Press, New York, 1991.
8. M. L. Sollenberger, E. C. Carlson, M. L. Johnson, J. D. Veldhuis, and W. S. Evans, *J. Neuroendocrinol.* **2**(6), 845 (1990).
9. A. Iranmanesh, G. Lizarralde, and J. D. Veldhuis, *J. Clin. Endocrinol. Metab.* **73,** 1081 (1991).
10. M. L. Hartman, A. CS. Faria, M. L. Vance, M. L. Johnson, M. O. Thorner, and J. D. Veldhuis, *Am. J. Physiol.* **260**(1), E101 (1991).
11. M. H. Samuels, J. D. Veldhuis, C. Cawley, R. J. Urban, M. Luther, R. Bauer, and G. Mundy, *J. Clin. Endocrinol. Metab.,* in press.
12. W. C. Nunley, R. J. Urban, J. D. Kitchen, B. G. Bateman, W. S. Evans, and J. D. Veldhuis, *J. Clin. Endocrinol. Metab.* **72,** 287 (1991).
13. J. D. Veldhuis, A. Iranmanesh, M. L. Johnson, and G. Lizarralde, *J. Clin. Endocrinol. Metab.* **71,** 452 (1990).
14. S. L. Alexander and C. H. G. Irvine, *J. Endocrinol.* **114,** 351 (1987).

15. J. D. Veldhuis, A. B. Lassiter, and M. L. Johnson, *Am. J. Physiol.* **259,** E351 (1990).

16. J. D. Veldhuis, W. S. Evans, J. P. Butler, and M. L. Johnson, *in* "Methods in Neurosciences" (P. M. Conn, ed.), Vol. 10, p. 241, Academic Press, San Diego, 1992.

17. J. D. Veldhuis and M. L. Johnson, *Am. J. Physiol.* **255,** E749 (1988).

18. R. J. Urban, M. L. Johnson, and J. D. Veldhuis, *Am. J. Physiol.* **257,** E88 (1989).

19. R. J. Urban, M. L. Johnson, and J. D. Veldhuis, *Endocrinology* (*Baltimore*) **124,** 2541 (1989).

20. R. J. Urban, M. L. Johnson, and J. D. Veldhuis, *Endocrinology* (*Baltimore*) **128,** 2008 (1991).

21. V. Guardabasso, G. De Nicolao, M. Rocchetti, and D. Rodbard, *Am. J. Physiol.* **255,** E775 (1988).

22. D. K. Clifton and R. A. Steiner, *Endocrinology* (*Baltimore*) **112,** 1057 (1983).

23. E. Van Cauter, *Am. J. Physiol.* **254,** E786 (1988).

24. J. D. Veldhuis, A. Iranmanesh, I. Clarke, D. L. Kaiser, and M. L. Johnson, *J. Neuroendocrinol.* **1,** 185 (1989).

25. D. J. Dierschke, A. N. Bhattaracharya, L. E. Atkinson, and E. Knobil, *Endocrinology* (*Baltimore*) **87,** 850 (1970).

26. T. F. Gallagher, K. Yoshida, H. D. Roffwarg, D. K. Fukushida, E. D. Weitzman, and L. Hellman, *J. Clin. Endocrinol. Metab.* **36,** 1058 (1973).

27. D. C. Parker, L. G. Rossman, and E. F. Vanderlaan, *J. Clin. Endocrinol. Metab.* **36,** 1119 (1973).

28. T. Bick, M. B. Youdim, and Z. Hochberg, *Endocrinology* (*Baltimore*) **125,** 1711 (1989).

29. C. Monet-Kuntz and M. Terqui, *Int. J. Androl.* **8,** 129 (1985).

30. G. W. Randolph and A. R. Fuchs, *Am. J. Perinatol.* **6,** 159 (1989).

31. D. S. Weigle, W. D. Koerker, and C. J. Goodner, *Am. J. Physiol.* **247,** E564 (1984).

32. P. A. Jansson, *in* "Deconvolution Methods in Spectrometry," p. 99. Academic Press, San Diego, 1984.

33. M. L. Johnson and S. G. Frasier, *in* "Methods in Enzymology" (C. H. W. Hirs and S. N. Timasheff, eds.), Vol. 117, p. 301. Academic Press, San Diego, 1985.

34. P. R. Bevington, T. Bick, M. B. Youdim, and Z. Hochberg, *in* "Data Reduction and Error Analysis for the Physical Sciences," p. 118. McGraw–Hill, New York, 1969.

35. P. L. Toutain, M. Laurentie, A. Autefage, and M. Alvinerie, *Am. J. Physiol.* **255,** E688 (1988).

36. R. P. McIntosh and J. E. A. McIntosh, *J. Endocrinol.* **107,** 231 (1985).

37. K. E. Oerte, V. Guardabasso, and D. Rodbard, *Comput. Biomed. Res.* **19,** 170 (1986).

38. A. Pilo, E. Ferrannini, and R. Navalesi. *Am. J. Physiol.* **233,** E500 (1977).

39. R. Rebar, D. Perlman, F. Naftolin, and S. SC. Yen, *J. Clin. Endocrinol. Metab.* **37,** 917 (1973).

40. E. Van Cauter, *Am. J. Physiol.* **237,** E255 (1979).

41. J. D. Veldhuis, V. Guardabasso, A. D. Rogol, W. S. Evans, K. Oerter, M. L. Johnson, and D. Rodbard, *Am. J. Physiol.* **252,** E599 (1987).

42. J. D. Veldhuis and M. L. Johnson *in* "Advances in Neuroendocrine Regulation of Reproduction" (S. S. C. Yen and W. W. Vale, ed.), p. 123. Plenum, Philadelphia, 1990.

43. R. P. McIntosh, J. EA. McIntosh, and L. Lazarus, *J. Endocrinol.* **118,** 339 (1988).

44. W. J. Jusko, W. R. Slaunwhite, Jr., and T. Aceto, Jr., *J. Clin. Endocrinol. Metab.* **40,** 278 (1975).

45. R. C. Turner, J. A. Grayburn, G. B. Newman, and J. DN. Nabarro, *J. Clin. Endocrinol. Metab.* **33,** 279 (1972).

46. J. D. Veldhuis, A. Faria, M. L. Vance, W. S. Evans, M. O. Thorner, and M. L. Johnson, *Acta Paediatr. Scand.* **347,** 63 (1988).

47. J. D. Veldhuis, A. Iranmanesh, M. L. Johnson, and G. Lizarralde, *J. Clin. Endocrinol. Metab.* **71,** 1616 (1990).

48. J. D. Veldhuis, F. Fraioli, A. D. Rogol, and M. L. Dufau, *J. Clin. Invest.* **77,** 1122 (1986).

49. R. L. Wolf, M. Mendlowitz, L. J. Soffer, J. Roboz, and S. E. Gitlow, *Proc. Soc. Exp. Biol. Med.* **119,** 244 (1965).

50. A. CS. Faria, J. D. Veldhuis, M. O. Thorner, and M. L. Vance, *J. Clin. Endocrinol. Metab.* **68,** 535 (1989).

51. R. J. Urban, V. Padmanabhan, I. Beitins, and J. D. Veldhuis, *J. Clin. Endocrinol. Metab.* **73,** 818 (1991).

52. R. J. Urban, D. L. Kaiser, E. Van Cauter, M. L. Johnson, and J. D. Veldhuis, *Am. J. Physiol.* **254,** E113 (1988).

53. J. D. Veldhuis, J. C. King, R. J. Urban, A. D. Rogol, A. Evans WS, L. A. Kolp, and M. L. Johnson, *J. Clin. Endocrinol. Metab.* **65,** 929 (1987).

54. W. S. Evans, E. Christiansen, R. J. Urban, A. D. Rogol, M. L. Johnson, and J. D. Veldhuis, *Endocr. Rev.* **13,** 81 (1992).

55. J. D. Veldhuis, A. Iranmanesh, K. KY. Ho, G. Lizarralde, M. J. Waters, and M. L. Johnson, *J. Clin. Endocrinol. Metab.* **72,** 51 (1991).

56. J. D. Veldhuis, R. M. Blizzard, A. D. Rogol, P. M. Martha Jr, J. L. Kirkland, B. M. Sherman, and Genentech Collaborative Group, *J. Clin. Endocrinol. Metab.* **74,** 766 (1992).

57. J. W. Finkelstein, H. P. Roffwarf, R. M. Boyar, J. Keam, and L. Hellman, *J. Clin. Endocrinol. Metab.* **36,** 665 (1972).

58. G. S. Tannenbaum and J. B. Martin, *Endocrinology* (*Baltimore*) **98,** 562 (1976).

59. S. L. Davis, D. L. Ohlson, J. Klindt, and M. S. Anfinson, *Am. J. Physiol.* **233,** E519 (1977).

60. R. A. Steiner, J. K. Stewart, J. Barber, D. Koerker, C. J. Goodner, A. Braown, P. Illner, and C. C. Gall, *Endocrinology* (*Baltimore*) **102,** 1587 (1978).

61. J. Isgaard, L. Carlsson, O. G. P. Isaksson, and J. O. Jansson, *Endocrinology* (*Baltimore*) **123,** 2605 (1988).

62. R. G. Clark and I. C. A. F. Robinson, *Nature* (*London*) **314,** 281 (1985).

63. K. Y. Ho, J. D. Veldhuis, M. L. Johnson, R. Furlanetto, W. S. Evans, K. GMM. Alberti, and M. O. Thorner, *J. Clin. Invest.* **81,** 968 (1988).

64. W. S. Evans, A. CSA. Faria, E. Christiansen, K. Y. Ho, J. Weiss, A. D. Rogol, M. L. Johnson, R. M. Blizzard, J. D. Veldhuis, and M. O. Thorner, *Am. J. Physiol.* **252,** E549 (1987).

65. S. Eden, *Endocrinology (Baltimore)* **105,** 555 (1979).

66. J. D. Veldhuis, M. L. Johnson, L. M. Faunt, M. Mercado, and G. Baumann, *J. Clin. Invest.* **91,** 629 (1993).

67. N. M. Wright, F. J. Northington, J. D. Miller, J. D. Veldhuis, and A. D. Rogol, *Pediatr. Res.* **32,** 286 (1992).

68. K. Albertsson-Wikland, S. Rosberg, E. Libre, L. O. Lundberg, and T. Groth, *Am. J. Physiol.* **257,** E809 (1989).

69. J. D. Veldhuis and M. L. Johnson, *Am. J. Physiol.* **250,** E486 (1986).

70. A. R. Feinstein, *Clin. Pharmacol. Ther. (St Louis)* **17,** 104 (1975).

71. B. M. Bennett, *Biometrics* **28,** 793 (1972).

72. I. Z. Beitins, A. Barkan, A. Klibanski, N. Kyung, S. M. Reppert, T. M. Badger, J. D. Veldhuis, and J. W. McArthur, *J. Clin. Endocrinol. Metab.* **60,** 1120 (1985).

73. J. D. Veldhuis, M. L. Johnson, and E. Seneta, *J. Clin. Endocrinol. Metab.* **73,** 569 (1991).

[16] Analysis of the Temporal Coincidence of Hormonal Pulses

George R. Merriam and Kenneth W. Wachter

Introduction

Many hormonal series present the appearance of simultaneity or near-simultaneity in the timing of pulses of two or more different hormones (Fig. 1). This synchronization is of interest because it suggests a causal relationship or a common mechanism driving the two hormones. In some cases the mechanism is well known and the copulsatility is fully expected, such as in the profiles of ACTH and cortisol, where secretion of the former stimulates secretion of the latter; or of luteinizing hormone (LH) and follicle-stimulating hormone (FSH), where secretion of both is stimulated by gonadotropin-releasing hormone (GnRH). In these cases the presence or absence of the anticipated concordance serves as a check on the method of sampling or analysis, or demonstrates the limitations in the precision of pulse detection due to long half-lives or other obscuring factors.

In other cases a linkage is expected but not proven, as with profiles of LH and prolactin (PRL), or only hypothesized, and one desires some measure of whether the visual appearance of synchronization can be objectively confirmed. To do this requires both a standardized procedure for measuring coincidence and near-coincidence and also a means of testing whether these rates exceed those which might be present due to chance alone.

Methods

Cross-Correlation Analysis

One approach is to determine whether the two series are mathematically correlated. Cross-correlation analysis, for which there is a large literature, assesses the tendency for two time series to deviate upward or downward simultaneously from their respective means. Alternatively, that comovement may not be simultaneous, but rather be offset by a lag or advance time (1, 2). The Pearson correlation coefficient r_j

$$r_j = \frac{\sum (x_i - \bar{x})(y_{i-j} - \bar{y})}{\sqrt{\sum (x_i - \bar{x})^2 \sum (y_i - \bar{y})^2}}$$

Methods in Neurosciences, Volume 20

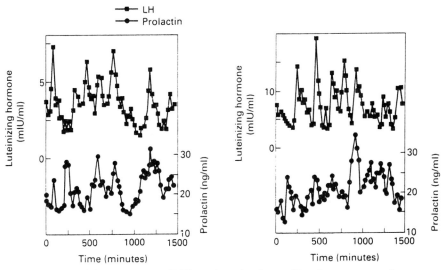

FIG. 1   Luteinizing hormone (LH) and prolactin profiles in two normal men as sampled at 20-min intervals for 24 hr (1440 min). [Adapted with permission from (4).]

provides a measure of the degree of correlation at lag j, and based on the size of the series a probability of that occurrence can be calculated if the series obey assumptions of independence and stationarity (uniformity over time). To the extent that simultaneous pulses cause a simultaneous upward or downward trend in both series, synchronized pulses will increase the correlation coefficient.

However, there are significant limitations to this approach; the most glaring are that many features of the series besides pulses, such as circadian variations in baseline levels, may contribute to the correlation and that the correlation coefficient does not specify what features of the series make this contribution. Also, the assumptions underlying the nominal probability values are frequently not observed: successive points are usually not independent but rather highly correlated, and circadian variations make most series nonstationary. For an accurate analysis of correlation at the frequencies usually encountered in pulsatile series, very frequent sampling (at least five to six times the interpulse interval) is needed to prevent aliasing (3).

These drawbacks are not necessarily fatal. For example, it is possible to measure the cross-correlation coefficient as a function of frequency (1) or to filter the series prior to cross-correlation analysis to remove circadian trends and retain only ultradian rhythms. Difficulties in calculating appropriate probability values for significance of a correlation can to some extent be circumvented by using some of the series "mismatching" techniques described below. However, in practice cross-correlation analysis has had limited utility.

Pulses as Discrete Events

A reason why correlation analysis seldom provides very helpful information is that pulses are usually viewed not as trends in the data but as discrete events, albeit events with an amplitude. And while one may wish to tally pulse amplitude, the usual question is occurrence—did the pulses occur simultaneously—rather than did the larger pulses of hormone A occur together with the larger pulses of hormone B, for which correlation is an appropriate measure. Since the primary question is usually the former one, methods aimed at treating pulses as discrete events occurring at a fixed time yield more insight than correlations.

This view suggests that one assess pulse synchronization by identifying and flagging the peaks in the two or more series being compared and then evaluating the extent of simultaneity in the marked events (4). Peak identification can be performed by any preferred method, e.g., Pulsar, Cluster, Detect, Ultra, or other available procedures (5–7). Since in practice it is unrealistically stringent to expect that the identified maxima of two different hormones with possibly different clearance half-times and volumes of distribution will occur exactly simultaneously, near-matches are also of interest.

A straightforward method which has proved useful closely approximates what the eye might do by inspection, but does so in a reproducible and quantitative fashion (4). Figure 2 outlines the procedure:

1. *Step one:* Identify and mark the peaks in both series.
2. *Step two:* Identify the point in the second series corresponding to the time of each peak in the first series. Record simultaneity if this point also marks a peak, and tally the total number and fraction of peaks so matched.
3. *Step three:* To assess near-simultaneity, open a "window" of ±1, 2, or more data intervals around each peak in the first series, and record a match if there is a peak within this window. The fraction of peaks matched will be higher as the window is widened.

Thus with a group of 11 LH and PRL data series drawn from normal young adults (Fig. 1), there was a 25% rate of exact synchrony, a 50% rate of peaks occurring within ±1 point, and 60% ±2 points (Fig. 3, upper curve).

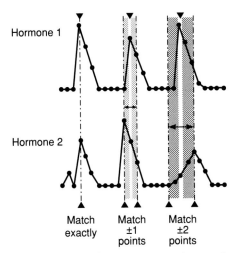

FIG. 2 Procedure for enumerating simultaneous and near-simultaneous peaks in different hormonal profiles. Positioning a marker atop each peak in the series of Hormone 1, one searches for peaks in Hormone 2 which occur either at precisely the same time or in a defined time window.

Background Rates of Random Synchronization

By themselves, however, these coincidence rates provide no information about the physiological significance of the correlation, because of the possibility that peaks may happen to coincide by chance. Thus the observed coincidence rates must be assessed against an estimate of the random background rate, and some measure of what constitutes a significantly enhanced degree of synchronization must be used. This background rate depends on several factors, most notably the event rate (peak frequency) and the distribution of that rate over the sampling period (stationarity).

Assuming a uniform peak rate, a first-order assessment of background coincidence rates is simple to estimate. In a series of m points containing n peaks, the probability that any given point chosen at random will be occupied by a peak is n/m. If there are n_1 peaks in the first series, then on average $n_1 n_2/m$ will find exact matches. Thus the rate of random coincidences goes up with the number of peaks in both series.

Also to first-order, if the window width is opened to ±1 point, there will be approximately three times as many matches because the window is 3 points wide; for ±2 points the increase is fivefold. Thus in two series of 100 points, each containing 10 peaks, one might expect about 10% exact matches, about 30% ±1 point, and about 50% ±2 points. A group of series could be

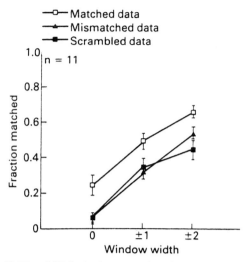

FIG. 3   Fraction of LH and PRL peaks occurring simultaneously or near-simultaneously in 11 hormonal series. The curves assess the rates of synchrony in the original "matched" data sets; in series in which the LH data from one subject have been mismatched to PRL data from a different subject; or in which the series of interpeak intervals have been rearranged ("scrambled"). In this series the two rearranged series do not significantly differ from each other, while the original data show a significantly higher rate of synchronization; $p < 0.001$. [Adapted with permission from (4).]

said to show significant correlation if the rates of synchrony exceed this rate by standard statistical testing.

This first-order assessment is inexact for several reasons, including the possibility of two or more peaks in the window (2) and minimum spacing requirements between the peaks; i.e., since peaks cannot occur in two successive data points and still be distinguished as separate events, the occurrence of peaks (their temporal dispersion) is not truly random. Thus actual background coincidence rates may differ from these very simple estimates. Combinatorial analysis provides a powerful means of calculating expected coincidence rates. This method is described in Chapter 17 (8).

Nonstationary Series

Such a calculation is possible in closed form based on the assumption that the event rate is uniform throughout the sampling period, i.e., that peaks are as likely in the daytime as at night in a typical 24-hr profile. Nonstationarity powerfully alters the background coincidence rate, as an example may illustrate. In the two hypothetical series of 10 peaks and 100 points, uniform expected event rates yield an expected coincidence rate of 10%, as derived above. However, if all peaks in series 1 occur during the first half of the series (e.g., "daytime") and all peaks in the second occur during the second half ("night"), the expected coincidence rate is zero. If all peaks in both series occur at night, the expected coincidence rate is 20%, since all 10 peaks occur within a span of 50 points. Less extreme distributions of event rates lead to intermediate values.

In theory, if one can model these changes in event rate probabilities, one can still calculate the expected coincidence rates—either by breaking the series into subseries for which the assumption of stationarity is valid or more practicably by a Monte Carlo method using large numbers of randomly generated series obeying the known event frequency distribution. Both approaches rely on the ability to construct an accurate model of the diurnal variability in the expected peak rate, which may not be available.

Empirical Assessment of Random Coincidence

We suggest as a practical alternative the much easier process of comparing the peak coincidence rate in the data series with the rate in a group of derived series which are as similar as possible in event rate and temporal dispersion, but in which there is no possibility of direct synchronization. This can be done by rearranging the original series in "mismatched" or "scrambled" form.

Mismatched series pairs compare the profile of the first hormone (e.g., LH) from one individual with that of the second hormone from a *different* subject selected at random. One proceeds to calculate the number of simultaneous and near-simultaneous peaks in the mismatched pairs exactly as with the original data pairs and compares the results. As shown in Fig. 3, the number of synchronized and nearly synchronized peaks in the mismatched data is lower than that in the original series, suggesting a significant excess of synchronization in the original data.

Even this degree of randomization does not destroy all possibility of peak synchronization. Specifically, mismatching does not factor out those determinants of pulses which may affect all subjects in a group, such as circadian rhythms in peak frequency, or external events which may trigger peaks. For example, if cortisol pulses are triggered by meals and all subjects eat their meals on the same schedule, one might expect at least some of the cortisol peaks to occur at close to the same time in all subjects, and so the rate of coincidence would be increased even in the mismatched series. Thus the rate of peak coincidence in the mismatched series may still be higher than

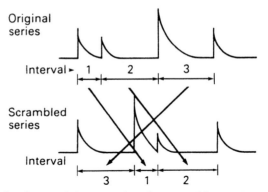

FIG. 4   Schematic of part of the procedure for scrambling and reassembling series of peaks. Not shown in the figure: the time of the first peak in the series must also be chosen at random and the series wrapped around to place any points extending beyond the end of the original data set at the beginning of the series.

a truly random rate. Whether this poses a problem depends on the specific objective of the study.

Scrambled Series

A way to eliminate the effects of those external cues and circadian variations, but still preserve the number and temporal dispersion of the peaks, is to scramble the interpeak intervals. After identifying the peaks in the original data, the series of interpeak segments is broken up and then reassembled in random order. The time of onset of the first peak is also randomized to avoid leaving the first and last peaks aligned, and parts of the reassembled series which extend beyond the end of the original data are wrapped around to the beginning. This process is shown schematically in Fig. 4. The reassembled series can then be compared and the matches tabulated in the usual fashion. As graphed in Fig. 3, the coincidence rate in the scrambled series is again lower than that in the original data. The scrambling procedure can be repeated many times, each time with a different random ordering of the segments. If the match rate is different for the original data than for all but, say, 5% of the scrambled cases, then the match rate is statistically significant at the 5% level.

In using this approach one must be aware that scrambling explicitly destroys ordering due to circadian and to cued ultradian signals. Thus if one finds no excess of peaks in the original vs the scrambled series, it provides strong evidence against physiological peak synchrony; but if an excess is observed this could be due either to internal synchronization or to external factors acting on the group as a whole. Since these external (circadian, cued) effects are preserved in the mismatched but destroyed in scrambled data sets, it is tempting to speculate that any differences between the results in mismatched vs scrambled data represent these group effects, while differences between original and mismatched data show the contribution of internal synchronization within the individual. This speculation, however, has not been directly tested.

Application

An application of these methods can be found in studies of synchronization in LH and PRL pulses (9, 10). Numerous authors have speculated on the possibility that GnRH might cue both hormones or that LH or α-subunit secretion might stimulate PRL. Liu and colleagues (9) measured LH, PRL, cortisol, and other hormones in groups of normal men and in patients with Kallmann's syndrome, in whom endogenous GnRH secretion is absent, in the untreated state and when treated with either pulsatile GnRH or with testosterone. Samples were collected at 20-min intervals for 24 hr and assayed, and peaks identified by Pulsar analysis (5). Simultaneous and near-simultaneous peaks were enumerated in original data sets and in mismatched and scrambled data sets. No significant linkage was found between LH and cortisol peaks in either normal men or patients, i.e., synchronization rates were no higher in matched than in mismatched or scrambled data.

A significant excess of linked LH and PRL peaks was found in both normal men and in Kallmann patients treated with pulsatile GnRH; the results summarized in Fig. 3 are those of the normal subjects. In patients treated with testosterone, who therefore still lacked GnRH and LH secretion, spontaneous PRL patterns were still present, and both the mean PRL and the pulse frequency in those men did not differ from those treated with GnRH. From these results it was concluded that GnRH/LH could entrain otherwise spontaneous PRL pulses, but that GnRH was not essential to maintain a normal PRL rhythm.

Summary

The optimal method(s) used to assess the correlation between hormonal profiles depends on whether one views pulses as part of a continuum of data or as discrete event markers. Cross-correlation analysis may be appropriate in the former but not the latter instance.

An intuitive and simple procedure for enumerating and evaluating synchronization in pulse profiles follows these steps:

1. Identify pulses in the different series using any preferred method.

2. In each series, count the number of synchronized and near-synchronized peaks. This can be performed automatically by computer, but the process is simple and straightforward enough to be done by hand (and should certainly be done manually for the first few cases to gain insight into the procedure).

3. Match the series of one hormone from a given subject with those of the other hormone from a different, randomly selected subject, and repeat the counts (mismatched series).

4. Compare the rates of coincidence in the original vs the mismatched data. (t testing, while not exact, is a serviceable approach.)

5. If desired, scramble the interpeak intervals and repeat the counts. (Automation is useful for this laborious step). Compare with original and with mismatched data.

6. If differences are observed, attempt to separate synchronizing factors which may be acting on the group as a whole from those occurring within individual subjects. This last step is more a consideration of physiological insight than of analytic methodology.

Acknowledgments

We thank Eric Libre, Linda Liu, Ning Ma, and Richard Sherins for their contributions to the work described here and to the collection of the data sets studied. A computer program, ''Synchrony,'' has been written to implement the procedure described and is available upon request.

References

1. J. E. A. McIntosh and R. P. McIntosh, ''Mathematical Modelling and Computers in Endocrinology,'' Chaps. 2 and 7. Springer-Verlag, Berlin, 1980.
2. C. Chatfield, ''The Analysis of Time Series: Theory and Practice.'' Chapman & Hall, London, 1975.
3. A. H. Vagnucci, A. K. C. Wong, and T. S. Ciu, *Comput. Biomed. Res.* **7,** 513 (1974).
4. G. R. Merriam, N. Ma, L. Liu, K. W. Wachter, and E. Libre, *Acta Paediatr. Scand. Suppl.* **349,** 167 (1989).
5. G. R. Merriam and K. W. Wachter, *Am. J. Physiol.* **243,** E310 (1982).
6. W. F. Crowley, Jr., and J. G. Hofler, eds., ''The Episodic Secretion of Hormones.'' Wiley, New York, 1987.

7. R. J. Urban, Chap. 14, this volume.
8. J. D. Veldhuis, M. L. Johnson, L. M. Faunt, and E. Seneta, Chap. 17, this volume.
9. N. Ma, L. Liu, and G. R. Merriam, *Endocrinology* (*Baltimore*) **124A,** 448 (1989).
10. G. R. Merriam, K. W. Wachter, N. Ma, and L. Liu, *Acta Paediatr. Scand. Suppl.* **372,** 63 (1991).

[17] Assessing Temporal Coupling between Two or among Three or More Neuroendocrine Pulse Trains

Johannes D. Veldhuis, Michael L. Johnson,
Lindsay M. Faunt, and Eugene Seneta

Introduction

Neuroendocrine systems typically communicate via a pulsatile mode of intermittent signaling (1–6). Moreover, feedback regulation is common within a system as well as between systems, sometimes resulting in significant temporal synchrony (7–20). Temporal coupling of pulse generators or their modulators is of considerable physiological interest, since it offers insights into a more complex order of regulation. We present three principal approaches to assessing the temporal relationship between two distinct neuroendocrine pulse trains and offer a more general solution to the analysis of linkage among three or more neuroendocrine pulse trains. In general, our approaches fall into three categories: (i) *cross-correlation analysis* with autoregressive modeling (a technique that does not pay any special attention to the presence or location of specific pulses in the data) (14, 15, 17, 18); (2) *computer simulations,* designed to emulate closely the temporal distribution of randomly dispersed pulses in the data (16, 21); and (3) *discrete conditional probability analysis* (9, 11, 13, 17, 19, 20), in which assumptions regarding a specific probability structure can be employed to yield a particular algebraic solution to the question of nonrandom pulse coincidence (the solutions involve binomial or hypergeometric probability distributions or higher-order combinatorial algebra that can be calculated within seconds on personal computers). We illustrate the application of these three complementary strategies to neuroendocrine data consisting of pulsatile luteinizing hormone (LH), testosterone, estradiol, progesterone, follicle-stimulating hormone (FSH), and prolactin measurements in the human. We also provide specific examples of calculations to allow readers to carry out their own computations, and we direct the investigator to relevant software to perform pertinent analyses.

Methods in Neurosciences, Volume 20

Cross-Correlation Analysis with Autoregressive Modeling

A classical approach to evaluating the general relationship between two temporally concurrent series of (paired) measurements is linear regression analysis. Linear correlation can also be applied across a range of individual lags (times separating samples of interest in the two series), in which case it is termed cross-correlation analysis (14, 15, 18). Linear correlation at any particular lag (e.g., zero lag, which involves comparisons of simultaneous measurements of two hormones) is a standard parametric statistical tool for evaluating the general association of tendencies toward high or low values in a given series with either corresponding (positive correlation coefficient) or inverse (negative correlation coefficient) tendencies in a second series. Indeed, linear correlation is merely a subset of cross-correlation analysis in its simplest form applied to any particular pairing of the data. For example, the data in the two series can be paired at zero lag (simultaneous samples) or at any particular positive or negative lag in which measured values in series A are consistently compared with measurements in series B that lag or lead by one or more samples.

Cross-correlation analysis typically provides useful insights into the overall coordinate behavior of two series of concurrent measurements, such as serum LH and testosterone concentrations, as illustrated in Fig. 1. For example, in Fig. 1A the upper profile represents pulsatile serum LH concentrations over 36 hr in a healthy young man in whom blood was collected at 10-min intervals, whereas the lower panel gives the corresponding testosterone measurements in the same blood samples (14). Visually there is an apparent general agreement between the tendencies of serum LH concentrations to increase or decrease and the parallel increases or decreases in serum testosterone concentrations at approximately the same time as well as somewhat later. Cross-correlation analysis of these two series and four others in similarly studied volunteers is shown in Fig. 1B. Note that the cross-correlation coefficients in the five men range in value between 0 and approximately 0.7 and are uniformly positive at various lags between 0 min (simultaneous LH and testosterone concentrations) and 100 min. In the last circumstance, correlated testosterone concentrations are permitted to lag LH concentrations by 100 min. The cross-correlation coefficients for the five men have median values that are well above the $p = 0.05$ level of significance over the lag times shown.

The level of significance for a cross-correlation coefficient can be approximated by estimating the standard error for the cross-correlation coefficient. The standard error is given by $1/(N - k)^{-1/2}$, where N denotes the number of samples measured and k the particular lag (14, 22). For example when blood is sampled at 10-min intervals for 36 hr, a total of 217 samples is

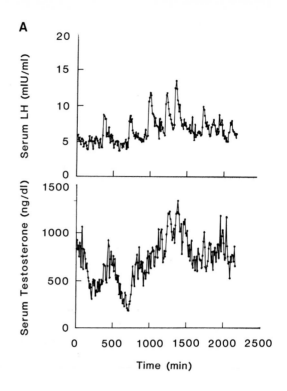

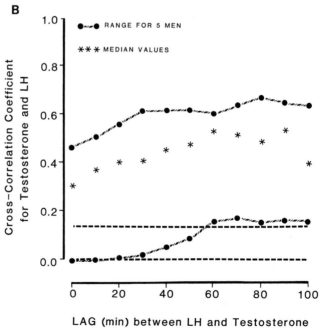

generated. When cross-correlation is carried out at zero lag, then $k = 0$, and the standard error of the resultant cross-correlation coefficient equals $1/(217)^{-1/2}$ or approximately 0.068. For $p < 0.05$, the absolute value of r must exceed approximately 1.96 standard errors, or a value of 0.13. In a similar manner, one can calculate the significance of the cross-correlation coefficient at some other lag k, such as $k = 10$, that is, when testosterone measurements lag behind those of LH by 10 sampling units, or 10×10 min in the case of 10-min blood sampling. Of interest, in normal men, LH and testosterone cross-correlation coefficients are highly significantly nonzero at all lags between 0 and 100 min, when the median values are considered. The absolute range for the five men is significantly nonzero and positive at lags between 60 and 100 min. This means that serum testosterone concentrations tend to vary in parallel with serum LH measurements in the same sample (zero lag) or when testosterone is considered as much as 100 min after the LH concentration changes (14).

The above initial approach to cross-correlation analysis is useful in providing general information about the tendency of the two series to covary in the same or opposite directions, when considered at various lags with respect to each other. However, in the case of hormone data particularly, each hormone series often exhibits strong internal correlation, i.e., the value of any given serum hormone measurement is a predictor of its predecessor and

FIG. 1   (A) Illustrative profile of serum LH (top) and testosterone (bottom) concentrations in a normal young man sampled at 10-min intervals for 36 hr. These profiles visually illustrate a general qualitative similarity and directional correspondence in the changes in serum LH and testosterone concentrations over time. (B) Cross-correlation coefficients for serum testosterone and LH concentrations at various lags assessed in five normal young men. Five healthy young men underwent blood sampling at 10-min intervals for 36 hr. The subsequent sera were submitted to LH and testosterone radioimmunoassay (RIA). The two time series were then subjected to cross-correlation analysis. The cross-correlation coefficient, r, values are shown as a range for the five men (upper and lower curves) and as median values for the group (asterisks). Each cross-correlation coefficient is given for a particular lag, which is the time in minutes separating the LH and testosterone concentration that are correlated. Note that the median cross-correlation coefficient is consistently above $p = 0.05$ random expected values (shown by the interrupted line) over the range of lags 0–100 min. As discussed further in the text, this traditional cross-correlation analysis should be followed by autoregressive modeling in order to remove the otherwise spurious effects of autocorrelation in each individual series, which can engender sustained apparent cross-correlation between the two series. [Adapted with permission from J. D. Veldhuis et al. (14).]

successor. This is because hormone secreted into the bloodstream tends to remain in the circulation for a number of minutes due to delayed metabolic clearance. This property of so-called *autocorrelation* can introduce spurious cross-correlation values. Consequently, a mathematical technique of *autoregressive modeling* is employed to identify the *partial* cross-correlation coefficients at various lags. The partial cross-correlation coefficient at some particular lag k is determined by stepwise autoregressive fitting, such that the influences of prior $(k - 1)$ correlations are removed (14, 22). When cross-correlation analysis with autoregressive modeling is applied to serum LH and testosterone concentration time series, we obtain significantly positive partial cross-correlation coefficients at much earlier lag times, namely, 0–30 min, compared to 60–100 min. Indeed, most men showed significant LH and testosterone partial cross-correlation coefficients within 0 to 30-min lag times. Of considerable interest, there are also *negative* cross-correlations observed at considerably longer lags, namely, at a median lag of 340 min. This observation indicates that approximately 340 min after testosterone concentrations tend to decrease, LH concentrations increase, and vice versa. This may indicate the presence of negative feedback within the LH–testicular axis.

In summary, most statistical software packages make provision for conventional cross-correlation analysis between paired values in two series of interest, such as the two hormones LH and testosterone illustrated above (14), LH and progesterone (15), and LH and prolactin (18). More sophisticated statistical analysis of neuroendocrine time series requires the use of autoregressive modeling combined with cross-correlation analysis, in order to determine significant partial cross-correlation coefficients at various lags. Autoregressive modeling is necessary to remove the otherwise artifactual effects of autocorrelation existing within each neurohormone series alone, in which successive hormone values tend to be correlated. In general, the use of autoregressive modeling with cross-correlation analysis reduces the calculated time lag connecting the changes of interest. In the case of our analysis of LH and testosterone, simple cross-correlation showed a lag of 60–100 min, whereas autoregressive modeling revealed that the true coupling between LH and testosterone changes occurred within 0–30 min.

As intimated above, cross-correlation analysis assesses the relationship between all appropriately paired serum hormone concentrations, without any attention to, knowledge of, or specific correction for discrete peaks or pulses within the data. Indeed, whether the data contain any peaks at all is irrelevant to the mathematical structure of cross-correlation analysis. Consequently, this tool provides a sweeping inference regarding similar directional and quantitative changes in the two series, but cannot answer the question: "Are *individual* discrete events in the two series nonrandomly associated in

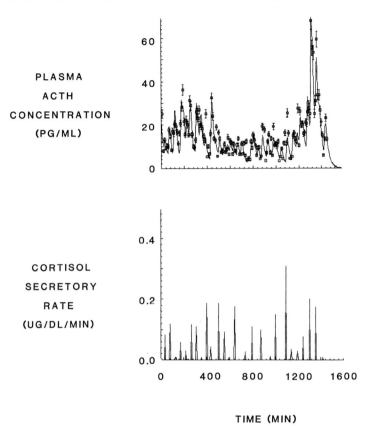

FIG. 2 Temporal relationships between plasma *ACTH concentrations* measured in blood collected at 10-min intervals over 24 hr in a healthy young man and the deconvolution-estimated sample *cortisol secretion rates* in the same individual. Cortisol secretion rates were estimated by deconvolution analysis of the corresponding 24-hr serum cortisol concentration profile (26). As suggested by the close visual coordination between plasma ACTH concentrations and calculated cortisol secretory rate, cross-correlation analysis with autoregressive modeling can be employed to quantitate the temporal linkage between the plasma trophic hormone *concentration* bathing the adrenal gland and the *secretory response* of the adrenal gland, as estimated from its calculated secretory rate (see text for further discussion). [J. D. Veldhuis and A. Iranmanesh, unpublished data.]

time?'' To address the query, simulations or probability calculations should be employed as discussed below.

Although not yet carried out in the literature to our knowledge, an important and relevant application of cross-correlation analysis is to relate serial hormone concentrations bathing a target gland to the calculated rates of hormone secretion by the target tissue. Indeed, as noted above, as in the case of cross-correlation between serum LH and testosterone concentrations, usually the correlation is applied to *concentrations* of both hormones. However, the concentration of testosterone is of less interest than the secretion rate of testosterone, particularly when the secretion rate is compared to the concentration of LH bathing the testis. Accordingly, we recommend that deconvolution analysis be used to calculate the actual sample secretion rates from the target tissue and that cross-correlation analysis with autoregressive modeling then be employed to relate the ambient hormone concentration bathing the target tissue to the time course of actual secretion. This is illustrated in Fig. 2 in the case of ACTH and cortisol, where the concentration of ACTH bathing the human adrenal glands is related very strongly to the calculated cortisol secretion rate in the same subject. This comparison is of greater physiological interest than that involving the serum ACTH and cortisol concentrations, or the ACTH secretion profile and the serum cortisol concentration profile.

Computer Simulations of Temporal Coupling between Two or among Three or More Neuroendocrine Pulse Trains

Since neuroendocrine time series typically exhibit sudden bursts, peaks, or pulses in the data, and since physiological regulation of the number and timing of such bursts is a prominent component of normal neuroendocrine communication, methods are necessary to quantitate the extent of temporal linkage between the individual discrete episodes in the two pulse trains. For example, an important question is, "Given two or more pulse trains (successions of randomly distributed secretory bursts) each independently regulated, what is the probability of observing on the basis of chance alone at least the number of coincident events actually found in the experimental data?" The null hypothesis of no temporal coupling would state that the observed number of coincident pulses between the two series does not exceed that anticipated on the basis of random associations alone. Accordingly, to test the null hypothesis, one must calculate the expected mean number of random coincidences on the basis of chance alone, estimate the variance inherent in that mean value, and construct a relevant probability distribution

(16, 19). This information will allow the investigator to calculate the *p* value for purely random associations between the two series of pulse episodes. If this *p* value is extremely small, then one may conclude that the observed degree of concordance between the pulses in the two series is extremely unlikely to be due solely to chance peak assortment. If chance associations alone are unlikely to account for the observed data, then some kind of temporal coordination or coupling can be inferred. Experiments can then be designed to disrupt this coupling selectively so as to ascertain its critical determinants.

Specific Computer Simulations

Pulse trains can be simulated in a number of ways that may be useful. For example, after identifying individual peaks or pulses in the data, the locations of some specific feature of the peak can be used to quantize or discretize the data. Useful features of a pulse might be the time of its maximal value, the time of the midpoint of the pulse, or the time of the first significant increase above baseline. We have used the time of the peak maximum as a simple way to discretize the timing of individual pulses. For example, if blood samples are collected at 10-min intervals for 24 hr, the resulting serum hormone concentration series first are submitted to pulse detection (either discrete peak detection or deconvolution analysis, etc.). When all significant peaks are idenitifed in the 24-hr measurements, samples containing the individual peak maxima are marked to discretize the maximal peak locations in time. If *n* peaks occur in the data, then *n* samples will be identified as the corresponding peak maxima. The remaining samples form another subset that is "peakless." One can then assign a true or false code, or a binary (0 or 1) code to each sample, where a "true" or a "1" denotes the presence of a peak maximum, and a "false" or a "0" denotes its absence. This discretization approach reduces the otherwise complex original neurohormone concentration series to binary or dichotomous information. Such binary series are relatively easy to simulate by one or more means.

After discretizing the neurohormone concentration data, computer simulations can be carried out. Indeed, as also discussed in Chapter 15 in this volume, simulations can require that the distribution of interpeak intervals be left intact or randomly reordered and relevant and irrelevant pairs of neurohormone series tested for coincidence. Irrelevant pairing can be used to provide an estimate of the background or chance rate of association between pulses in unrelated series. The *random pairing* of irrelevant series without reordering preserves the individual interpulse intervals in the manner observed, but is potentially limited by the investigator's ability to obtain only a relatively small number of series for irrelevant pairing. The pairing of randomly *reordered* series, on the other hand, could disrupt diurnal variations in interpulse intervals.

When pulse frequencies do not vary systematically over the total sampling session, we suggest a more exhaustive randomization and simulation of chance coincidences that consists of inserting true or false values in paired theoretical pulse series in a random manner to match the pulse frequencies in the original experimental data pair. Simulations are unconstrained or constrained, for example, only by the inability to insert peak maxima in the first, last, or immediately consecutive samples (such peaks could not be resolved by most pulse-detection methods) (16, 19). In such a randomization strategy, large numbers of synthetic appropriately paired pulse trains with desired pulse frequencies can be generated. For example, in a group of five men, in each of whom serum LH and testosterone concentrations were measured in blood collected at 10-min intervals for 24 hr, the resultant hormone series first would be submitted to peak detection or deconvolution analysis. After determining the numbers of pulses of LH and testosterone in each man's paired series, one can create 10,000 simulated paired pulse series containing randomly inserted peaks matching the observed frequencies, e.g., 18 LH pulses and 14 testosterone pulses for man A. Another set of simulations of 10,000 paired series might consist of 21 LH and 18 testosterone pulses for man B, etc. To evaluate the *p* values for coincidence findings in the individual men, the *cumulative probability distribution* of expected numbers of purely random coincidences defined by the simulations is used. The expected (mean) number of random coincidences is also found by simulation and can be compared to the observed number of coincidences in that individual. Moreover, a group *p* value can also be obtained (see below).

The only constraints reasonably imposed on the randomization of peak locations in the simulated series, we believe, are that peak maxima do not occur in consecutive samples or in the first or last sample of the series. These constraints arise since one cannot demonstrate definitively the occurrence of consecutive peak maxima, or a peak maximum in the first or last sample, without knowing that both flanking samples contain lower values (16, 23). Accordingly, the assigned locations of the peaks are pseudorandomized, subject to the two constraints of nonconsecutiveness and the absence of peak maxima in the first or last sample. As shown in Fig. 3, these constraints have little impact on the number of observed coincidences due to chance alone, so long as the peak density in the data is not extremely high. The number of (randomly) coincident peaks within each of the 10,000 simulated pairs is simply enumerated by the computer program at the various lags of

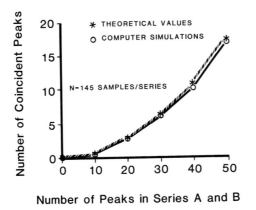

FIG. 3   Lack of significant effect of pseudorandomization on expected numbers of randomly coincident events in paired neurohormone pulse series. The two lines represent numbers of randomly coincident peaks in relation to peak density in computer simulations constrained, or not constrained, by the assumption that peak maxima cannot be assigned to immediately consecutive blood samples. [J. D. Veldhuis and M. L. Johnson, unpublished data.]

interest. For example, one can count all coincidences at zero lag, which would require peak maxima in the same sample. Alternatively, peaks separated by unit lag (one sampling interval) or higher lags can be tabulated. From the 10,000 simulated pairs of pulse trains, the expected number of random coincidences is determined with a mean, variance and standard deviation, and cumulative probability distribution. The mean, variance, and cumulative probability distribution will be relatively well determined from this number of simulations. Accordingly, for any given subject's pair of pulsating hormone series, we can state and test a null hypothesis: "The number of concordant pulses observed between the paired hormone series is no more than that expected on the basis of chance associations alone."

Simulations will provide an *expected* mean value, which can be compared with the observed number of coincidences. As importantly, an individual p value is obtained from the cumulative probability distribution, in order to estimate the probability that the null hypothesis is true in that individual, namely, that no association exists between peak locations in the two series beyond that due to chance assortments. This p value is interpreted from the expected cumulative probability distribution's right-hand tail.

Of interest, the above computer simulations can also be applied to triple pulse series and group behavior (16, 19). For n subjects, we generate 10,000 sets each consisting of *n* paired (or triple) randomly pulsating time series. Each of the *n* pairs (or triplets) of randomly pulsating synthetic time will contain exactly the number of peaks recognized in the corresponding test subject's physiological data. For example, in evaluating triple copulsatility, let us suppose subject 1 had LH, FSH, and prolactin pulse frequencies of 18, 14, and 21 peaks/24 hr determined in samples collected at 10-min intervals for 1 day, and subject 2 had 15, 17, and 16 peaks/24 hr, respectively, etc. Our *group simulations* would consist of 10,000 sets of triply pulsating series. In each set, subset 1 for subject 1 would contain a triplet of pulsating series with 18, 14, and 21 peaks distributed randomly over 145 samples; subset 2 would contain 15, 17, and 16 randomly distributed peaks, etc. For each of the 10,000 sets of *n* triple randomly pulsating series, the total number of triple coincidences in the group is counted. Based on 10,000 such as enumerations for random assortments, a group mean, variance, and cumulative probability distribution are estimated for the total number of randomly coincident events in the group. We have extended these simulations to four contemporaneous pulse trains (16, 19).

Relevance of Computer Simulations

As discussed further below, the above simulations provide predictions of the algebraic values for means, variances, and cumulative probability distributions very close to those we obtain by assuming in essence a particular binary series for the first hormone (each sample either does or does not contain a peak maximum) and another binary series for the second (or third and fourth) hormone(s). These specific algebraic probability calculations are given next.

Discrete Conditional Probability Calculations

Of considerable physiological importance is the extent to which discrete events in contemporaneous but distinct neurohormonal time series are synchronized. One general approach to this problem entails the use of cross-correlation analysis, which quantitates the degree of correlation observed between simultaneous or successive hormone concentrations (see above). This procedure does not identify discrete events (peaks, bursts, or pulses) in the data nor make any distinction about the temporal relationships between or among such individually identifiable events. In this section, we present methods for approximating expected numbers of randomly coincident discrete events contained in *two or more* independently regulated series. This explicitly defined algebra offers a statistical basis for calculating relevant means, variances, and (cumulative) probability distributions for random coincidence rates. Such calculations offer a formal basis for evaluating available simulations as well as published reports on putatively coupled physiological events. Indeed, we can test the null hypothesis that the timing of discrete events in *two or more* contemporaneous series is statistically independent. Our statistical formalism has been validated by computer modeling (16, 19, 21, 24) and then applied to physiological experiments designed to assess temporal coupling between and among two or more neuroendocrine pulse trains *in vivo* (9, 11, 13, 17, 20).

Definition of Discrete Peak Coincidence

For the purposes of enumerating individual pulse concordance, "exactly" coincidence peaks can be defined as pulses whose maxima are contained in the same sample. Lagged coincidence is defined as peak maxima in two or more series separated by some specified time lag (e.g., peak maxima separated by 10 min). For example, at a lag of ± 10 min, three possible coincident behaviors could occur, i.e., the peak maxima in series A could (i) coincide exactly with those in series B (lag of zero); (ii) precede those in series B by 10 min (+ 10-min lag); or (iii) follow those in series B by 10 minute (−10-min lag).

Conditional Probability Formulation

We initially assume that the occurrence of discrete neurohormonal events (e.g., pulses, bursts, or peaks) in any given samples in any given time series can be represented by a binomial distribution, subject to the following assumptions that characterize Bernoulli processes:

1. Any given observation unit (or sample) in the series either contains or does not contain an event (e.g., a burst or peak maximum). These two outcomes are mutually exclusive.
2. The probability of a given outcome (e.g., that a burst or peak maximum is, or is not, contained in a particular sample) is essentially constant from sample to sample.
3. The tests (e.g., detection of a burst or hormone pulse) or whether an event is identified in a sample are independent of prior or future results in

the same series. This condition is essentially true at expected physiological peak densities (see Fig. 3).

Our computer simulations (above) demonstrate that the preceding assumptions are reasonable, except when very high pulse frequencies occur, such as would cause virtually alternate samples to contain peaks.

Two Pulsatile Neuroendocrine Series*

If m and n designate the number of individual discrete events (e.g., bursts or peaks) identified in hormone time series A and B, respectively, and z, the total number of observation unit (samples) in each series,† then the binomial probability density functions of interest for each of the two neurohormone series can be specified as shown in Eqs. (1) and (2).

For series A

$$P(m) = \binom{z}{m} P_a^m (1 - P_a)^{z-m}, \qquad m = 0, 1, \dots z \tag{1}$$

and for series B

$$P(n) = \binom{z}{n} P_b^n (1 - P_b)^{z-n}, \qquad n = 0, 1, \dots z \tag{2}$$

where P_a and P_b are the individual probabilities that any given sample in series A and B, respectively, contains a peak.

---

* Symbol definitions: z, number of samples (observation units) in each series; m, number of events (e.g., peaks) in series A; n, number of events (e.g., peaks) in series B; k, number of events (e.g., peaks) in series C; l, number of events (e.g., peaks) in series D; x_d, number of coincident events observed between a pair of series (double coincidences); x_t, number of coincident events observed between a set of three series (triple coincidences); x_{go}, total number of *observed* coincidences in a *group* of subjects or experiments; x_{ge}, *expected* total number of (random) coincidences in a *group*; P_a, probability that any given sample in series A contains a peak; P_b, probability that any given sample in series B contains a peak; P_c, probability that any given sample in series C contains a peak; N, number of subjects studied in a group; N_a, number of peaks in the entire group of series A; N_b, number of peaks in the entire group of series B; N_c, number of peaks in the entire group of series C; $x Cy$, combinatorial notion; $P(x_d$ or $x_t)$, probability of observing exactly "x_d" two-way or "x_t" triple coincidences; $P(>x_d$ or $>x_t)$, probability of observing at least "x_d" two-way or "x_t" triple coincidences.

† If peaks cannot occur or be detected in the first and last samples of the series, then the term "z" is replaced by "$z - 2$."

The statistical properties that characterize x_d, the number of randomly coincident peaks between two time series (coincident peak maxima contained in the same samples) conditional on the number of peaks in series A and B fixed at m and n, respectively, are described by the conditional probability Eq. (3).

$$\Pr(X_d = x_d) = \frac{\binom{m}{x_d}\binom{z-m}{n-x_d}}{\binom{z}{n}}, \qquad x_d = 0, 1, \ldots \min(m, n) \qquad (3)$$

The mathematical proof of the above formulation follows by calculating the conditional probability required from (1) and (2) above. Note that the above distribution of coincident peak numbers is hypergeometric, with the expected mean, $E(X_d)$, and variance, $\mathrm{Var}(X_d)$, shown in Eqs. (4) and (5).

$$E(X_d) = \frac{m \times n}{z} \qquad (4)$$

$$\mathrm{Var}(X_d) = \frac{m \times n}{z}\left(1 - \frac{m}{z}\right)\left(1 - \frac{n-1}{z-1}\right) \qquad (5)$$

To calculate exact conditional (hypergeometric) probability values from combinatorial Eq. (3), we use logarithmic transformation and Stirling's formula (19, 25) for factorials greater than 15, i.e., $n!$ is approximately the product of the square root of the quantity two π times n, and (e/n) to the n power. Otherwise, large factorial computations result in values exceeding 10^{300}, which are not readily manipulated in many computing systems.

Equation (3) specifies the probability of observing exactly x coincident events, given m events in series A, n events in series B, and z observations in each series.

As presented above, Eq. (3) applies to any individual subject. For a *group* of N subjects, a similar formulation can be applied, in which the following considerations apply: Denote by N_a and N_b the number of peaks in series A and B, respectively, considered over all N subjects, so that the total number of samples for each series is

$$N \times z \qquad (6)$$

Then, if the probability of observing a total of exactly x_{go} coincident peaks in the group as a whole can be viewed to reflect a concatenation of the individual series, it can be given as shown in Eq. (7):

$$\Pr(X_{go} = x_{go}) = \frac{\binom{N_a}{x_{go}} \binom{N_z - N_a}{N_b - x_{go}}}{\binom{N_z}{N_b}} \tag{7}$$

for which the expected group mean number of coincident peaks x_{ge}, is

$$X_{ge} = E(X_{go}) = \frac{N_a \times N_b}{N_z} \tag{8}$$

and the variance is

$$\mathrm{Var}(X_{go}) = \frac{N_a \times N_b}{N_z} \left(1 - \frac{N_a}{N_z}\right) \left(1 - \frac{N_b - 1}{N_z - 1}\right) \tag{9}$$

Alternatively, since the hypergeometric distribution for large values approaches normal, the probability distribution of x_{go} can be approximated for large groups by z-score transformation, i.e.,

$$z = \frac{X_{go} - X_{ge}}{\sqrt{\mathrm{Var}(X_{go})}} \tag{10}$$

The statistical implications of the calculated z-score can then be inferred from the unit normal (Gaussian) zero mean distribution. The resultant p value offers a measure of the probability that the particular total number of coincident peaks observed in a group of subjects can be attributed to random peak associations alone.‡

‡ To assess the probability that *at least* the observed number of coincident events d (for double coincidences) and t (for triple coincidences) could be attributed to chance alone, one must calculate the following:

$$\Pr(X_d > x_d) = \left(1 - \sum_{i=0}^{d} P(x_i)\right) \tag{A1}$$

$$\Pr(X_t > x_t) = \left(1 - \sum_{i=0}^{t} P(x_i)\right)$$

where d or t are integral numbers of coincident events, and $P(x_i)$ is the conditional probability of observing exactly i coincident peaks.

Three Neurohormone Series

For three contemporaneous pulsatile series each comprising z observations, and containing respectively m, n, and k discrete events, the expected number of random triple coincidences can be given as shown in Eq. (11).

$$E(X_t) = \frac{m \times n \times k}{z^2} \tag{11}$$

The variance of the number of triple coincidences is

$$\text{Var}(X_t) = \frac{m \times n \times k}{z^2}\left(1 + \frac{(m-1)(n-1)(k-1)}{(z-1)^2} - \frac{mnk}{z^2}\right) \tag{12}$$

and the corresponding probability density function is

$$\Pr(X_t = x_t) = \sum_{y=0}^{k} \frac{\binom{y}{x_t}\binom{z-y}{n-x_t}}{\binom{z}{n}} \frac{\binom{m}{y}\binom{z-m}{k-y}}{\binom{z}{k}}, \qquad x_t = 0, 1, \dots k \tag{13}$$

where y is an indexing term, k is the number of peaks in the most slowly pulsating of the three series, m and n are the numbers of pulses in the other two series, and $(yCx_t) = 0$ for all $X_t > y$.

For a group of N individuals, formulas (11), (12), and (13) apply with z replaced by Nz, and m, n, and k replaced by N_a, N_b, and N_c, where k is the fewest number of peaks among all series. Thus, for example, the group mean is

$$u = \frac{N_a N_b N_c}{(N_z)^2} \tag{14}$$

Using Eq. (13) (written with values reflecting concatenation of all individual series within the group), one can estimate an exact group probability value that the observed total number of coincident events is attributable to chance alone. The Poisson Eq. (15), using the mean from (14), provides a good approximation of group behavior for three or more contemporaneous series:

$$\Pr(X_{go} = x_{go}) = \frac{e^{-u}\, u^{x_{go}}}{x_{go}!}, \qquad x_{go} = 0, 1, \ldots \tag{15}$$

Generalization to Four or More Contemporaneous Series

Let s be the number of distinct contemporaneous time series in each subject and $k_1, k_2, \ldots k_s$ be the number of discrete peaks, pulses, or events in each time series. Then, the expected number of coincidences among all s series, where x_r is the number of coincidences among the first r series, and the probability distribution are given as shown in Eqs. (16) and (17).

$$E(X_s) = \frac{(k_1 k_2 \cdots k_s)}{z^{s-1}} \tag{16}$$

$$\Pr(X_s = x_s) = \sum_{y=0}^{(k_1^{\min}, \ldots k_{s-1})} \frac{\binom{y}{x_s}\binom{z-y}{k_s - x_s}}{\binom{z}{k_s}} \Pr(X_{s-1} = y) \tag{17}$$

The group mean (with obvious notation) is

$$u = \frac{N_1 N_2 \cdots N_s}{(N_z)^{s-1}} \tag{18}$$

and the group probability distribution can be approximated by the Poisson Eq. (15), i.e., the variance approximates the mean.

Comparisons of Simulations and Probability Algebra

Paired Neurohormone Series

To determine expected coincident behavior between any particular two contemporaneous but randomly and independently pulsating time series containing discrete events, we formulated an algebraically explicit model of conditional probability deriving from two binomial distributions and leading to a hypergeometric probability density function (Eqs. 1–5 above). The relevant hypergeometric probability density function specifies exact conditional probabilities that the observed number of coincident peaks or events in any given pathophysiological setting is attributable to chance associations alone. This mathematical formalism offers a means to test the null hypothesis that two pulsating hormone series are temporally uncoupled, i.e., are statistically independent in the timing of their hormone pulses. Theoretically predicted probability values (means, variances, and cumulative probability distributions) can be compared to results of computer simulations of pulsatile hormone time series.

The theoretically expected *mean* numbers of randomly coincident events based on the predicted hypergeometric probability distribution are statistically indistinguishable from those of the computer simulations of paired independently pulsating synthetic time series (Fig. 4). The *variances* calculated from the hypergeometric distributions and estimated by computer simulations also correlate closely over a wide range of pulse frequencies ($r = + 0.9993$, $p < 0.0001$) (Fig. 4B). Absolute values of the variances in the computer simulations are not distinguishable from those of a corresponding hypergeometric distribution. The slope of the regression of theoretically predicted variance on computer-simulated variance is 1.0041 [±0.0075 SE]. Moreover, the *cumulative probability distributions* generated theoretically and by computer simulation are statistically indistinguishable by the Kolmogorov–Smirnov test (Fig. 4C).

Both the conditional probability algebra and the computer simulations project high rates of random coincidence even between independently pulsating time series at high peak densities. High peak densities can result from either increased pulse frequency or the same pulse frequency dispersed over fewer samples (reduced sampling intensity). For example, at an invariant sampling rate (e.g., blood samples withdrawn at 10-min intervals for 24 hr), a higher pulse frequency in one or both series results in a larger number of (randomly) coincident peaks. Conversely, at any given pulse frequency (e.g., 12 peaks per 24 hr), a smaller number of samples (e.g., 20-min versus 10-min sampling) among which the peaks are distributed yields a higher chance coincidence rate. Such observations help explain the vast range of coincidence rates reported in the neuroendocrine literature, in which varying sampling intensities and varying pulse frequencies are represented.

Example of Calculations for Paired Hormone Series

On the basis of the foregoing formulation of expected random coincidence rates between two temporally uncoupled neuroendocrine time series, we can examine the statistical significance of physiological coincident behavior. Consider LH and FSH pulse series in 14 normal men each studied on two

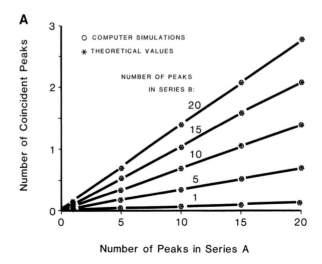

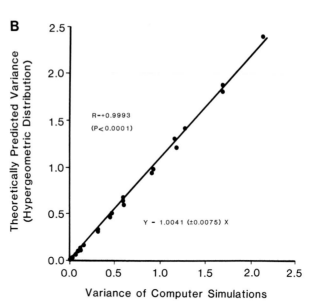

FIG. 4   (A) Influence of event (e.g., hormone peak) frequencies in two independently regulated (e.g., pulsating endocrine) time series on the *mean* number of purely random coincidences. Theoretical predictions of expected numbers of random coincidences based on a hypergeometric probability distribution are compared with computer-simulation estimates. Note the strong concordance between the conditional probability model ("theoretical value") and the empirical computer-based estimates over a

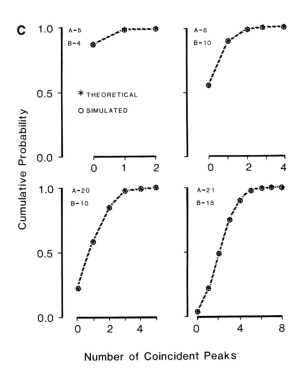

Number of Coincident Peaks

wide range of discrete (pulse) frequencies in each time series (here designated series A and B). For each point shown, 10,000 simulated pairs of randomly and independently pulsating synthetic hormone series comprising 145 "samples" were generated containing the indicated numbers of discrete events (peak maxima). (B) Correlation between theoretically predicted *variance* based on a hypergeometric distribution and variance estimates derived from computer-simulated hormone time series. Ten thousand randomly and independently pulsating synthetic time series were generated by computer simulations to estimate the variance about the mean number of coincident peaks. (C) Theoretical (hypergeometric) and computer-simulation-based *cumulative probability distributions* for numbers of randomly coincident hormone peaks between two temporally uncoupled (independently pulsating) endocrine time series. For illustrative purposes, a range of physiological pulse frequencies in the two series (denoted A and B) is given. [J. D. Veldhuis, M. L. Johnson, and E. Seneta, unpublished data.]

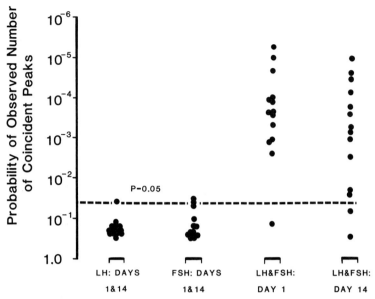

FIG. 5   Individual exact conditional probabilities of observing on the basis of chance at least the numbers of coincident pulses identified between physiological gonadotropin (LH and/or FSH) pulse series in 14 normal men. Subjects each underwent blood sampling at 10-min intervals for 24 hr on two occasions at least 14 days apart to generate serum-immunoactive LH and FSH pulse profiles, each comprising 145 samples. LH and/or FSH peaks were identified by Cluster analysis (23) and then examined for coincidence in four circumstances: (i) LH peaks in Day 1 were tested for coincidence (peak maxima occurring in the same sample) with LH peaks on Day 14 in the same subject; (ii) FSH peaks in the two separate sessions (Days 1 and 14) were also assessed for coincidence in the same subject; and (iii) and (iv) LH and FSH peaks in any given subject were evaluated for coincidence during each sampling session, i.e., Day 1, as well as Day 14. The exact conditional probabilities shown for each subject were calculated from the appropriate hypergeometric probability density function (Eq. 3). [Adapted with permission from J. D. Veldhuis *et al.* (19).]

separate occasions, in whom we can test several null hypotheses, e.g., that (i) LH and FSH peaks in any given subject are randomly associated on any given day; and (ii) LH (or FSH) peaks in any given subject studied on one particular occasion (i.e., first sampling session) are not coupled temporally to peaks of the same gonadotropin (LH or FSH) identified on another date (e.g., second sampling session 2 weeks later). As illustrated in Fig. 5, the first null hypothesis can be rejected at an α level of 0.05 in 13 of 14 men in their first sampling session and in 12 of 14 men in their second sampling

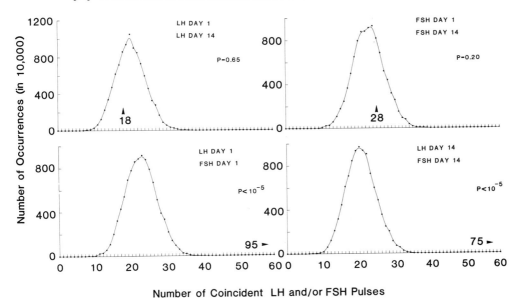

Number of Coincident LH and/or FSH Pulses

Fig. 6 Group probability of observing on the basis of chance alone at least the indicated total number of coincident LH and/or FSH peaks observed in 14 normal men studied as described in the legend of Fig. 5. The solid curve denotes the theoretically expected total numbers of coincident peaks assuming the null hypothesis that any given pair of pulsatile gonadotropin time series is random and independent. Numerical values denote the total number of *observed* coincident LH and FSH peaks in the group of 14 normal men studied on two occasions (Day 1 and Day 14, as noted). *p* values derive from the corresponding cumulative conditional probability distribution defined from 10,000 computer simulations of families of 14 pairs of independently and randomly pulsating hormone time series with the observed frequencies. [J. D. Veldhuis, M. L. Johnson, and E. Seneta, unpublished data.]

session. In contrast, the second null hypothesis cannot be rejected at $p < 0.05$ in 12 of the 14 men (LH) or in 14 of 14 men (FSH). Consequently, we can infer that LH and FSH copulsate (exhibit a high degree of nonrandom peak coincidence) in any given subject on any given day, but that LH (or FSH) pulses are not temporally synchronized with the same hormone in normal men on different study days.

Further analysis of coincident behavior for the group of 14 men considered in aggregate (Fig. 6) reveals that the null hypothesis of random associations between LH and FSH peaks in the same man on the same day can be rejected at a probability level of $p < 10^{-5}$ using simulations. In particular, a total of 95 (first session) and 75 (second session) coincident LH and FSH peaks

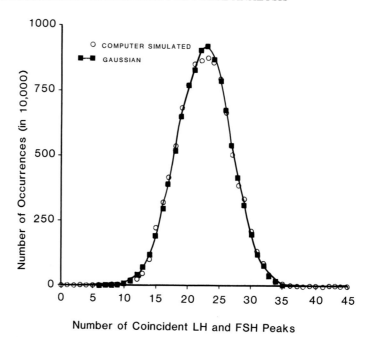

Number of Coincident LH and FSH Peaks

FIG. 7   Comparison of computer-simulated frequency distribution of expected numbers of randomly coincident LH and FSH peaks in a group of 14 men (studied as defined in the legend of Fig. 5) with a Gaussian (standardized normal deviate) z-score approximation. Computer simulations were performed to emulate random and independent LH and FSH pulse generators in 14 men having the individual LH and FSH pulse frequencies identified on the second sampling session (Day 14), when a total of 75 coincident LH and FSH peaks were counted in the group. The expected total number of randomly coincident peaks (mean of the indicated distributions) was 23 ± 4.3 (SD). [J.D. Veldhuis, M. L. Johnson, and E. Seneta, unpublished data.]

occurred in the group of 14 men, compared to an expected total of 23 ± 4.3 (SD) assuming independently pulsating hormone series. As shown in Fig. 7, even the lesser value of 75 total (group) coincidences markedly exceeds chance expectations, the distribution of which is well represented by a Gaussian approximation in which the number of observed total coincidences correspond to standardized normal deviates (z-scores) in excess of $+15$. However, significant LH and FSH coincidences for the group of 14 men considered on any given day should be distinguished from the behavior of LH (or FSH) peaks on separate days, when gonadotropin peaks were dissociated temporally ($p = 0.65$ and 0.20).

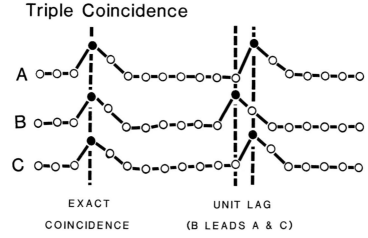

FIG. 8   Suggested definition of *triply* coincident events in three series, A, B, and C. Note that exact triple coincidence requires discrete events in all three series to occur in the same observation unit. Lagged coincidence would allow distinct events in the three series to bear a finite and constant relationship to one another (e.g., events in series B lead those in series A and C by one time unit). Many such possible lagged relationships can be stated. Only one is illustrated.

Triple Neurohormone Series

The preceding formulation of the coincident peak problem can be extended to triple time series. Triple coincidences can be defined as schematized in Fig. 8. Exact three-way coincidences would require peak maxima from all three series to occur in the same sample. The concept of "lagged" coincidence data at a finite, fixed lag (number of time units separating peak maxima) can also be introduced for two or more series.[2] Note that a variety of possible lags can be considered including a "diagonal" lag, in which the three events are found in immediately successive samples.

As shown in Fig. 9A, Eq. (11) describes very well the computer-predicted number of random triple coincidences expected among three independently pulsating hormone time series ($r = +0.9997$, $p < 0.0001$). Equation (12) closely approximates the computer-simulation estimates of the standard deviation for random triple coincidence (Fig. 9B). Moreover, Eq. (13) provides a good definition of the cumulative probability distributions expected for chance triple coincidences, as shown in Fig. 9C.

Physiological experiments in the human allowed us to evaluate two- or three-way concordance between and among discrete LH, FSH, and prolactin

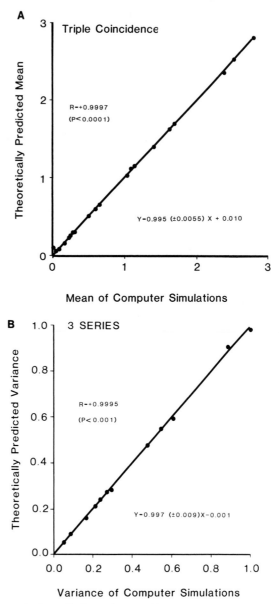

FIG. 9   (A) Theoretical predictions (by combinatorial algebra) of expected numbers of *triply* coincident events among three independently regulated time series compared to estimates made by computer simulations. The latter comprised 10,000 subsets of

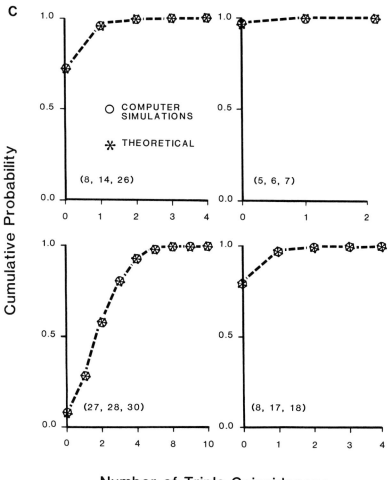

Number of Triple Coincidences

three randomly and independently pulsating synthetic series. Triple coincidence was defined as the simultaneous occurrence of an event from each of the three series in any given sample, or any other fixed *a priori* lag. (B) Predicted and computer-simulated variances of numbers of random triple coincidences. (C) Illustrative predicted and computer-stimulated cumulative probability distributions for the expected number of random triple coincidences among three series with the indicated individual event frequencies. Simulations were carried out as described (19), except that triplets (rather than pairs) of randomly pulsating time series were created. [J. D. Veldhuis, M. L. Johnson, and E. Seneta, unpublished data.]

pulses, as illustrated in Fig. 10. Figure 10B shows the various exact conditional probabilities of pairwise pulse coincidence in individual subjects for the hormones LH and FSH, LH and prolactin, and FSH and prolactin. The individual probabilities that the observed number of triple coincidences (LH, FSH, and prolactin) can be attributed to chance associations alone are shown for each subject in Fig. 10A.

The total (group) number of paired coincident peaks observed in the six postmenopausal subjects is given in Figure 10B, e.g., 21 for prolactin and LH ($p = 0.023$), 23 for prolactin and FSH ($p = 0.0003$), and 55 for LH and FSH ($p < 10^{-4}$). The corresponding expected (random) numbers of paired coincidences ($\pm$SD) are also noted. The distributions illustrated were generated from 10,000 computer stimulations of relevant groups, each containing six pulsating pairs of synthetic LH and/or FSH and/or prolactin series with appropriate frequencies.

Computer simulations for all three series of hormones considered together are shown in Fig. 10C. For exact three-way coincidence (all three hormone peak maxima occur in the same observation unit or sample), we observe a total of 13 events compared to an expected number of 1.6 ± 1.2 (SD) ($p < 10^{-5}$). If LH and FSH are both considered to lead prolactin by 10 min (i.e., prolactin peaks lag those of both gonadotropic hormones by 10 min), a total of 8 lagged triple coincidences are observed [expected value 1.6 ± 1.2 (SD)] ($p < 10^{-4}$). Conversely, if both LH and FSH peak maxima lag prolactin peak maxima by 10 min, then a total of five lagged triple coincidences is observed [expected value 1.6 ± 1.24 (SD)] ($p < 0.05$). Such temporal linkage is specific, since none of six various other lags tested among LH and/or

---

FIG. 10   (A) Individual exact conditional probabilities of observing at least the number of coincident peaks identified between *paired* physiological series (LH and FSH, FSH and prolactin, prolactin and FSH) and among the *triply* pulsating series (LH, FSH, and prolactin) in six postmenopausal women. The exact individual conditional probability for each subject's paired series was calculated from the appropriate hypergeometric probability density function (Eq. 3) and for the triple coincidences from the higher-order summed combinatorials (Eq. 12). (B) Predicted (random) versus observed (physiological) numbers of coincident prolactin and LH (top), prolactin and FSH (middle), and LH and FSH (bottom) peaks. Six postmenopausal estrogen-unreplaced women each underwent blood sampling at 10-min intervals for 24 hr. The subsequent sera comprising 145 samples were subjected to immunoassay for the measurement of prolactin, LH, and FSH. Discrete pulses of LH, FSH, and prolactin were identified by Cluster analysis (23). The total numbers of coincident peaks observed in this group of six subjects were 21 [prolactin and LH, versus expected 14 ± 3.4 (SD)], 23 (prolactin and FSH, versus 12 ± 3.1), and 55 (LH and FSH, versus 12 ± 3.1). The indicated p values were determined from 10,000 computer simulations of each relevant group of pairs of independently pulsating synthetic time series,

(*continues on page 365*)

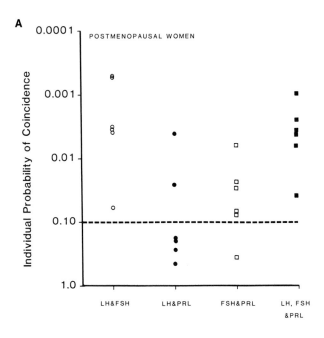

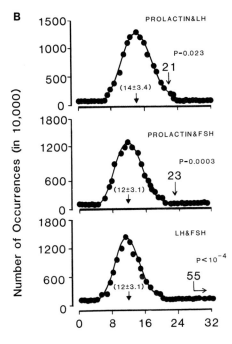

Fig. 10

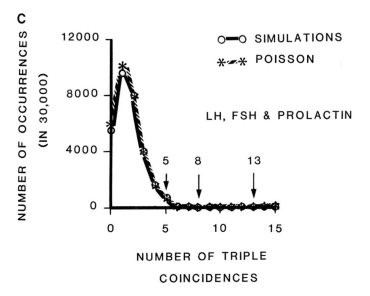

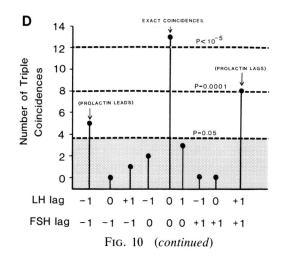

FIG. 10 (*continued*)

FSH and/or prolactin (Fig. 10D) exceed chance expectations. Therefore, LH, FSH, and prolactin copulsate to a degree highly unexpected on the basis of chance associations alone. Moreover, prolactin peaks are more likely to follow than to precede the LH and FSH peaks to which they are temporally coupled at a fixed, finite (e.g., 10-min) lag. This temporal coupling is illustrated for one subject in Fig. 11A.

Lagged and "Window" of Coincidence

The occurrence of significant lagged coincidence can also be examined statistically. For example, coincidence at any single fixed lag (e.g., peak maxima in series A are stipulated to lead peak maxima in series B by a designated number of time units) has the same probability of occurrence as exact (zero lag) coincidence. Conversely, if coincidence is defined within some "window" of time (e.g., 10-min separating peaks in series A and B), the probability of such lagged coincident events can also be calculated. In this circumstance,

---

FIG. 10 (continued)
which yielded the indicated frequency distributions predictive of random (uncoupled) pulsatile behavior. (C) Triple coincidence among LH, FSH, and prolactin peaks in a group of postmenopausal women. We observed a total of 13 exact (unlagged) triple coincidences, compared to an expected number of 1.6 ± 1.24 (SD). When prolactin peaks were considered to *lag* both LH and FSH by one time unit (10 min) a total of 8 lagged triple coincidences was observed. Conversely, when prolactin peaks were considered to *lead* both LH and FSH by one time unit (10 min), a total of 5 lagged triple coincidences was observed. The distribution of group coincidences demonstrated by computer simulations (solid curve) was approximated closely by a Poisson distribution (interrupted curve). (D) Specificity of the significant lagged triple coincidences among LH, FSH, and prolactin. Various lags of LH and/or FSH compared to an arbitrarily stationary prolactin pulse series were tested for triply coincident pulses. A lag of "+1" indicates that the indicated series leads the prolactin series by one time unit (10 min), whereas "−1" denotes that the indicated series follows the prolactin series by 10 min. For example, at a lag of "−1" for both LH and FSH (i.e., prolactin leads both other time series by one time unit), 5 triple coincidences were observed. At zero lags for both LH and FSH (all three peaks are simultaneous), 13 triple coincidences were recognized. And, at LH and FSH lags of "+1" (prolactin lags both other time series by one time unit), there were 8 triple coincidences. None of the other various combinations of lags shown resulted in a significant number of triple coincidences. Horizontal interrupted lines denote $p = 0.05$, $p = 0.0001$, and $p < 10^{-5}$ α levels for random triple coincidences based on the relevant distribution of expected coincidences in 30,000 groups of six triply pulsating independent hormone time series, each comprising the relevant number of synthetic LH, FSH, and prolactin peaks. [Adapted with permission from J. D. Veldhuis *et al.* (19).]

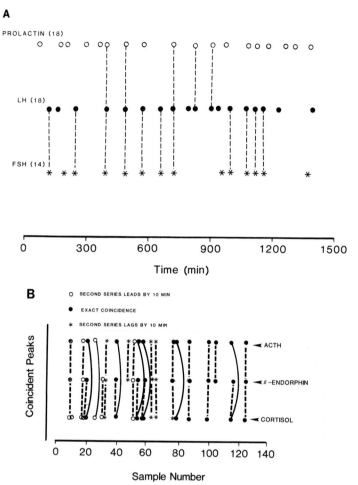

FIG. 11   Illustrative schematized profiles of doubly and triply coincident pulsations in (A) Schematized coincidences among prolactin, LH, and FSH peaks. 24-hr LH, FSH, and prolactin time series in one estrogen-unreplaced postmenopausal woman. The volunteer underwent blood sampling at 10-min intervals for 24 hr. The subsequent 145 serum samples were subjected to radioimmunoassay to quantitate LH, FSH, and prolactin concentrations. The resulting time series were evaluated by Cluster analysis (23) to mark individually significant pulses of hormone release. The number of discrete peaks per series is given in parentheses. Coincident events (zero lag) are noted by interrupted vertical lines. (B) Coincidence data derived from ACTH, β-endorphin, and cortisol measurements in a normal man sampled as subject in A. Coincident pulse pairs and triples are shown. [J. D. Veldhuis, M. L. Johnson, and E. Seneta, unpublished data.]

the apparent number of peaks in the series with fewer peaks is increased by a factor equal to the number of possible "locations" a peak can occupy (e.g., for a 10-min window, three locations are generated).§ The latter concept helps explain why very high coincidence rates often have been reported in the literature, when a *window* of coincidence is considered. Thus, we emphasize that presumptively significant coincidence rates within a window of peak overlap must be interpreted with special caution unless the appropriate statistical limits for random peak overlap have been calculated.

Coincidence of Actual Secretory Events

Under conditions in which secretory events per se can be discerned, e.g., by deconvolution analysis, the foregoing statistical concepts will also be relevant to understanding the temporally coordinated behavior of endocrine *secretory* bursts. The latter must be investigated directly or estimated by deconvolution methods [see Chapter 18 in this volume, and (24, 26)]. Such studies can examine the physiological mechanisms subserving significant synchrony of secretory events whether controlled at the level of the secretory gland, nerve terminal, or target organ.

Specific Concordance Index

A complementary way to evaluate concordance between two neurohormone pulse series is the so-called specific concordance index (27). This important strategy has been described in detail elsewhere and applies well to paired

§ For a lag of ±one time unit (e.g., a "window" of ±1 sample, in which the two coincident events may occur in any order), the probability of observing exactly x_d coincidences is

$$\Pr(X_d = x_d) = \frac{\binom{3m}{x_d}\binom{z - 3m}{n - x_d}}{\binom{z}{n}}, \qquad x_d = 0, 1, \ldots \min(3m, n) \tag{A2}$$

The expected number of two-way coincidences can be given as

$$E(X_d) = 3mn/z \tag{A3}$$

with variance

$$\mathrm{Var}(X_d) = \frac{3mn}{z}\left(1 - \frac{(n - 1)}{(z - 1)}\right)\left(1 - \frac{3m}{z}\right) \tag{A4}$$

series. At present, no one has generalized this methodology to three or more series, in contrast to the specific hypergeometric and higher-order combinatorial algebra given above.

Statistical Power Analysis

An important question that the experimentalist confronts is the statistical power of his analysis. By power, we mean 1-β, where β is the probability of a type II statistical error, or the probability of falsely accepting a null hypothesis of no effect (or a null hypothesis of purely random associations in the case of coincidences). Thus, power is a measure of the expectation that, when no significant copulsatility is identified, significant copulsatility was indeed not overlooked. To our knowledge the literature contains no data to aid the investigator in calculating the power of his coincidence analysis. In general, a desired level of statistical power is in the range of 0.85 or higher (85% power or greater). We have recently applied computer simulations to the question of power analysis in coincidence studies. This important predictive information is summarized below.

To address the statistical power question, we can simulate paired pulsatile hormone series of defined peak frequencies and sample numbers. We assume that an investigator has some initial data available consisting of a particular sampling schedule (and hence a known number of samples over the time interval) with pilot measurements from several animals or subjects with individually enumerated peak frequencies for the two hormones. We then ask the question, "What group size is required for any particular power to demonstrate nonrandom coincidence at some particular α-level (or p value), assuming that the observed numbers of peaks and coincidences in the pilot data are generally representative of expectation for the larger series being planned?" By α-level, we mean the probability of falsely rejecting the null hypothesis of no significant coincidence. Thus, in order to estimate the statistical power, the investigator must obtain pilot data that include estimates of the pulse frequency of the two hormones and the number of coincidences detected in a small group of animals or volunteers. As shown in Fig. 12, given starting estimates of pulse frequency and numbers of coincident pulses in preliminary experiments, the number of subjects required for a given statistical power (1-β) can be estimated. These so-called power curves are generated with or without assuming a normal approximation to the hypergeometric probability distribution of the expected number of random peak associations between concentrated pairs of pulse trains in the group of subjects (19, 28). The algebraic estimate of the statistical power inherent in a given experimental context is given by Eq. (19).

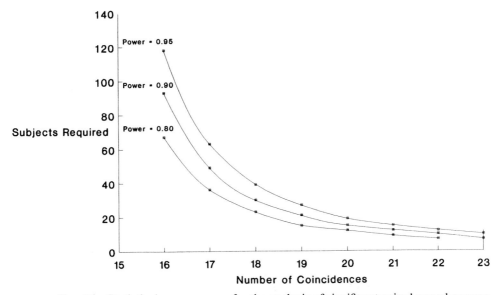

FIG. 12   Statistical power curves for the analysis of significant paired neurohormone pulse coincidence rates given initial pilot observations on the basal pulse frequencies in the two series and their apparent coincidence rates in a subset of six subjects or animals. The curves are given for three different statistical powers $(1-\beta,$ where β is the probability of a type II error of falsely accepting the null hypothesis of purely random concordance). The vertical axis denotes the number of subjects or animals required in the final study in order to achieve the indicated statistical power. The latter is a measure of the expectation of not overlooking significant coincidences between the two series. The horizontal axis stipulates the total number of coincidences observed in the concatenated pilot series, which we assume here consist of 144 blood samples/24 hr and 18 peaks (mean) in each series. An α-level of 0.05 is assumed. [J. D. Veldhuis, M. L. Johnson, and L. M. Faunt, unpublished data.]

$$x^* \approx \frac{N}{143}\left(\frac{m_0}{N_0}\right)\left(\frac{n_0}{N_0}\right) + 1.645\sqrt{\frac{N}{143}\left(\frac{m_0}{N_0}\right)\left(\frac{n_0}{N_0}\right)\left(1 - \frac{m_0}{143\,N_0}\right)\left(1 - \frac{n_0}{143\,N_0}\right)}$$

$$x^* \approx NA + 1.645\,B\sqrt{N}$$

$$A = \frac{1}{143}\left(\frac{m_0}{N_0}\right)\left(\frac{n_0}{N_0}\right) \qquad B = \sqrt{A\left(1 - \frac{m_0}{143\,N_0}\right)\left(1 - \frac{n_0}{143\,N_0}\right)}$$

$$m = \frac{N}{N_0}m_0 \qquad n = \frac{N}{N_0}n_0 \qquad\qquad (19)$$

$$\beta = \frac{\displaystyle\sum_{x \leq 0}^{x} \frac{\binom{m}{x}\binom{143\,N - m}{n - x}}{(143\,N)} p_c^x (p_1 - p_c)^{m-x} (p_2 - p_c)^{n-x} (1 - p_1 - p_2 + p_c)^{143\,N - n - m + x}}{\displaystyle\sum_{\substack{0 \leq x}}^{m \leq n(m,n)} \frac{\binom{m}{x}\binom{143\,N - m}{n - x}}{\binom{143\,N}{n}} p_c^x (p_1 - p_c)^{m-x} (p_2 - p_c)^{n-x} (1 - p_1 - p_2 + p_c)^{143\,N - n - m + x}}$$

$$p_1 = \frac{m_0}{143\,N_0} \qquad p_2 = \frac{n_0}{143\,N_0}$$

$$p_c = \frac{C_0}{143\,N_0}$$

$$\Pr_0(x^* \geq x) \approx \alpha = 0.05$$

Where variables are defined as follows (assuming 145 samples/series): N_0, number of subjects in pilot study; $m_0\ n_0$, total number of peaks in each of the two concatenated pilot study series; c_0, total number of coincidences between peaks in the two concatenated pilot study series; N, total number of subjects needed in final study; m, n, total number of peaks in each of the two concatenated final study series; x, total number of coincidences in final study; x^*, number of coincidences such that null hypothesis is rejected at α-level $p = 0.05$; p_1, p_2, a priori probabilities, based on the pilot study, of observing a peak at a particular position in one of the two concatenated final study series; p_c, a priori probability, based on the pilot study, of observing a coincidence at a particular position, between peaks in the two concatenated final study series.

Note that the normal approximation to the hypergeometric distribution is

$$x^* = NA + 1.645\,B\sqrt{N}$$
$$= \left(\frac{N}{143}\right)\left(\frac{m_0}{N_0}\right)\left(\frac{n_0}{N_0}\right) + 1.645\,B\sqrt{N} \tag{19A}$$
$$= 143\,N p_1 p_2 + 1.645\,B\sqrt{N}$$

which is of the form

$$x^* = \mu + 1.645\,\sigma \tag{19B}$$

which holds if

$$\mu = 143\,N p_1 p_2 \qquad \frac{\sigma^2}{\mu} = (1 - p_1)(1 - p_2) \tag{19C}$$

TABLE I   Estimates of Statistical Power of Coincidence Testing[a]

Conditions	Power = 0.80 (β = 0.20)	Power = 0.90 (β = 0.10)	Power = 0.95 (β = 0.05)
145 samples/subject (No. = 11)	7 (7)	10 (10)	14 (12)
289 samples/subject (No. = 18)	7 (12)	10 (15)	20 (20)
6 pilot subjects (No. = 19)	11 (15)	16 (21)	21 (27)
A: 14 peaks B: 18 peaks (No. = 9)	6 (7)	16 (21)	21 (27)

[a] Comparison of the (Eq. 19) algebraic estimates of the number (in parentheses) of study subjects required for an indicated statistical power with those of computerized (Monte-Carlo) simulations for typical midrange numbers of coincidences between the concatenated series A and B in a group of subjects. We assumed a pilot group size of three subjects or six where indicated above, in which there are 145 blood samples collected in series A and B, and a mean of 18 peaks per subject in series A and 18 peaks per subject in series B, except as noted. An α (p value)-level of 0.05 is assumed.

As summarized in Table I, the computer simulations and the algebraic predictions behave relatively congruently over a range of tested pilot conditions; i.e., variable numbers of observed peaks and coincidences in small study groups. The above algebraic predictor of statistical power for paired coincidence testing is available as a short program that will run on most personal computers.

Group Probability Estimates

We suggest several approaches to address the query, "Is the coincident behavior of the paired, triple, or quadruple neurohormone pulse series, considered for the group of subjects as a whole, significantly nonrandom?"

i. A χ^2 test of the observed versus expected (Eqs. 4, 11, or 14) numbers of coincidences for the N subjects or a χ^2 statistic equal to the sum of the natural logarithms of the individual p values

ii. A concatenation of all individual series, as suggested in Eqs. (7)–(9) (above)

iii. A normal (z-score) approximation for a large group, see Eq. (10) (above)

iv. A Poisson approximation for smaller groups, see Eq. (15) (above)

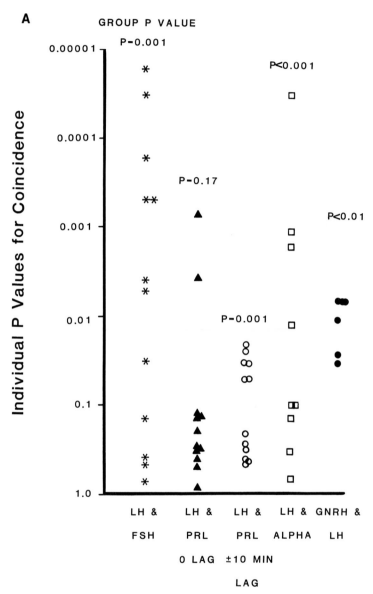

FIG. 13   (A) Individual p (α) values for individual subjects (LH, FSH, α-subunit) or sheep (GnRH, LH), in whom nonrandom coincidence was evaluated. The group p

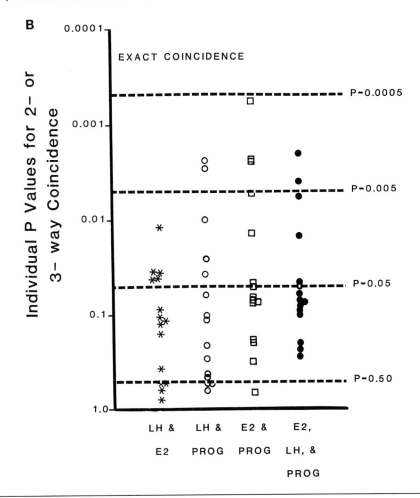

values by concatenation Eqs. (7)–(9) are given at the top of each column, assuming the null hypothesis that p values are distributed randomly and uniformly between zero and unity. [Adapted with permission J. D. Veldhuis, *et al.* (16).] Individual p values in women for the (nonrandom) coincidence of estradiol (E_2), progesterone (PROG), and LH pulses identified by Cluster analysis following blood sampling at 15-min intervals for 24 hr in the luteal phase of the menstrual cycle. All group p values were significant statistically when tested as in A. [Unpublished figure adapted from data presented in W. G. Rossmanith *et al.* (11).]

v. A Kolmogorov–Smirnov test of the null hypothesis that the N individual p values in the group are randomly and uniformly distributed between zero and unity

We tend to favor choices (i) and (v) above. Choice (ii) is illustrated in Fig. 13. Choice (ii) assumes a similar structure in individual and group data, whereas our simulations suggest that concatenation tends to produce somewhat smaller p values perhaps overestimating the odds against randomness. Choices (iii) and (iv) are nominal approximations that appear to yield reasonable estimates of group p values.

Summary

We have reviewed classical cross-correlation analysis as modified with autoregressive modeling to correct for intrinsic autocorrelation in neuroendocrine time series as a robust and useful complementary tool for assessing the coupling between two neuroendocrine pulse trains. However, cross-correlation analysis cannot be applied to three series evaluated simultaneously, but rather must be applied pairwise. Moreover, cross-correlation analysis does not account for the occurrence of discrete and delimited events in the data or address the question of how often such individual events occur together compared to expected coincidence based on chance associations alone. Such discrete coincidence testing can be approached using computer simulations, as reviewed here and elsewhere. In addition, we show that explicit conditional probability analysis can be applied assuming binary, hypergeometric, or higher-order combinatorial algebra (reviewed above). All calculations can be carried out in a few seconds on a personal computer. We emphasize that probability analysis that assumes a random uniform distribution of peak locations over time would be inappropriate when there are strong systematic variations in pulse frequency throughout the sampling session. In those circumstances, we recommend the use of computer-stimulation methods. Finally, specific concordance values (27) can be calculated on microprocessors, so as to estimate the extent of concordance observed beyond that expected on the basis of chance assortment of the pulses. Of considerable practical importance to the experimental neuroscientist, we show that power analysis can be carried out to make preliminary estimates of the group sizes required for detecting a given degree of nonrandom concordance between two neurohormone series. Finally, we emphasize that no concordance testing is more accurate or valid than the sampling paradigm and the pulse-detection methodology applied to enumerate the number and location of discrete neurohormonal release episodes in the data (1, 21, 24, 27, 29–32).

Acknowledgments

We thank Patsy Craig for her skillful preparation of the manuscript, Paula P. Azimi for the artwork and laboratory assistance, Sandra Jackson and the expert nursing staff at the University of Virginia Clinical Research Center for conduct of the clinical research protocols, and Drs. Alan D. Rogol and Randall J. Urban for sharing their gonadotropin data. This work was supported in part by NIH Grant No. RR00847 to the University of Virginia Clinical Research Center, RCDA No. 1 K04 HD00634 (J.D.V.), NIH Grants AM-30302 and GM-28928 (M.L.J.), Diabetes Endocrinology Research Center Grant No. 5 P60 AM 22125-05, NIH-supported Clinfo Data Reduction Systems, Baxter Laboratories (Round Lake, IL), and the National Science Foundation Science Center for Biological Timing (J.D.V., M.L.J., L.F.).

References

1. R. J. Urban, W. S. Evans, A. D. Rogol, D. L. Kaiser, M. L. Johnson, and J. D. Veldhuis, *Endocr. Rev.* **9,** 3 (1988).
2. W. S. Evans, E. Christiansen, R. J. Urban, A. D. Rogol, M. L. Johnson, and J. D. Veldhuis, *Endocr. Rev.* **13,** 81 (1992).
3. L. A. Frohman, T. R. Downs, I. J. Clarke, and G. B. Thomas, *J. Clin. Invest.* **86,** 17 (1990).
4. D. T. Krieger and W. Allen, *J. Clin. Endocrinol. Metab.* **10,** 675 (1975).
5. P. M. Plotsky and W. Vale, *Science* **230,** 461 (1985).
6. S. L. Alexander and C. H. G. Irvine, *J. Endocrinol.* **114,** 351 (1987).
7. N. S. Cetel and S. S. C. Yen, *J. Clin. Endocrinol. Metab.* **56,** 1313 (1983).
8. D. L. Clifton, S. Aksel, W. J. Bremner, *et al., J. Clin. Endocrinol. Metab.* **67,** 832 (1988).
9. S. N. Pavlou, J. D. Veldhuis, J. Lindner, K. H. Souza, R. J. Urban, J. E. Rivier, W. W. Vale, and D. J. Stallard, *J. Clin. Endocrinol. Metab.* **70,** 1472 (1990).
10. C. R. Pohl, R. I. Weiner, and M. S. Smith, *Endocrinology (Baltimore)* **123,** 1591 (1988).
11. W. G. Rossmanith, G. A. Laughlin, J. F. Mortola, M. L. Johnson, J. D. Veldhuis, and S. S. C. Yen, *J. Clin. Endocrinol. Metab.* **70,** 990 (1990).
12. P. H. Rowe, P. A. Racey, G. A. Lincoln, M. Ellwood, J. Lehane, and J. C. Shenton, *J. Endocrinol.* **64,** 17 (1975).
13. M. H. Samuels, J. D. Veldhuis, P. Henry, and E. C. Ridgway, *J. Clin. Endocrinol. Metab.* **71,** 425 (1990).
14. J. D. Veldhuis, J. C. King, R. J. Urban, A. D. Rogol, A. Evans WS, L. A. Kolp, and M. L. Johnson, *J. Clin. Endocrinol. Metab.* **65,** 929 (1987).
15. J. D. Veldhuis, W. S. Evans, L. A. Kolp, A. D. Rogol, and M. L. Johnson, *J. Clin. Endocrinol. Metab.* **66,** 414 (1988).
16. J. D. Veldhuis, A. Iranmanesh, I. Clarke, D. L. Kaiser, and M. L. Johnson, *J. Neuroendocrinol.* **1,** 185 (1989).

17. J. D. Veldhuis, A. Iranmanesh, M. L. Johnson, and G. Lizarralde, *J. Clin. Endocrinol. Metab.* **71,** 452 (1990).
18. J. D. Veldhuis and M. L. Johnson, *J. Clin. Endocrinol. Metab.* **67,** 116 (1988).
19. J. D. Veldhuis, M. L. Johnson, and E. Seneta, *J. Clin. Endocrinol. Metab.* **73,** 569 (1991).
20. J. D. Veldhuis, M. L. Johnson, E. Seneta, and A. Iranmanesh, *Acta Endocrinol. (Copenhagen)* **126,** 193 (1992).
21. J. D. Veldhuis, A. B. Lassiter, and M. L. Johnson, *Am. J. Physiol.* **259,** E351 (1990).
22. C. Chatfield, p. 60, Chapman & Hall, New York, 1984.
23. J. D. Veldhuis and M. L. Johnson, *Am. J. Physiol.* **250,** E486 (1986).
24. J. D. Veldhuis and M. L. Johnson, *in* "Methods in Enzymology," (L. Brand and M. L. Johnson, eds.), Vol. 210, p. 539. Academic Press, San Diego, 1992.
25. R. C. Weast, "Standard Mathematical Tables," p. 382. Chemical Rubber Co., Cleveland, OH, 1964.
26. J. D. Veldhuis, M. L. Carlson, and M. L. Johnson, *Proc. Natl. Acad. Sci. USA* **84,** 7686 (1987).
27. V. Guardabasso, A. D. Genazzani, J. D. Veldhuis, and D. Rodbard, *Acta Endocrinol. (Copenhagen)* **124,** 208 (1991).
28. W. V. R. Vieweg, J. D. Veldhuis, and R. M. Carey, *Am. J. Physiol.* **262,** F871 (1992).
29. R. J. Urban, M. L. Johnson, and J. D. Veldhuis, *Am. J. Physiol.* **257,** E88 (1989).
30. J. D. Veldhuis and M. L. Johnson, *Am. J. Physiol.* **255,** E749 (1988).
31. J. D. Veldhuis, W. S. Evans, M. L. Johnson, and A. D. Rogol, *J. Clin. Endocrinol. Metab.* **62,** 881 (1986).
32. R. J. Urban, M. L. Johnson, and J. D. Veldhuis, *Endocrinology (Baltimore)* **128,** 2008 (1991).

[18] Estimating Thyrotropin Secretory Activity by a Deconvolution Procedure

Klaus Prank and Georg Brabant

With the improvement of assay systems for hormone determinations and frequent blood sampling methods episodic hormone secretion has been established as a physiological phenomenon and the importance of time-dependant processes for the regulation of endocrine systems has been described (see references 1–3 for an overview). Attempts to differentiate biologically relevant hormone pulses from assay noise led to the development of a number of algorithms for computer-assisted analysis of these time series. None of the currently available techniques is able to reliably detect the underlying "true" secretory pattern of the endocrine gland under study, but many of these programs provide a tool to objectively compare different time series with identical criteria.

Prerequisites for the Analysis of Pulsatile Hormone Secretion

Blood Sampling

To minimize sampling noise it is important that blood be collected by highly standardized methods. This is achieved either by punctually sampling blood at fixed intervals or by continuously withdrawing blood with the help of an automatic pump system. The latter method does not provide hormone levels at a certain time but the integral of the hormonal concentrations over a time segment. With high frequency of blood sampling considerable amounts of blood are lost, thus limiting the duration of the sampling. A method to reduce this problem was proposed by T. O. F. Wagner of our group using a miniplasmapheresis capsule to collect plasma instead of whole blood (4). Even though technical problems like convection within the capsule were solved the system appeared too complicated to be reliably used on a routine basis.

Assay Systems

The development of sensitive methods for hormone determinations allows better differentiation of small alterations of hormone concentrations. The determination of the inter- and intraassay coefficient of variance (CV) is a prerequisite for the analysis of a hormonal time series as only assay systems with a low CV may be used for computer-assisted evaluation of episodic hormone secretion. To avoid the higher interassay CV, all samples of one time series should be measured in one assay, if possible, by the assay characteristics. The hormone concentrations of one or more samples in the expected range of the experiment are measured repetitively to evaluate variations due to measurement errors. This allows one to estimate the rate of false-positive peaks by the pulse-detection algorithm under study and to adjust the characteristics of the analytical methods to a projected level. The rate of false-negative peaks in a time series can be estimated by generating a model set of data with a given number of pulses and estimating the number of peaks detected by the pulse-detection algorithm.

Pulse-Detection Methods

Basically there are two different approaches for the detection of episodic hormone secretion: heuristic methods, describing the hormonal time series by characteristics of the pulse shape, duration, and velocity of increase or decrease (5–9), and methods based on a model assumption as the power spectrum analysis of a Fourier transformation of the data or deconvolution techniques (10–13).

Heuristic Methods

To distinguish true hormone pulses in the circulation from noise resulting from the blood sampling procedure and from the detetction systems used in measuring hormone concentrations, the expected noise for a certain hormone level is calculated or estimated by these programs. Assuming certain characteristics for pulse shape, duration, or velocity of up- and downstroke, a peak in the hormonal time series is accepted as a true hormone pulse when the threshold set by the noise calculation is exceeded.

Santen and Bardin Program, Baird Program, and the "Ultra" Method

The method of Santen and Bardin first published in 1973 (5) formed the basis for the development of a number of more elaborate approaches. According to the original description a pulse is defined as an increase of hormone concentration of at least 20% compared to the preceding point in the time series of the hormone concentration under study. The hormone level of the succeeding point has to be smaller than or equal to that of the pulse. Three times the coefficient of variation of the intraassay variance [of the original luteinizing hormone (LH) time series] was used alternatively as a threshold criterion. This method has some obvious disadvantages: assumption of a fixed coefficient of variation for all ranges of hormone concentration within a 24-hr rhythm and the "one-point" test for increases and decreases.

Important improvements of the Santen and Bardin algorithm were implemented in the algorithms of Baird (6) and in the Ultra method proposed by van Cauter (7). The program of Baird uses four times the assay standard deviation and two points for the detection of decreases in the hormone concentration time series, which decreases the susceptibility of the analysis for false-positive peaks.

The Ultra method introduced by van Cauter creates a time series free of assay noise by using a concentration-dependant coefficient of variation. The generated "noise-free" time series is then analyzed by the technique of Santen and Bardin.

Cluster Program

The most elaborate heuristic method for pulse detection based on the original method of Santen and Bardin was published by Veldhuis and Johnson (9). This algorithm iteratively scans the time series for significant increases and decreases of hormone concentration assuming certain criteria for the shape of a hormone pulse (peak). It must be surrounded by two valleys, which do not have any significant variations and are limited by a significant increase. A pooled t statistic is used to test a cluster of m data points versus a preceding cluster of n data points for significant increases as well as decreases. The size of the peak/valley cluster and the thresholds for the t values can be chosen freely to define a significant increase or decrease. Comparison to a noise series allows estimation of the rate of the detection of false-positive pulses.

After significant increases are detected, the time series is scanned for significant decreases. The measurement error necessary for calculating the t statistic is obtained from the duplicates or triplicates of the hormonal time series under study or by one of nine variance models. It has been shown that the Cluster program works very well for a hormone concentration time series with a large signal-to-noise ratio as, e.g., LH (14). As the t values, the threshold for an upstroke and a downstroke, can be set independently, the detection of pulses, especially in a time series of hormones with a pronounced circadian rhythm such as TSH, is much better compared to those obtained with the Santen and Bardin approach. However, hormonal pulses occurring with high frequency may not be detected as separate peaks but fused to large pulses.

Pulsar Program

The Pulsar program (8) uses a different approach for pulse detection than the methods discussed above. It first removes long-term trends as the circadian rhythm from the time series by using a smoothing procedure to calculate a baseline. In a second step, the difference between the smoothed time series and the original time series is calculated for each time step and scanned for the presence of peaks. Then, the time series of residuals (differences) is scaled in units of the standard deviation which is calculated for each point of the time series. Peaks are identified by the combined criteria of length and height. The residuals of all points belonging to a peak of length n must exceed the value $G(n)$, which is the threshold criterion for a pulse of length n scaled in units of the standard deviation. Thus the Pulsar program is able to select both narrow high peaks and broader peaks with a lower amplitude. The threshold criteria $G(n)$ can be chosen based on different types of distribution of assay noise or on theoretical considerations. Points meeting the threshold criteria are detected as pulses. After the detection of pulses a new baseline is obtained by the smoothing procedure, assigning a smaller weight to points belonging to peaks. This pulse-detection procedure is repeated iteratively until a fixed number of iterations is reached or until no further changes in the analyzed pulsatile pattern occur.

The "window" used for the smoothing procedure is important for the application of the Pulsar program to the analysis of hormones with a circadian pattern of secretion. Selecting a window that is too long only allows detection of a single peak for the circadian variation. Selecting a too small window leads to a variable baseline which obscures peak detection.

Model-Based Methods

Analysis of the Power Spectrum

One model-based approach is the analysis of the power spectrum using Fourier transformation (15). In this analysis the time series is modeled by the assumption of periodic phenomena, namely, the sum of sine and cosine waves. Characteristic frequencies of oscillation and their intensity in the time series under study are determined. However, no information about the temporal location of the characteristic oscillations is provided by this method.

Deconvolution Techniques

Other model-based approaches for pulse detection are deconvolution techniques estimating the secretory activity of the gland under study. They assume a compartmental model in which a hormone is secreted into one or multiple compartment(s) from which it decays with one or two half-lives (decay rates). The method of the discrete (stepwise) deconvolution estimates

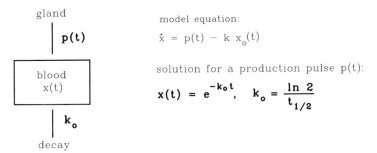

FIG. 1 One-compartment model for hormone secretion.

the secretory activity of the gland from information contained in the hormone concentration time series. The decay rate of the hormone under study or two decay rates in the case of a two-compartment model have to be defined experimentally or to be estimated.

"Detect" Program The "Detect" program (10) developed from techniques used in chromatographic peak detection (16) was the first to introduce discrete deconvolution in the analysis of hormonal time series. This method is a mixture of heuristic and model-based approaches, since hormone peaks are determined by a heuristic approach using curve-fitting techniques and *t* statistic for pulse detection. Detect uses discrete deconvolution to obtain an estimate of the secretory activity (instantaneous rate of secretion) of the gland under study. The time series of the secretory activity is then evaluated for peaks, again using the heuristic pulse-detection method described briefly above.

DESADE Program (Detection of Episodic Secretory Activity by Discrete Deconvolution) In contrast to the Detect program, the DESADE program, which was developed by U. Ranft of our group (12, 13), uses the assay noise (measurement error) and its propagation to the values of the secretory activity for separating significant signals from those in the range of the assay noise.

The DESADE algorithm is based on a simple model assumption. A gland secretes its hormone into the blood (one compartment) from where it decays with one half-life. This one-compartment model is described by a first-order differential equation (Fig. 1).

A two-compartment model better adapted to physiological situations describes the hormonal clearance as a process with two phases. In this approach the hormonal storage (compartment) is separated into a primary storage, the blood, and a secondary storage, the interstitium. A prerequisite for two significantly different decay rates is that the hormonal clearance from the secondary storage (interstitium) be much slower than the main clearance from the primary storage (blood). One major advantage of the one-compartment model compared to the two-compartment model is that the one-compartment model depends on one parameter only, whereas the two-compartment model requires three parameters (the two half-lives and the fraction of the fast to the slow component of decay).

Discrete Deconvolution   Discrete deconvolution is used to obtain an estimation of hormone production from the secretory gland. Since we are dealing with a hormone concentration time series with discrete, equally spaced measurements we cannot use a deconvolution applying the Laplace transformation for an exact solution. Only an approximate solution can be provided by using the discrete deconvolution:

$$f(i) = x(i) - \sum_{j=1}^{\infty} f(i-j) g(j)$$

$g(j)$ being the solution of the model equation (Fig. 1) at time j and $f(i) \geq 0$.

Since the length of the time series is finite, in our cases 24 hr, the autoregressive expression must be replaced by an approximation. However, the error induced by this approximation is much smaller than that induced by the step from the continuous to the discrete form of the solution:

$$f(i) = x(i) - x(i-t-1) g(t+1) - \sum_{j=1}^{t} f(i-j) g(j)$$

where $t = 5\, t_{\mathrm{HL1}}$ with t_{HL1} being the larger half-life of the model; $x(-i) = x(n+1-i); f(-i) = f(n+1-i); i = 1, \ldots, n; f(i)$, instantaneous secretory activity (ISA) or hormone production function; $x(i)$, hormone concentration time series; and $g(j)$, solution of the model equation (Fig. 1).

$$g(j) = e^{-kt}$$

with $k = \ln 2/t_{\mathrm{HL}}$ being the decay rate (one-compartment model).

$$g(j) = A e^{-k_1 t} + (1 - A) e^{-k_2 t}$$

with $k_1 = \ln 2/t_{\mathrm{HL}_1}$, $k_2 = \ln 2/t_{\mathrm{HL}_2}$ (two-compartment model) A, fraction of the fast component of decay; k_1, decay rate for the fast component; k_2, decay rate for the slow component.

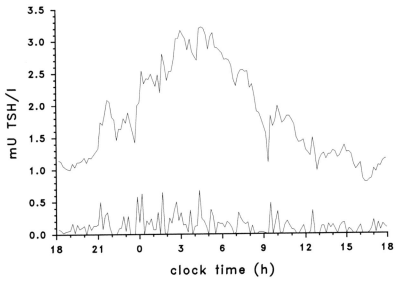

FIG. 2   Twenty-four-hour TSH time series and instantaneous secretory activity (ISA). Negative values of the ISA are cut off.

The secretory activity $f(i)$ of the gland is determined for each time step i of the hormone concentration time series $x(i)$ applying this recursive equation until $j = 5\ t_{HL}$ (Fig. 2).

Significant Secretory Activity   The time series of the secretory activity reveals shorter pulses than the original data set as the smoothing by the half-life of the hormone is removed by discrete deconvolution. In principle, one of the above-mentioned heuristic programs can be used to detect pulses within the time series of the secretory activity. For the analysis of the secretory pattern of TSH secretion we have developed another very simple heuristic approach for detecting significant pulses. A global threshold is calculated which separates significant from nonsignificant secretory activities. This approach is based on the assumption that the calculated values of the secretory activity comprise three components: a basal activity of the gland (in the sense of noise), a significantly higher activity, and a propagation of the assay noise. A fourth component might be considered comprising a systematic violation of the model assumption, where negative secretory activities occur. We assume in our approach that the basal secretory activity of the gland under study and the assay noise are of similar orders of magnitude. Secretory pulsatile activities of the gland, however, are of different

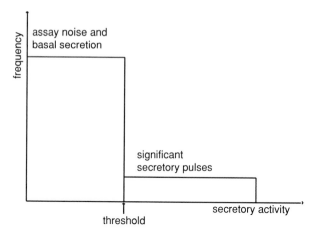

FIG. 3   Frequency distribution of the secretory activity.

orders of magnitude and can be detected by using an appropriate threshold. Two different approaches have been implemented into the DESADE program to determine this threshold value: estimating the threshold by error propagation or by a distribution model of the error.

Estimating the threshold by error propagation   Duplicates or triplicates of the hormone concentration measurement allow an estimation of the assay noise and the propagation of the measurement error by discrete deconvolution. The time series of duplicates or triplicates is split into individual time series of single determinations which are separately analyzed by discrete deconvolution, and the standard error of the secretory activity is determined for each time step. The threshold is estimated from the histogram of the propagated standard error of the secretory activity freely choosing a certain percentage. This percentage may be regarded as an error probability for the detection of significant secretory activity.

Estimating the threshold by a distribution model of the error   It is possible to create a simple model for the distribution of the secretory activity assuming that this activity is composed of different components as shown above. The propagated measurement error and the basal secretory activity, on one hand, as well as the significant activity, on the other, overlap. This leads to a "step"-like frequency distribution (Fig. 3). The step defines the threshold separating significant from nonsignificant secretory activity. For practical purposes, a distribution function is better suited for finding the threshold than a histogram. An iterative procedure scans for a significant change of slope of a regression line, which runs through those parts of the distribution

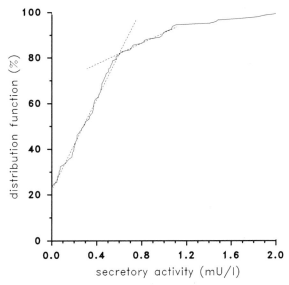

FIG. 4   Determination of the threshold for significant secretory pulses.

function which belong to the basal secretion and the measurement error (Fig. 4). The procedure starts at the secretory activity with the value zero. DESADE contains two different methods for determining this point of slope change, both of which need two parameters. The slope of the regression line (to the current point of search on the distribution function) is compared to the slope of the regression line running through a fixed number of succeeding points.

The difference between both methods is that one method uses a freely chosen factor for the slope difference and the other uses a t statistic for correlation coefficients with an adjustable error probability to test for different slopes.

Multiple-Parameter Deconvolution Model   Veldhuis *et al.* (11) have proposed a multiple-parameter deconvolution model which allows an even more subtle estimation of the parameter of secretion using nonlinear least-square parameter estimation. The deconvolution procedure which is used following a preliminary detection of significant hormone pulses by the Cluster program affords the estimation of a high number of variables.

Performance of Different Heuristic or Model-Based Algorithms in the Detection of Pulsatile TSH Secretion

Twenty-one healthy male volunteers were investigated for pulsatile TSH secretion by sampling blood every 10 min over 24 hr via an indwelling venous catheter. TSH was measured by a sensitive immunoradiometric assay (IRMA) system with an inter- and intraassay CV of less than 8%. Pulsatile secretion of TSH was measured by the power spectrum of the Fourier-transformed series, by Cluster and Pulsar analysis, and by the DESADE technique. Two points were chosen for scanning significant increases and decreases in the hormone concentration time series by the Cluster program using a pooled t statistic. The threshold for the t values was defined as 5.0 for an upstroke and 1.0 for a downstroke. To fit the assay variation from the hormone concentration data a linear model was chosen.

To overcome the problem of the Pulsar program analyzing pulses despite the marked circadian variation of TSH secretion, the width of the smoothing window was reduced to 4 hr (24 data points). The G parameters used for pulse detection were $G(1) = 3.98$; $G(2) = 2.40$; $G(3) = 1.68$; $G(4) = 1.24$; $G(5) = 0.93$.

For the DESADE analysis a one-compartment model with a single half-life [100 min. assumed for TSH (17)] was applied.

Statistical evaluation was performed by the Student's paired or unpaired t test. Data are given as the mean ± SD.

Comparing the results of the pulse-detection analysis by the deconvolution procedure DESADE with those of the heuristic approaches Cluster and Pulsar, we found a significantly higher number of pulses within 24 hr with the DESADE program than with the Cluster or the Pulsar program in any subject under study (Table I, Fig. 5). These pulses clustered during the evening rise of TSH suggesting that an increased activity of the pituitary gland is responsible for the higher nightly TSH levels. The TSH pulse amplitude appeared to be similar, but one has to bear in mind that all programs define the pulse amplitude differently.

Investigating the pulsatile pattern of TSH secretion in three 8-hr segments (2000 to 0400, 0400 to 1200, 1200 to 2000 hr) the impact of pulsatile TSH secretion for the circadian pattern of TSH could be analyzed. Systematic differences between the three methods were seen. The DESADE and Cluster algorithms detected most of the pulses in the nightly segment between 2000 and 0400 hr whereas the Pulsar program revealed an almost uniform distribution of pulses over the three 8-hr segments (Table II). The deconvolution technique DESADE compared to the Cluster method provided an even more

TABLE I   Analysis of the 24-hr Pulsatile Pattern of TSH Secretion in 21 Healthy Male Subjects with the DESADE, Cluster, and Pulsar Methods as Well as the Power Spectrum

Method of analysis	Number of pulses in 24 hr	Mean pulse amplitude (mU TSH/liter)
DESADE	14.0 ± 4.5^a	0.51 ± 0.21
Cluster	10.8 ± 1.6^b	0.52 ± 0.20
Pulsar	6.9 ± 2.2^c	0.54 ± 0.20
Power spectrum	Characteristic frequencies: 24 hr 133 min 33 min	

[a] $p < 0.01$, DESADE vs Cluster.
[b] $p < 0.0001$, DESADE vs Pulsar.
[c] $p < 0.0001$, Cluster vs Pulsar.

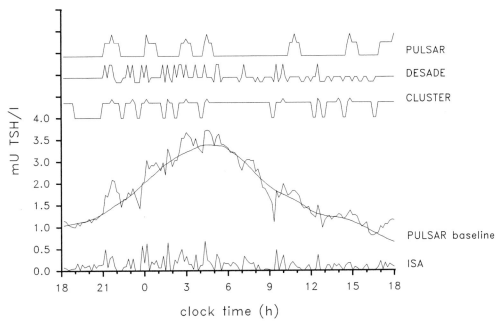

FIG. 5   Twenty-four-hour TSH secretion in one healthy male subject. Original 24-hr TSH serum concentration time series; baseline computed by the Pulsar method; instantaneous secretory activity (ISA); pulse-detection analysis with the DESADE, Cluster, and Pulsar programs.

TABLE II　Analysis of Pulsatile TSH Secretion in 8-hr Segments in 21 Healthy Male Subjects

Method	2000–0400 hr	0400–1200 hr	1200–2000 hr
DESADE			
Number of pulses/8 hr	7.1 ± 2.9	4.1 ± 2.4	2.8 ± 1.6
(% of 24 hr total)	$(51)^a$	$(29)^b$	(20)
TSH secreted/pulse (mU/liter)	0.57 ± 0.34^c	0.45 ± 0.17^d	0.40 ± 0.15
Total TSH (mU/liter) secreted in	4.0 ± 2.9	1.9 ± 1.3	1.2 ± 1.2
pulses (% of 24 hr total)	$(56)^e$	$(27)^b$	(17)
Cluster			
Number of pulses/8 hr	4.5 ± 1.0	3.2 ± 1.3	3.2 ± 0.9
(% of 24 hr total)	$(42)^e$	$(29)^d$	(29)
Pulse amplitude (mU TSH/liter)	0.68 ± 0.43^c	0.45 ± 0.19^d	0.39 ± 0.17
Total area under TSH pulses	204 ± 104	152 ± 82	68 ± 48
(mU/TSH/liter, % of 24 hr total)	$(48)^f$	$(36)^g$	(16)
Pulsar			
Number of pulses/8 hr	2.3 ± 1.2	2.3 ± 1.6	2.4 ± 1.5
(% of 24 hr total)	$(33)^f$	$(33)^d$	(34)
Pulse amplitude (mU TSH/liter)	0.60 ± 0.39^c	0.42 ± 0.26^d	0.44 ± 0.23

[a] $p < 0.001$, vs 0400–1200 hr.
[b] $p < 0.05$, vs 1200–2000 hr.
[c] $p < 0.05$, vs 0400–1200 hr.
[d] ns, vs 1200–2000 hr.
[e] $p < 0.01$, vs 0400–1200 hr.
[f] ns, vs 0400–1200 hr.
[g] $p < 0.001$, vs 1200–2000 hr.

pronounced circadian variation of the pulse frequency in the 8-hr segments, showing a significantly higher number of pulses between the second (0400–1200 hr) and third 8-hr segment (1200–2000 hr). A circadian variation of the mean pulse amplitude was detected in the analysis of the 8-hr segments by all three methods. The total amount of hormone secreted in TSH pulses varied significantly in the Cluster and DESADE analysis, but not in the Pulsar approach.

Visual inspection of the 24-hr TSH rhythms agrees with the results found by the Cluster and DESADE analysis. In contrast, the Pulsar program systematically revealed a lower number of TSH pulses and no clear circadian pattern of secretion. The close concordance between the Cluster and the DESADE program in the proportion of pulsatile secreted TSH during the various time segments suggests that these methods may be capable of providing a fair estimate of the underlying physiological TSH pulsatility. Deconvolution of the time series using the DESADE program seems to distinguish more clearly small secretory activities occurring within a short time of the previous activity than does the Cluster evaluation. This impression is supported by the investigations of Veldhuis *et al.* (11) using a multicompartment model and estimation of the plasma half-life of the hormone in various time series under study. Despite considerable efforts of various groups in validating these programs and optimizing the estimates, none of the current approaches is capable of evaluating the true secretory pattern. The programs may however confidently be used to analyze distribution patterns of pulses as shown here and to objectively compare pulsatile secretion before and after manipulation as shown by many groups (18–22). New approaches using adaptive self-organized feature detectors which make fewer assumptions about the shape of a pulse or the mechanism of hormone secretion might be closer to the pattern "biologically seen" by the target cell. Further developments rest on better systems for collecting samples and measuring hormone concentrations, ideally by a biosensor for the "on-line" determination of hormone concentrations. With the knowledge of the true temporal pattern of hormone secretion new methods may be developed and standardized to extract important information from a smaller number of data points. As shown by the development of glucose biosensors, this hope may be realized in the not too distant future and may switch the analysis of temporal hormonal patterns from purely research tools to a routine diagnostic procedure.

References

1. G. Brabant, K. Prank, and C. Schöfl, *TEM* **3**, 183 (1992).
2. G. Leng, "Pulsatility in Neuroendocrine Systems." CRC Press, Boca Raton, FL, 1988.
3. W. F. Crowley, Jr., and J. G. Hofler, "Episodic Secretion of Hormones." Churchill–Livingstone, New York, 1987.
4. T. O. F. Wagner, A. Göhring, A. Prechtel *et al.*, *in* "Episodic Hormone Secretion: From Basic Science to Clinical Application." (T. O. F. Wagner and M. Filicori, eds.), p. 61. TM-Verlag, Hameln, Germany, 1987.
5. R. J. Santen and C. W. Bardin, *J. Clin. Invest.* **52**, 2617 (1973).
6. D. T. Baird, *Biol. Reprod.* **18**, 359 (1978).
7. E. van Cauter, *in* "Human Pituitary Hormones: Circadian and Episodic Variations," (E. van Cauter and G. Copinschi, eds.), p. 1. Nyhoff, The Hague, 1981.
8. G. R. Merriam and K. W. Wachter, *Am. J. Physiol.* **243**, E310 (1982).
9. J. D. Veldhuis and M. L. Johnson, *Am. J. Physiol.* **250**, E486 (1986).
10. K. E. Oerter, V. Guardabasso, and D. Rodbard, *Comput. Biomed. Res.* **19**, 170 (1986).
11. J. D. Veldhuis, M. L. Carlson, and M. L. Johnson, *Proc. Natl. Acad. Sci. U.S.A.* **84**, 7686 (1987).
12. U. Ranft, K. Prank, and G. Brabant, *Acta Endocrinol.* **117**(Suppl. 287), 79 (1988).

13. G. Brabant, K. Prank, U. Ranft, T. Schuermeyer, T. O. F. Wagner, H. Hauser, B. Kummer, H. Feistner, R. D. Hesch, and A. von zur Mühlen, *J. Clin. Endocrinol. Metab.* **70,** 403 (1990).
14. R. J. Urban, W. S. Evans, A. D. Rogol, D. L. Kaiser, M. L. Johnson, and J. D. Veldhuis, *Endocr. Rev.* **9,** 3 (1988).
15. W. J. Dixon, "BMDP Statistical Software; Program 1T: Univariate Spectral Analysis." University of California Press, Berkeley, 1981.
16. D. Rodbard, B. R. Cole, and T. Murakami, *Steroids* **34,** 1 (1979).
17. A. Law, G. W. Jack, M. Tellez, and C. J. Edmonds, *J. Endocrinol.* **110,** 375 (1986).
18. G. Brabant K. Prank, C. Hoang-Vu, R. D. Hesch, and A. von zur Mühlen, *J. Clin. Endocrinol. Metab.* **72,** 145 (1991).
19. H. J. Balks, A. Schmidt, K. Prank, F. Hemmer, A. von zur Mühlen, and G. Brabant, *J. Clin. Endocrinol. Metab.* **75,** 1198 (1992).
20. M. L. Hartmann, J. D. Veldhuis, M. L. Johnson, M. M. Lee, K. G. Alberti, E. Samojlik, and M. O. Thorner, *J. Clin. Endocrinol. Metab.* **74,** 757 (1992).
21. M. L. Vance and M. O. Thorner, *J. Clin. Endocrinol. Metab.* **68,** 1013 (1989).
22. S. N. Pavlou, J. D. Veldhuis, J. Lindner, K. H. Souza, R. J. Urban, J. E. Rivier, W. W. Vale, and D. J. Stallard, *J. Clin. Endocrinol. Metab.* **70,** 1472 (1990).

Modeling Techniques for Pulsatile Systems

[19] Modeling Modulatory Effects on Pulsatility

Jeppe Sturis, Erik Mosekilde, and Eve Van Cauter

Introduction

The observation that many hormones are secreted in a pulsatile fashion has fundamentally changed our perception of hormonal secretion and action (1–4). Clearly, stable equilibrium concentrations of hormones do not exist in general. Instead, the secretion and action of individual hormones are controlled by complicated regulatory processes, the nature of which brings about the pulsatile or oscillatory secretory patterns. For hormones that are under direct hypothalamic control, such as the gonadotropins, pulsatile release usually ultimately reflects phasic neural activation. However, these hormones are also peripherally regulated by feedback loops which could themselves cause oscillatory behavior. For hormones that are part of peripheral endocrine systems, such as insulin, oscillatory secretion is generally caused by the dynamic properties of the local regulatory network.

Modulatory effects on pulsatility may occur at various levels. First, the experimental conditions themselves, i.e., the interval of blood sampling, the precision of the assay, and the procedure for pulse detection, may markedly modulate the detection of the pulses or oscillations in peripheral blood levels. Second, independently of these experimental factors, the pattern of peripheral concentrations reflects the combination of the process of pulsatile or oscillatory secretion and clearance with presumably constant kinetics. The kinetics of hormonal clearance may result in major differences between the pattern of secretion and that of peripheral concentrations. Third, long-term periodicities controlled by the central nervous system, such as intrinsic circadian rhythmicity and sleep–wake transitions, may modulate the expression of pulsatility in the ultradian or circhoral range. Finally, in many cases, the individual neural and/or regulatory processes responsible for the generation of pulsatility interact and modulate each other's behaviors. Recent progress in the theory of nonlinear systems predicts that such interactions can lead to a variety of complex dynamic phenomena which are qualitatively different from those occurring in linear systems. Among these phenomena are mode-locking between the pulsatile subsystems, deterministic chaos, and coexisting stationary solutions. It is also possible that coupling between a slow and a rapid oscillation can lead to changes in the behavioral characteristics (amplitude and frequency) of the rapid oscillation in dependence on the phase of the slow oscillation.

Both the individual mechanisms causing pulsatility and the way in which they may be modulated by peripheral or central effects are still incompletely understood. Mathematical modeling is a tool which can be used to understand in qualitative terms the nature of the mechanisms which could be involved in the generation and modulation of pulsatility. In this chapter, we use deterministic models represented by ordinary differential equations. A fundamental feature of this approach is the assumption that essential aspects of the pulsatile behavior are systematic, i.e., the occurrence of pulses is the product of well-defined cause-and-effect relationships associated with explainable physiological processes in the individual hormone-producing cells, in the interaction between these cells, and in the interaction between the hormone production and other regulatory mechanisms in the organism. Conceptually, this is in contrast to stochastic models which assume that certain processes occur at random and/or are due to factors outside the system itself. In addition to the systematic behavior, hormonal systems may, of course, still exhibit random components.

Pulsatile hormonal systems are inherently nonlinear. Although aspects of such systems (such as, for instance, the kinetics of a particular hormone after it has been secreted) may be linear, others, including threshold and saturation mechanisms, are clearly nonlinear. In the following sections, we therefore model pulsatile or oscillatory hormonal systems using sets of nonlinear differential equations. The solution to a set of nonlinear differential equations can be a stable limit cycle, that is a self-sustained periodic oscillation which exists for certain ranges of parameter values. Characteristic of a stable limit cycle is its attracting behavior which means that the system will respond to an external perturbation by settling back into oscillatory behavior with the same period and amplitude as before the perturbation. If parameter values are modified, the simple self-sustained oscillation may become unstable and other more complex dynamical behaviors may arise through a variety of different bifurcations, i.e., qualitative changes in stationary behavior (5). It is also possible for a nonlinear system to have several coexisting stationary solutions so that the initial conditions determine the final state of the system which may thus be viewed as history dependent.

In the following sections, we briefly illustrate modulatory influences of experimental conditions, hormonal clearance kinetics, and diurnal changes using simple computer simulations. We then use deterministic nonlinear models to exemplify the type of processes that may cause pulsatile or oscillatory secretion and the various types of behaviors that may result from interactions between ultradian oscillators. Following a brief introduction, the various types of dynamic behaviors of coupled oscillators are illustrated by computer simulations and an example of a hormonal system where such behaviors may arise is given.

Modulatory Effects of Experimental Conditions

In vivo estimations of pulsatile hormonal secretion are usually based on discrete measurements of hormonal concentrations in the blood. A number of factors can influence the way in which the actual pulsatile secretory signal is recognized in the concentration profile. Among these are assay precision and methodology of pulse detection. The influences of these factors on the estimation of the pulsatile pattern are discussed in detail in Chapter 14. Another important factor which can markedly affect the observed profile is the frequency of blood sampling. Sampling rates from 1 to 20 min and lengths of sampling ranging from 1 to 24 hr have been used to characterize hormonal pulsatility. Not surprisingly, widely different results have been obtained for the same hormone depending on the sampling protocol chosen. Considerations on the total amount of blood withdrawn and on the amount of plasma needed to assay the hormones under study are obviously essential to the definition of an adequate sampling protocol. The intuitive notion that more frequent sampling will unmask more rapid episodic fluctuations has been shown to hold true for hormones such as adrenocorticotropin (ACTH), growth hormone (GH), luteinizing hormone (LH), and insulin (6–9). The definition of an optimal sampling protocol thus depends on the type of phenomenon under study. Aliasing occurs when sampling is too infrequent to ensure that all pulses are adequately represented in the profile, thus leading to an overestimation of the pulse period and/or an incorrect estimation of pulse amplitude. An example of this phenomenon is illustrated in Fig. 1 using simulated data generated by a simple nonlinear model of hormonal pulsatility which is described later. The actual pattern (dashed curve) is regular, with a strictly periodic oscillation, but because sampling was performed less frequently than twice each period, the apparent regular period of the observed profile (solid curve) is much longer than the actual. Analogously, if the

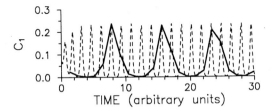

FIG. 1   Demonstration of the effects of aliasing on a periodic signal. Dashed line, actual oscillations in peripheral concentration of hormone C_1. Solid line, observed oscillations in peripheral concentration of hormone C_1.

pulsatile pattern is aperiodic (e.g., pulsatile but not strictly periodic), aliasing may also give rise to an incorrect estimation in pulse number and/or amplitude. It is thus essential that the sampling interval is appropriate compared to the expected pulse characteristics.

Modulatory Effects of Hormonal Clearance Kinetics

Even if problems related to aliasing are avoided, the kinetics of a particular hormone can markedly affect the interpretation of the secretory activity. For instance, if the pulse frequency varies systematically with time of day, pulses of secretion may be masked by the kinetics of the hormone. Figure 2 shows such an example. The assumed secretory profile is shown in the top panel. The secretory pulses are all identical in terms of shape and duration and occur, on average, every 2 hr, but there is a systematic slow variation in the interpulse interval. In the middle panel, the corresponding concentration profile is shown. Here, a simple two-compartment model with a short half-life of 5 min and a long half-life of 30 min is assumed to represent the kinetics of this particular hormone. These values are representative of, for instance, the kinetics of C-peptide (10). Evidently, during the phase in which the pulses occur frequently, the pulses are difficult to see in the concentration profile due to the fact that they represent the combined result of secretion, distribution, and degradation. A circadian variation has been produced, solely due to the variation in interpulse interval. By use of deconvolution, one can in theory derive the actual secretion rates. Thus, if the exact kinetic parameters used in the simulations are used to calculate secretion rates by deconvolution of the measurements shown in the middle panel of Fig. 2, the secretion profile can be relatively accurately reconstructed. However, with addition of noise, this becomes more problematic. If we assume an intraassay coefficient of variation of 8% and add random noise to the simulated time series to represent this (lower panel of Fig. 2), a number of false-positive and false-negative pulses occur. One may be able to partial circumvent this problem by using various noise reduction techniques and/or formal pulse-detection programs. These techniques are discussed in Chapter 14. However, the varying signal-to-noise ratio throughout the time series because of the changing interpulse intervals poses a serious problem. This example illustrates

FIG. 2   Modulation of a pulsatile pattern by the kinetic properties of the hormone. (Top) Pattern of pulsatile secretion; each pulse is represented by a rectangular pulse. (Center) Resulting concentration pattern if the hormone clearance kinetics are described by a two-compartmental model with a short half-life of 5 min, a long half-

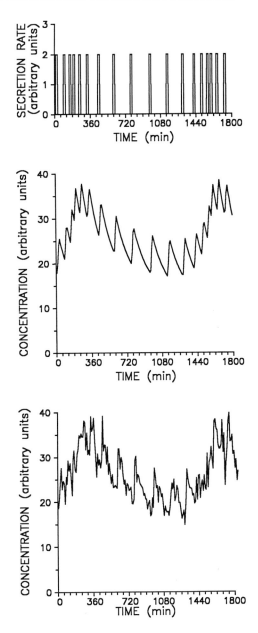

life of 30 min, and a fraction of decay associated with the short half-life of 75%. (Bottom) Concentration pattern with the addition of 8% random measurement error at each time point.

how the hormone kinetics can strongly influence the way pulsatile secretion is reflected in the peripheral circulation.

Modulatory Effects of Circadian Rhythmicity and Sleep

Among the most important modulatory effects on hormonal pulsatility are those of circadian rhythmicity and sleep. Virtually all hormonal secretions vary with time of day, and the overall diurnal variation generally reflects the combined influences of the central circadian signal and of the wake–sleep and sleep–wake transitions. Even glucose tolerance varies with time of day, and the 24-hr pattern is also dependent on both sleep and circadian rhythmicity (11). While the roles of circadian rhythmicity, i.e., intrinsic effects of time of day independent of the sleep or wake state, and sleep, i.e., intrinsic effects of the sleep state irrespective of the time of day when it occurs, on hormonal pulsatility have long been recognized, the dissociation between circadian effects and sleep effects and the nature of the modulatory mechanisms have been, however, more difficult to establish. In the discussion which follows, it is assumed that the coupling between the long-term periodicities and hormonal pulsatility is unidirectional, i.e., the mechanisms generating pulsatility are influenced by circadian rhythmicity and/or sleep but the hormonal levels do not affect the circadian or sleep signals.

Under these conditions, the modulation of hormonal release by circadian rhythmicity and sleep could theoretically be achieved by two distinct types of mechanisms, schematically represented in Fig. 3. Circadian modulation could be achieved by modulation of pulse frequency, with more pulses occurring around the time of the daily maximum and fewer pulses occurring around the time of the daily minimum. An example is shown in Fig. 2. Alternatively, circadian modulation could be achieved by modulation of pulse amplitude, with larger or smaller pulses occurring around the daily maximum or minimum, respectively. Similarly, modulatory effects of sleep on pulsatile release, whether stimulatory or inhibitory, could be exerted by either amplitude or frequency modulation. Importantly, to distinguish circadian effects from sleep effects, it is necessary to study circadian modulation in the absence of the confounding effects of sleep (i.e., during sleep deprivation) and sleep modulation at abnormal times of day, to avoid confounding circadian effects. These issues have only been examined in a handful of studies which used mathematical deconvolution to remove the effects of distribution and degradation on peripheral concentrations to reveal the temporal pattern of secretion. In the case of the corticotropic axis, several studies, based on different deconvolution techniques and underlying assumptions for hormonal kinetics, have concluded that the pronounced circadian variation of ACTH and cortisol secretion is achieved by modulation of pulse amplitude without changes in

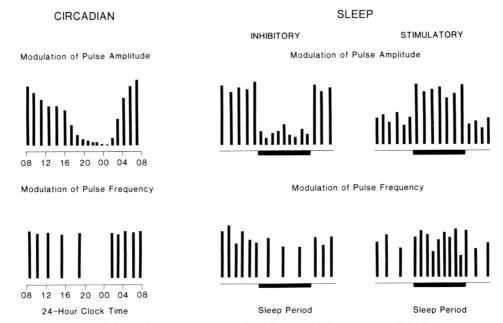

FIG. 3   Schematic representation of amplitude and frequency modulation of pulsatility by circadian rhythmicity and sleep.

pulse frequency (12–14). There is evidence to indicate that modulatory effects of sleep may be exerted on frequency or set the phase of the oscillation. For example, in the case of GH secretion, available evidence suggests that sleep has a phase-setting effect since a pulse of GH release is consistently associated with sleep onset, irrespective of the time of day (15–17). In normally menstruating women in the early part of the follicular phase, the frequency of LH pulses is markedly decreased during sleep (18–21). Sleep also exerts some control over the frequency of neuroendocrine release in the corticotropic axis, with a clear inhibition of pulsatility during the first few hours after sleep onset (22).

Modulatory Effects of Interacting Pulsatile Systems

A Simple Model of Oscillatory Hormone Secretion

To illustrate the various types of dynamic behaviors arising in interacting oscillating systems, we start by formulating a simple model for oscillatory hormone secretion, represented schematically in Fig. 4A. Assume that the

A

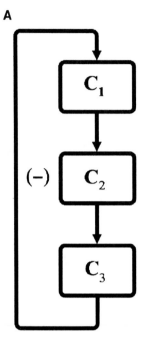

FIG. 4   (A) Negative feedback regulatory system involving three components C_1, C_2, and C_3.

hormonal system has three main components, C_1, C_2, C_3. The endocrine gland producing C_1 has a natural tendency to oversecrete. Because of this tendency, C_1 exerts more and more of its stimulatory effect on the target cells at the next level where C_2 is produced. Consequently, these cells also overproduce, and the presence of increasing amounts of C_2 stimulates the target cells at the following level to increase their production of C_3. This cascaded structure allows amplification to occur so that a few molecules at the first level can control the production of a very large number of molecules at the final functional level. Along with C_3, the target cells at the final level may produce a factor which feeds back to the endocrine gland and causes the gland to reduce its production. Thus, the overall structure is a negative feedback regulation, typical of several endocrine systems such as the gonadotropin-releasing hormone (GnRH)–LH–testosterone loop (23) and the corticotropin-releasing hormone (CRH)–ACTH–cortisol loop. A model with a similar structure has been proposed for observed oscillations in bacterial operons (24). This simple model may thus serve as an illustrative example, although other structures are possible as well. We use the System Dynamics

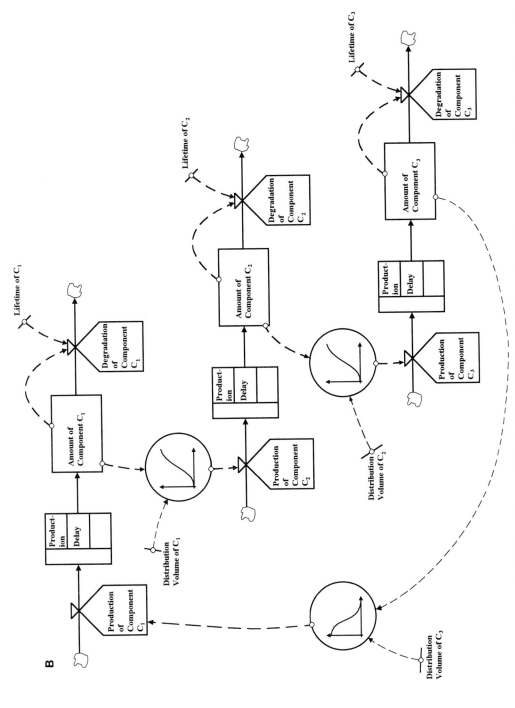

FIG. 4 (*continued*) (B) Flow diagram of the basic model. The model describes a three-stage cascaded system of hormonal production with negative feedback control.

methodology as developed by Forrester to obtain a detailed description of this model (25). With this approach, a set of coupled ordinary differential equations is illustrated by means of a flow diagram (Fig. 4B) in which box symbols represent the amounts of different compounds in particular compartments, and valve symbols represent the rates at which these compounds are produced, used, or degraded, or the rates at which they pass into other compartments. The solid lines connecting rate and box symbols represent conditions of continuity, i.e., they describe the fact that material quantities do not appear or disappear out of nothing. At any particular moment, the amounts of the various compounds in the system define its state. For this reason, the box variables are commonly referred to as state variables. The biochemical, pharmacokinetic, or physiological laws underlying this control are represented by the dashed lines. In many cases, it is practical to express these laws in terms of intermediate (or auxiliary) variables. These are represented as circles in the flow diagram. Intermediate variables could be pressures or concentrations of various substances. Such variables do not obey an equation of continuity.

The stability of the regulation depends on the number of stages in the cascade (here assumed to be three) and on the slopes of the regulatory functions which determine how much the production of one hormone is changed by a change in the concentration of the controlling hormone. For many systems, there are additional delays in the control, associated, for instance, with the response of the target cells to a given stimulation. In the flow diagram in Fig. 4B, a delay in the production of each component is included. Such delays tend to destabilize the system. On the other hand, the finite biological lifetimes of the hormones provide stabilizing dissipative mechanisms to the system. The shorter the lifetimes of the hormones, the stronger the stabilizing effects are.

In a particular modeling effort, it is clearly important to have good parameter estimations, i.e., estimates of the delay times associated with the production of the various components, of their lifetimes, as well as of the nonlinear relationships in the model. It is a virtue of the modeling concept described here that all parameters and relationships are defined so that, in principle, they can be determined independently of one another. However, our example is used only to illustrate various types of behaviors and does not relate to a particular system. Consequently, we do not discuss parameter values here. The set of ordinary differential equations corresponding to the flow diagram shown in Fig. 4B, the functional relationships, and base case parameters are given in the Appendix. The equations were solved numerically using a 5/6-order variable time step Runge–Kutta method (26).

The outcome of a simulation depends on the parameters and functional relationships in the model. It may also depend on the initial values of the

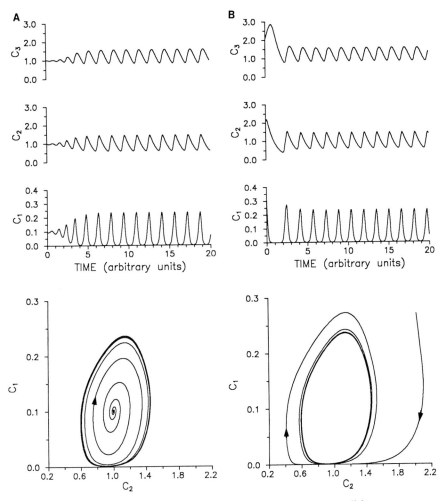

FIG. 5   Simulations with base case parameters. (A) The initial conditions were very close to equilibrium. (B) The initial conditions were far away from equilibrium. The same steady-state solution is obtained in both cases.

state variables. Figure 5 shows the result of two simulations with the same parameter values and initial conditions out of equilibrium. The stationary behavior is a self-sustained oscillation. The upper panels of Fig. 5 show the hormonal concentrations C_1, C_2, and C_3 plotted over a number of oscillatory periods. In both cases, after an initial transient period, the system settles in a regular limit cycle oscillation. Although in one simulation (upper panel of

Fig. 5A) the system was initiated close to equilibrium whereas in the other simulation (upper panel of Fig. 5B) it was started far away from equilibrium, the stationary behavior beyond the transient phase is identical, illustrating the attracting nature of the limit cycle. The lower panels of Fig. 5 show the corresponding phase plots of C_2 vs C_1. This representation is particularly illustrative in revealing the stable limit cycle nature of the oscillation.

The pulse shape is different from that often observed for some pituitary hormones where the concentration typically rises from nadir to peak very abruptly and thereafter decays exponentially with a time course corresponding to the metabolic clearance rate, suggesting the secretion of brief pulses into the circulation. More complicated models, but sharing some of the same basic features as those involved in the system illustrated in Fig. 4, could account for such pulse waveshapes.

An Introduction to Dynamic Behaviors of Coupled Oscillators

The use of nonlinear models has several advantages in the description of hormonal pulsatility. In particular, it allows modeling of interactions between different oscillatory processes. In contrast to linear systems, simple superposition of independent oscillatory modes does not occur in nonlinear systems. Instead, various pulsatile signals will interact and affect each other's periods and amplitudes in a variety of different manners. An important feature of the nonlinear interaction is that it tends to lock oscillations of two subsystems into an overall periodic motion. This is obtained when the oscillations have commensurate periods such that one subsystem completes precisely q cycles each time the other system completes p cycles, where p and q are integers. The simplest form of such frequency-locking (or entrainment) is synchronization, in which case the two subsystems adjust themselves until their periods are equal. A well-known example is the synchronization of the endogenous circadian rhythmicity of many living organisms to the external 24-hr day and night cycle. Other examples are synchronization of the menstrual cycles of women living in close contact or synchronization of the orbital and rotational motions of the moon (the same side of the moon always faces the earth). However, synchronization is a universal phenomenon which is likely to occur in many different biological situations. Moreover, since each oscillation in nonlinear systems generally is accompanied by a spectrum of harmonic overtones, entrainment can occur whenever the pth overtone of one oscillator is close to the qth overtone of the other.

Imagine that two hormonal systems have the structure outlined in Fig. 4. However, they have somewhat different parameter values. If the two systems exist completely independently of each other, oscillations with different

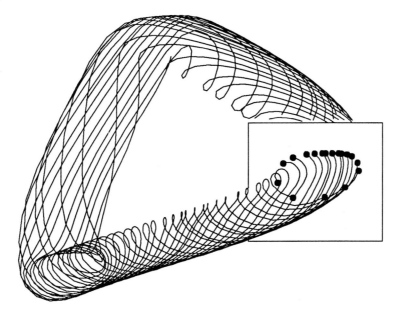

FIG. 6   Three-dimensional representation of the trajectory of two uncoupled oscillators. The trajectory lies on the surface of a torus. Intersection points between the trajectory and a plane defined by the phase of one of the oscillations form a circle.

periods will arise in each system. As illustrated in Fig. 6, the total trajectory can then be represented as a curve on a torus. For particular parameter combinations, namely, when the two periods are commensurate, the trajectory forms a closed orbit, and the overall motion is periodic. In general, however, the periods will be incommensurate (i.e., their ratio will be irrational), and the trajectory will fail to close onto itself. The motion is then said to be quasiperiodic, and the trajectory gradually covers the entire surface of the torus. If the torus is intersected by a plane (see Fig. 6), a periodic motion will give rise to a finite number of intersection points between the trajectory and the plane, whereas a quasiperiodic trajectory will cut the plane an infinite number of places. In either case, the intersection points will lie on a closed curve (which is topologically like a circle) defined by the intersection between the plane and the torus. By noting the angular position u_n along this curve of each subsequent point of intersection, we can define a map of the circle onto itself

$$\theta_{n+1} = f(\theta_n) \qquad\qquad (\text{mod } 1)$$

Here, $\theta_n = u_n/2\pi$ measures the phase of one of the oscillatory subsystems as obtained stroboscopically with the period of the other. If at a certain time the phase is θ_n, one period later it will be θ_{n+1}. With this procedure, the behavior of a complicated, multidimensional system is represented by a one-dimensional iterative map. Thus, if we know the phase of the system at one time, we can calculate this phase one period later, and by iterated use of the map we can continue to calculate the phase period by period. Moreover, we can use the map to determine the conditions under which the system exhibits stable periodic behavior and the conditions under which the behavior is aperiodic. Periodic behavior is obtained, of course, if θ_n after a number of iterations returns to precisely the same value again.

With no interaction between the two oscillators, the phase shift of one oscillator in each period of the other must always be the same, and thus, the map is linear

$$\theta_{n+1} = \theta_n + \Omega \qquad \text{(mod 1)}$$

where Ω measures the ratio between the two periods. In general Ω is irrational, and the linear map produces a never-repeating quasiperiodic motion. Only for specific parameters where Ω is rational is the overall motion periodic.

If interaction between the two modes is introduced, the phase shift of one mode during the period of the other may depend on the initial phase of the first mode, and the circle map becomes nonlinear. The map can then be expressed as

$$\theta_{n+1} = \theta_n + \Omega + g(\theta_n) \qquad \text{(mod 1)}$$

where $g(\theta_n)$ represents the nonlinear (phase-dependent) term. If Ω is close to 0 (or 1), the map may cut the diagonal of the (θ_{n+1}, θ_n) plane (i.e., where values of Ω and $g(\theta_n)$ are identical) and produce a stable fixed point toward which all trajectories will converge, independent of the initial conditions. This fixed point represents the synchronized solution in which the two oscillators have precisely the same period. More importantly, if Ω is changed slightly in either direction, the fixed point will continue to exist (even though it will move along the diagonal). In the nonlinear system, the stable phase-locked 1:1 solution therefore exists over a finite range of parameters. Similarly, for Ω close to $\frac{1}{3}$, the triply iterated map $f^3(\theta) = f(f(f(\theta)))$ may have three stable fixed points, and these fixed points will continue to exist under small changes in the model parameters. In general, one finds that frequency locking occurs in intervals around all rational ratios of the two periods. The interval in which a particular mode locking occurs is a measure of the strength of the nonlinear interaction in the model. The interval therefore tends to

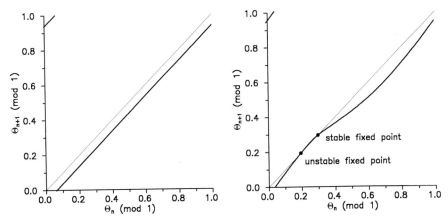

FIG. 7   Circle maps of two uncoupled (left) and two coupled (right) oscillators. In the uncoupled situation, the circle map is linear, whereas it is nonlinear in the coupled situation. In the coupled case, the map intersects the diagonal, producing a stable and an unstable fixed point.

widen with increasing coupling between the two hormonal oscillators. The interval also depends on the mode-locking ratio. Generally, entrainment between modes with simple period ratios and with period ratios of the order of 1 is more pronounced than entrainment between modes with more complicated winding numbers. Thus, 1:1 and 1:3 entrainments occur over wider parameter ranges than do, for instance, 1:10 and 4:9 entrainments.

Figure 7 illustrates the circle map of the two hormonal oscillators both when they are independent and when a coupling has been introduced. Iteration of the map is performed by entering θ_n on the x-axis and reading θ_{n+1} off as the y-coordinate of the corresponding point on the graph. This θ_{n+1} is then used as the next entry θ_n and so on. The fixed points of the map are the points where the map intersects the diagonal $\theta_{n+1} = \theta_n$. If the system has arrived at such a point, it will remain there. A fixed point is stable if the slope of the map in this point is numerically less than unity. Under this condition, iterations of the map starting in the neighborhood of the fixed point will converge toward the fixed point.

Quasiperiodicity and Frequency-Locking (Entrainment)

We now simulate the various types of behaviors that can occur in coupled oscillators using two systems as shown in Fig. 4, interacting as represented in Fig. 8. System 2 is almost identical to system 1, except that for a difference

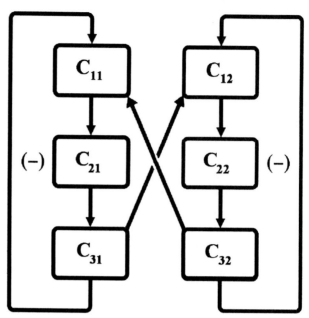

FIG. 8   Interaction between two negative feedback regulatory systems. The two systems are identical, except τ_{12} (τ_1 of system 2) is set to 0.14 in the base case (see Appendix for remaining parameters).

in value of a single parameter which characterizes the lifetime of component C_1 (τ_1; see Appendix and legend of Fig. 8). In addition, the two systems are coupled: the production of component C_{11} depends not only on C_{31} but also on component C_{32}. Similarly, the production of component C_{12} depends not only on C_{32}, but also on component C_{31}. Let us also assume that the effect of component C_{32} is proportional to the amount of component C_{31} and that the coupling is identical in both directions. Such a coupling can be expressed as $f_1(C_{31} + \sigma C_{31}C_{32})$ and $f_2(C_{32} + \sigma C_{32}C_{31})$, where σ measures the degree of coupling between the two systems. A vanishing value of σ corresponds to uncoupled systems. In all simulations, the equations are normalized so that, in equilibrium, the value of each functional relationship equals unity.

Figure 9 shows the dynamics of component C_{21} and C_{22} as the coupling between the two hormonal systems goes from $\sigma = 0$ to $\sigma = 0.3$ at time 10. With no coupling, the two systems oscillate in an unsynchronized or quasiperiodic fashion—they have incommensurate periods. After the coupling is activated, system 1 "slows down" while system 2 "speeds up," and the systems oscillate with the same period—they are entrained or synchronized. Synchronization is also referred to as 1 : 1 frequency locking, because

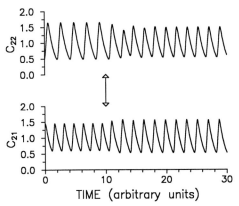

FIG. 9   Frequency locking of two oscillators. In the beginning, the two systems are uncoupled and each oscillates with its own period. At time = 10, a coupling is introduced ($\sigma = 0.3$), and both systems respond by adjusting their period so that the overall motion becomes periodic.

each system performs one full oscillation during the same time. As mentioned in the previous section, synchronization will occur not only at specific parameter values, but also in intervals of the model parameters. For instance, τ_{11} plays an important role in determining the period of oscillation for system 1. However, when the two systems are coupled and both oscillate with the same period, a slight change in τ_{11}, in either direction will not change the fact that the systems remain entrained, although the overall period may be affected.

If the two systems have very different periods, frequency locking may occur with a ratio different from 1 : 1. In other words, one system may perform one full oscillation while the other system goes through, say, three swings. This would be referred to as 1 : 3 frequency locking. An example of this type of motion is shown in Fig. 10. In principle, the systems entrain at all rational mode-locking ratios. If the interaction is strong enough, the parameter ranges for which some of these solutions occur may overlap the parameter ranges for which other solutions occur, and thus different periodic solutions may exist for the same model parameters. The initial conditions determine which of the stationary solutions the trajectory approaches, and thus the stationary state is history dependent.

A more complete picture of the entrainment process can be obtained by plotting the observed mode-locking ratio as a function of a parameter which influences the uncoupled period of one of the systems. Figure 11 shows an example of such a construction. Here, all parameters of system 1 are kept

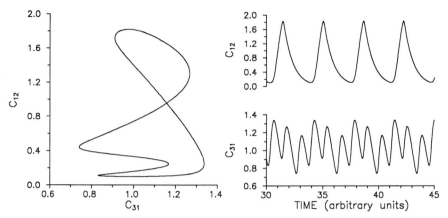

FIG. 10   Simulation with base case parameters, except $\tau_{11} = 0.06$, $\tau_{12} = 0.8$, and $\sigma = 0.1$. In this case, system 1 performs three swings for every oscillation of system 2. Note that the apparent intersection of the trajectory by itself observed in the phase plot is due to the fact that the system is multidimensional; although C_{12} and C_{31} are equal in the intersection point, other state variables are different. This comment holds true for all remaining phase plots shown in this chapter.

constant but one of the parameters determining the uncoupled period of system 2 (τ_{12}) is varied between 0.04 and 2.5 while the coupling between the two hormonal oscillators is kept constant ($\sigma = 0.05$). The left panel of Fig. 11 shows that, when parameter τ_{12} increases, and thus the uncoupled period of system 2 is lengthened, a series of $1:n$ frequency-locked solutions arise. Between these solutions, intervals with other rational winding numbers are observed. In the region from $\tau_{12} = 0.08$ to 0.22, shown in greater detail in the right panel of Fig. 11, we thus find intervals with $4:7$, $3:5$, $2:3$, $3:4$, $4:5$, and $5:6$ entrainment.

The structure depicted in Fig. 11 is often referred to as a devil's staircase (27, 28). By refining the calculations, one can continue to find more and more steps covering narrower and narrower parameter intervals. At least for small coupling strengths, i.e., below the level where the mode-locked intervals start to overlap, the phenomenon has a self-similar character which causes it to repeat itself ad infinitum at a smaller and smaller scale. In practice, the finer details, i.e., very narrow steps corresponding to complicated mode-locking ratios, will be washed out by noise; that is, the random external events which continuously influence the hormonal control will not allow the behavior to settle down into one of these more complex periodic solutions. Simpler examples of mode locking such as, for instance, $1:2$ or $1:3$ are more likely to be observed in the time series of hormonal concentrations. We

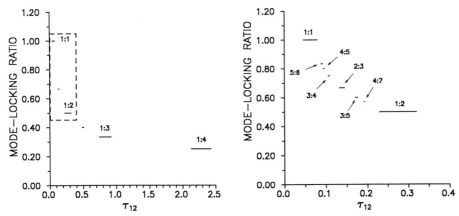

FIG. 11   (Left) Intervals of the parameter τ_{12} in which some of the main mode-locked solutions can be observed. (Right) Magnification of the region for lower values of τ_{12}. Between any pair of intervals with locked solutions, solutions with other rational winding numbers exist. The structure is often referred to as a devil's staircase.

suggest, however, that frequency locking in most cases will be undesirable, because, by locking their periods to one another, the individual hormonal systems lose part of their regulatory ability.

Although frequency locking is a general and pronounced phenomenon in coupled nonlinear oscillators, other types of dynamics are possible as well. As previously mentioned, quasiperiodicity is a motion that occurs if the periods of the two systems are incommensurate, and the coupling is insufficient to pull them together into a locked state. In this case, the system never repeats its own behavior exactly. In Fig. 12, an example of quasiperiodic behavior of the coupled system is shown.

Deterministic Chaos

Another possible type of motion is deterministic chaos. It resembles quasiperiodicity in that it is also aperiodic. However, important differences exist. One of the most striking contrasts is the fact that a chaotic solution is sensitive to the initial conditions. This is best illustrated by an example. In Fig. 13, four simulations are shown which were performed with four different values for the coupling parameter σ. In Fig. 13A, $\sigma = 0.12$, and the resulting system behavior is a $1:2$ frequency-locked solution. The upper panel of Fig. 13A shows the evolution of C_{22} and C_{21} over time, whereas the lower panel shows the corresponding phase plot. After an initial transient period, system 1 (as

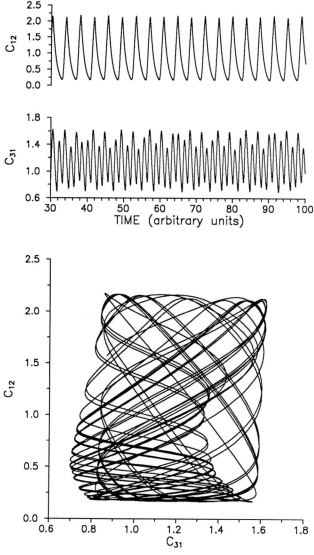

FIG. 12   A quasiperiodic solution obtained for $\tau_{12} = 1$ and $\sigma = 0.09$. This type of solution is characterized by the fact that it never repeats itself. The system continues to find new ways in phase space. Quasiperiodic behavior distinguishes itself from deterministic chaos by not showing sensitivity to the initial conditions.

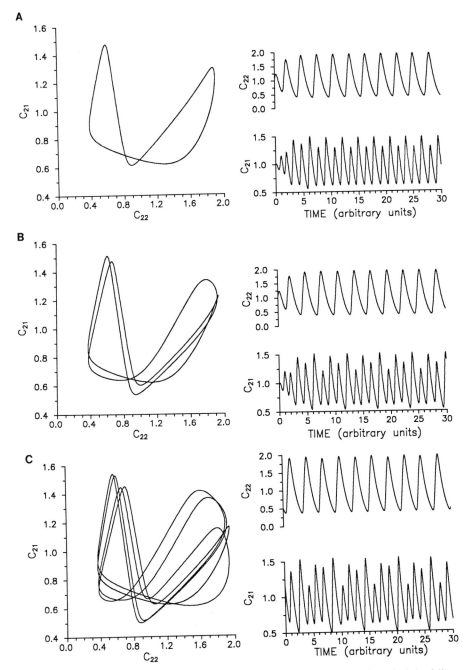

FIG. 13 Transition to chaotic dynamics by an infinite cascade of period-doubling bifurcations. (A) $\sigma = 0.12$, $1:2$ frequency locking; (B) $\sigma = 0.2$, $2:4$ frequency locking; (C) $\sigma = 0.24$, $4:8$ frequency locking.

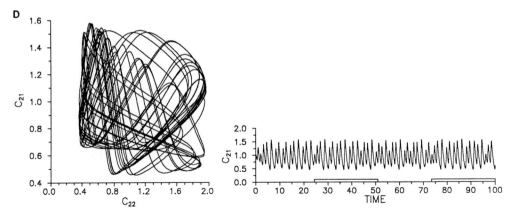

FIG. 13 (D) $\sigma = 0.34$, chaos.

represented by C_{21}) performs exactly two swings for each oscillation of system 2 (as represented by C_{22}). In the phase plot, the trajectory forms a closed loop after two maxima in C_{21} and one maximum in C_{22} have occurred. In Fig. 13B, $\sigma = 0.2$ and now system 1 goes through four oscillations of different amplitude for every two periods of system 2—a 2:4 frequency-locked solution. The system has undergone what is referred to as a period-doubling bifurcation (28). In the phase plot (shown in the lower panel of Fig. 13B), the trajectory appears to be "split." When σ is increased to 0.24, another period doubling has taken place, producing a 4:8 locked solution (Fig. 13C). As σ is further increased, the system passes through a cascade of period-doubling bifurcations, producing 8:16, 16:32, etc., frequency-locked solutions until its period finally becomes infinite. Thus, in Fig. 13D, $\sigma = 0.34$, and the system has become chaotic. The oscillations undergo continuous changes in period and amplitude, and the pattern never repeats itself. The motion almost appears to be random in certain intervals despite the fact that the equations of motion are purely deterministic—they contain no stochastic (i.e., random) element. During some periods of time, such as for examples during the two time segments highlighted on the x-axis of Fig. 13D, the behaviors may be similar for a while, but eventually they diverge and the patterns develop differently.

Figure 14 (top) illustrates this sensitivity to the initial conditions. The Euclidian distance D^* (i.e., the distance in phase space) between the trajectory at time $= t$ and time $= t + 49.9$ is plotted in the interval of t between 24.3 and 50.7 (corresponding to the two segments highlighted in Fig. 13D).

* $D = \sqrt{\Sigma_{i,j} (C_{i,j}(t) - C_{ij}(t + 49.9))^2}$

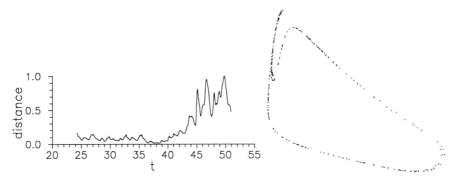

FIG. 14   (Left) Sensitivity of the chaotic solution shown in Fig. 13D on the initial conditions. (Right) The sensitivity on initial conditions is a consequence of the fact that the trajectory no longer lies on a torus. Use of the method illustrated in Fig. 6 reveals that the intersection between a plane and the trajectory no longer produces a circle.

In the beginning, the distance is short, but eventually the two segments of the trajectory move far away from each other. Regardless of how close the two trajectory segments are initially, as long as there is a finite distance, they will ultimately diverge. If the trajectory is intersected by a plane as illustrated in Fig. 6, the points of intersection no longer lie on a circle. As shown in Fig. 14 (right), the curve exhibits an infinite number of foldings (one of which can be clearly seen in the figure). In combination with a stretching mechanism [in Fig. 14 (right) seen where the density of intersection points is low], this produces the sensitivity to the inital conditions. This behavior is characteristic of a deterministic system operating in a chaotic mode and contrasts the behavior of the same system operating in a quasiperiodic mode. In the latter case, the distance between two trajectory segments that are initially close will remain close.

The development of deterministic chaos through a cascade of period-doubling bifurcations is only one of the ways in which a nonlinear dynamic system can become chaotic. Other routes to chaos also exist in our simple model of coupled hormonal oscillators. In particular, a quasiperiodic motion can become chaotic as the coupling between the two subsystems is sufficiently increased. Several of these routes have universal aspects. Thus it is one of the most important results of modern nonlinear systems theory (29) that the development deterministic chaos through a cascade of period doublings for a large class of systems proceeds in a universal manner, independent of the detailed form and origin of the describing differential equations. In fact, this development is characterized by two universal constants

$\alpha = 2.5029078...$ and $\delta = 4.6692016...$ which specify the asymptotic behavior of the bifurcation cascade as it approaches the threshold to chaos.

Example: Frequency-Locking in Forced Insulin Secretion

In man as well as in animals, insulin is secreted in a pulsatile fashion, containing both rapid 8- to 15-min pulses and slower oscillations with a period of approximately 2 hr (8, 30, 31). Although the precise mechanisms underlying the former pulses are unknown, much experimental evidence exists which shows that these pulses can be either very regular or quite irregular. Presumably, the same basic mechanism is responsible for both types of behavior. This is so much more plausible as both regular and irregular insulin secretory pulses can be observed in the same person under different experimental conditions (8). Typically, during fasting, the pulses are regular in approximately 50% of nondiabetic study subjects. Administration of intravenous glucose in the same subjects results in loss of regularity of the pulses which however persist. It thus appears that the administration of glucose in some people modulates insulin pulsatility so that the pulses become irregular. The exercises in this chapter have shown that the same deterministic system can easily produce both regular and irregular behavior depending only on a small change in as little as a single parameter.

The slow oscillations in insulin secretion appear to be regulated closely by the glucose concentration in normal man. Thus, during a constant intravenous administration of glucose, concomitant oscillations occur in glucose and insulin secretion with an approximate 2-hr periodicity. The oscillations are usually not completely regular, indicating that modulation from other systems occurs. It is also possible to experimentally modulate these oscillations. We have thus shown in normal man that when intravenous glucose is administered in an oscillatory fashion, the internally generated oscillations in insulin secretion can be entrained to the exogenous glucose infusion (31). Figure 15 shows an example from that study in which the same subject was studied on three occasions: once during constant and twice during oscillatory glucose infusion using periods 20% above and below the endogenous periods, respectively. These experimental results can be reproduced using a nonlinear dynamic model of the insulin–glucose feedback system (30, 32). This model was derived using the approach described above, and when a constant glucose infusion is simulated, self-sustained oscillations in glucose and insulin secretion occur. When the oscillatory glucose infusion experiments are simulated, entrainment occurs. Examples of these simulation results are shown in Fig. 16. In agreement with the model and the theory presented here, we have also experimentally demonstrated a more complicated mode of entrainment.

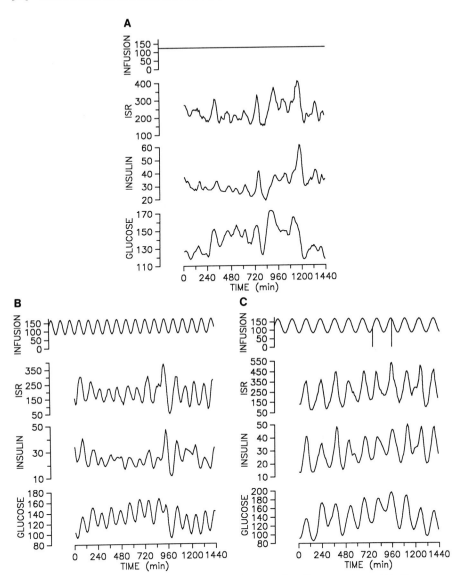

FIG. 15   Experimental entrainment of oscillatory insulin secretion. (A) Constant glucose infusion. (B) Oscillatory glucose infusion—period 96 min. (C) Oscillatory glucose infusion—period 144 min. These results which were obtained on separate occasions in the same normal subject have been redrawn from Sturis *et al.* (31).

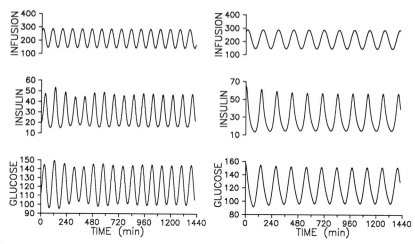

FIG. 16   Simulation of entrainment experiments shown in Fig. 15 by use of a nonlinear dynamic model constructed with the System Dynamics method (25, 30, 32). (Top) Rapid oscillatory glucose infusion. (Bottom) Slow oscillatory glucose infusion.

When the period of glucose infusion was increased to approximately twice the endogenous period, two full oscillations in the glucose and insulin secretion entrainment were observed for each oscillation in the infusion (31, 32). These results demonstrate the usefulness of computer modeling in examining the modulatory effects on insulin pulsatility brought about by exogenous means.

Discussion

In this chapter, we have shown how pulsatility may be modulated by a variety of mechanisms, including experimental conditions, hormonal clearance kinetics, circadian rhythmicity, sleep, and interactions between self-oscillating systems. These latter interactions are obviously ubiquitous throughout the endocrine system and can give rise to both periodic and aperiodic phenomena. Limited cycle behavior of one system and frequency locking between modes of several systems are examples of periodic behavior, whereas quasiperiodicity and deterministic chaos are examples of aperiodic behavior. It is important to realize that these phenomena are universal, and one can expect to encounter quasiperiodicity, frequency locking, and chaos in many biological circumstances besides those related to hormonal pulsatility. For instance, Glass *et al.* (33) have reported the observation of complicated patterns of frequency locking when chicken heart cells are excited by external periodic signals. Similarly, frequency locking and chaos have been found to influence the flow of information between coupled nerve cells (34). A detailed theoretical understanding of these phenomena has only emerged during the past decade (27, 28) and the implications for the understanding of the mechanisms and properties of oscillatory behaviors in living systems are just beginning to be appreciated. The examples shown here demonstrate in particular that the fact that pulsatile hormonal secretion is often irregular does not imply that it is due to random processes. The numerical exercises presented in this chapter have illustrated that random-like pulsatile behavior can easily arise from a nonlinear system that obeys precise deterministic laws. In particular, chaotic behavior easily arises when several systems are coupled.

It is presently unclear whether regular or irregular pulsatile hormonal secretion is preferable from a physiological point of view. It seems likely, however, that completely regular behavior brought about by frequency locking between all kinds of hormones would be undesirable, because such a mode would be very rigid and adaptation would be difficult. A certain degree of chaotic behavior, on the other hand, would give the system a chance to adapt to environmental changes. This view is supported by the fact that perfect frequency locking between modes is seldom observed experimentally.

Although the model used here to illustrate the behaviors that may arise from coupled pulsatile systems does not necessarily reflect the precise mechanisms of any one hormonal system, it serves as an example of a useful approach. Combining detailed analyses of experimental data and nonlinear dynamic modeling may provide insight into major biological mechanisms and generate testable working hypotheses.

Appendix

Transforming the flow diagram in Fig. 4B into a set of ordinary differential equations, we get

$$\frac{dC_1}{dt} = f(C_3) - \frac{C_1}{\tau_1}$$

$$\frac{dC_2}{dt} = g(C_1) - \frac{C_2}{\tau_2}$$

$$\frac{dC_3}{dt} = h(C_2) - \frac{C_3}{\tau_3}$$

In this formulation, the production delays illustrated in Fig. 4B have not been included. The functional relationships and base case parameters are chosen to be

$$f(C_3) = \frac{4}{1 + 3 \exp\left(\alpha\left(\frac{C_3}{\tau_3} - 1\right)\right)}$$

$$g(C_1) = \frac{4}{1 + 3 \exp\left(\beta\left(-\frac{C_1}{\tau_1} + 1\right)\right)}$$

$$h(C_2) = \frac{4}{1 + 3 \exp\left(\gamma\left(-\frac{C_2}{\tau_2} + 1\right)\right)}$$

$$\tau_1 = 0.1; \quad \tau_2 = 1; \quad \tau_3 = 1;$$

$$\alpha = 10; \quad \beta = 3; \quad \gamma = 6$$

We solve the equations numerically with a 5/6-order variable time step Runge–Kutta method (26).

Acknowledgment

Supported in part by Grant DK-41814 from the NIH and a NATO Scientific Exchange Programme—Collaborative Research Grant. Dr. Sturis was supported by a fellowship from the Juvenile Diabetes Foundation International.

References

1. W. F. Crowley and J. G. Hofler, eds., "The Episodic of Hormones." Wiley, New York, 1987.
2. T. O. F. Wagner and M. Filicori, eds., "Episodic Hormone Secretion: From Basic Science to Clinical Application." TM-Verlag, Hameln, FRG, 1987.
3. G. Leng, "Pulsatility in Neuroendocrine Systems." CRC Press, Boca Raton, FL, 1988.
4. E. Van Cauter and F. W. Turek, in "Endocrinology" (L. J. DeGroot, ed.). Saunders, Philadelphia, 1994 (in press).
5. D. K. Arrowsmith and C. M. Place, "An Introduction to Dynamical Systems." Cambridge Univ. Press, Cambridge, 1990.

6. A. Iranmanesh, G. Lizarralde, D. Short, and J. D. Veldhuis, *J. Clin. Endocrinol. Metab.* **71,** 1276, 1990.

7. W. S. Evans, A. C. S. Faria, E. Christiansen, K. Y. Ho, J. Weiss, A. D. Rogol, M. L. Johnson, R. M. Blizzard, J. D. Veldhuis, and M. O. Thorner, *Am. J. Physiol.* **252,** E549, 1987.

8. N. M. O'Meara, J. Sturis, J. D. Blackman, D. Roland, E. Van Cauter, and K. S. Polonsky, *Am. J. Physiol.* **264** (*Endocrinol. Metab.* **27**), E231, 1993.

9. J. D. Veldhuis, W. S. Evans, A. D. Rogol, C. R. Drake, M. O. Thorner, G. R. Merriam, and M. L. Johnson, *J. Clin. Endocrinol. Metab.* **59,** 96, 1984.

10. E. Van Cauter, F. Mestrez, J. Sturis, and K. S. Polonsky, *Diabetes* **41,** 368, 1992.

11. E. Van Cauter, J. D. Blackman, D. Roland, J.-P. Spire, S. Refetoff, and K. S. Polonsky, *J. Clin. Invest.* **88,** 934, 1991.

12. J. Veldhuis, A. Iranmanesh, G. Lizarralde, and M. Johnson, *Am. J. Physiol.* **257,** E6, 1989.

13. J. D. Veldhuis, A. Iranmanesh, M. L. Johnson, and G. Lizarralde, *J. Clin. Endocrinol. Metab.* **71,** 452, 1989.

14. E. Van Cauter, A. van Coevorden, and J. D. Blackman, *in* "Advances in Neuroendocrine Regulation of Reproduction" (S. Yen and W. vale, eds.), pp. 113–122. Serono Symposia USA, Norwell, 1990.

15. E. Van Cauter, *in* "Recent Advances in Endocrinology and Metabolism" (C. W. Edwards and D. W. Lincoln, eds.), No. 3, pp. 109–134. Churchill–Livingstone, Edinburgh, 1989.

16. E. Van Cauter, *Horm. Res.* **34,** 1990.

17. E. Van Cauter, M. Kerkhofs, A. Caufriez, A. Van Onderbergen, M. O. Thorner, and G. Copinschi, *J. Clin. Endocrinol. Metab.* **74,** 1441, 1992.

18. E. D. Weitzman *in* "Effect of Sleep–Wake Cycle Shifts on Sleep and Neuroendocrine Function," pp. 93–111. Plenum, New York, 1973.

19. M. Soules, R. Steiner, N. Cohen, W. Bremner, and D. Clifton, *J. Clin. Endocrinol. Metab.* **61,** 43, 1985.

20. M. Filicor, N. Santoro, G. R. Merriam, and W. F. J. Crowley, *J. Clin. Endocrinol. Metab.* **62,** 1136, 1986.

21. W. G. Rossmanith and S. S. C. Yen, *J. Clin. Endocrinol. Metabl.* **65,** 715, 1987.

22. E. D. Weitzman, J. C. Zimmerman, C. A. Czeisler, and J. M. Ronda, *J. Clin. Endocrinol. Metab.* **56,** 352, 1983.

23. W. R. Smith, *Bull. Math. Biol.* **42,** 57, 1980.

24. R. D. Bliss, P. R. Painter, and A. G. Marr, *J. Theor. Biol.* **97,** 177, 1982.

25. J. W. Forrester, "Principles of Systems." Wright-Allen Press, Cambridge, MA, 1963.

26. W. H. Enright, K. R. Jackson, S. P. Nørsett, and P. G. Thomsen, *ACM Trans. Math. Software* **12,** 193, 1986.

27. S. Ostlund, D. Rand, J. Sethua, and E. Siggia. *Physica D (Amsterdam)* **8,** 303, 1983.

28. M. H. Jensen, P. Bak, and T. Bohr, *Phys. Rev. A* **30,** 1960, 1984.

29. M. Feigenbaum. *Los Alamos Sci.* **1,** 4, 1980. Also *Physica D (Amsterdam)* **7,** 16, 1983.

30. J. Sturis, K. S. Polonsky, E. Mosekilde, and E. Van Cauter, *Am. J. Physiol.* **260** (*Endocrinol. Metab.* **23**), E801, 1991.
31. J. Sturis, E. Van Cauter, J. D. Blackman, and K. S. Polonsky, *J. Clin. Invest.* **87,** 439, 1991.
32. J. Sturis, K. S. Polonsky, J. D. Blackman, C. Knudsen, E. Mosekilde, and E. Van Cauter, *in* "Complexity, Chaos and Biological Evolution" (E. Mosekilde and L. Mosekilde, eds.), NATO ASI Series B: Physics Vol. 270, pp. 75–93. Plenum Press, New York, 1991.
33. L. Glass, M. R. Guevara, A. Shrier, and R. Perez. *Physica D* **7,** 89, 1983.
34. M. Colding-Jørgensen, *in* "Complexity, Chaos and Biological Evolution" (E. Mosekilde and L. Mosekilde, eds.) NATO ASI Series B: Physics Vol. 270, pp. 163–178. Plenum Press, New York, 1991.

[20] Modeling Pulsatile Hormone Stimulation of Cell Responses

Rosalind P. Murray-McIntosh and
James Edward Alister McIntosh

Introduction

It is now accepted that presentation of a hormone to a cell expressing specific receptors for that hormone causes characteristic changes in cellular functional activity. But presence of stimulant alone fails to fully explain most biological responses—dynamics also play an important part. The contribution made by time to both hormone signals and cellular responses must be taken into account in exploring efficiency of signal transmission during intercellular communication or pharmacological intervention (1, 2). We describe ways to investigate dynamic dimensions of control, and of mechanisms, in cell stimulation both *in vivo* and *in vitro*.

Using cultured cells (mainly from the pituitary), we have varied the dynamics of stimulation *in vitro* to investigate how different kinds of pulsatile hormone input signals alter cellular output and its patterns (3–7). (Uninterrupted application of hypothalamic releasing hormones *in vivo* and *in vitro* is well known to depress or terminate release of many pituitary hormones.) Investigated attributes of pulse amplitude, baseline level, pulse interval, duration, and rise rate which may interact with the dynamics of intracellular mechanisms to control cellular "output patterns" are shown in Fig. 1. We have also studied interactions in the dynamics of both different stimulants of the same response (7) and between multiple responses to the one stimulant (5, 6).

We have used modifiers of intracellular processes *in vitro* to assess their part in controlling the dynamics of cell responses (8, 9) and exploited pulsatile stimulation in perifusion to detect, clarify the mechanisms of action, or investigate dynamic interactions of natural and exogenously expressed receptors (10).

Where direct manipulation of hormones is impossible in humans *in vivo*, we have measured the naturally changing output patterns of the pituitary as revealed in the blood stream and, from a knowledge of the input effects of hypothalamic hormones, have drawn inferences on the dynamics of natural stimulatory signals (11, 12).

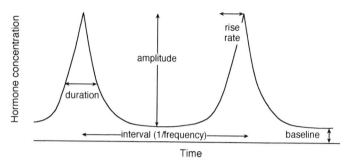

FIG. 1   Characteristics of a hormone pulse.

Methods

Preparation of Tissue

Pituitary Cells

Many of our studies concerned the effects of an input signal of gonadotropin-releasing hormone (GnRH) acting on anterior pituitary tissue to release luteinizing hormone (LH) or follicle-stimulating hormone (FSH). Isolating tissue from the body has allowed us to control and reproduce experimental conditions precisely. Choice of tissue preparation is determined by both theoretical and practical considerations. Biological relevance is essential, as are the experimental needs for reproducibility of results between experiments and the ability to vary several parameters of the stimulatory signal in a single experiment, while permitting replication on identical samples.

The large sheep pituitary is a convenient source of tissue, although we have also used rat, beef, and horse glands. Sheep anterior pituitary slices and pieces gave variable and unsatisfactory results. Passing finely chopped tissue through a coarse sieve to form uniformly sized pieces of naturally linked cells usually causes loss of responsiveness to GnRH despite the presence of protease inhibitors. We therefore routinely use dissociated cells which are aliquotted into multiple identical portions and cultured.

It was possible that the process of dissociation and culture altered the response dynamics of the cells. To determine whether attachment and formation of cellular contacts influenced the results, most experiments were performed after about 3 hr from completion of cell dissociation (when the unstimulated baseline "bleed" of released hormone had been shown to reach negligible levels), or after culture of cells on Cytodex beads (Pharmacia, Piscataway, NJ) for 2 days.

When studying endocrine systems by controlled variation of cell stimulation with specific hormones, account must be taken of the general hormonal milieu from which the tissue is withdrawn to minimize uncontrolled effects caused by change in the hormonal content of the culture medium.

Pituitaries are collected within 20 min of slaughter at the local abattoir from a minimum of four sheep for each experiment. Nonpregnant females are individually selected from absence of external urethra and after checking uterine state. We usually select animals 6- to 24-months old (from examination of teeth) because, in comparison with other sexual states, their pituitaries are consistently responsive to GnRH. Using sterilized instruments the median eminence and connective tissue are dissected away and the split, nonsterile pituitary pieces placed in Dulbecco's minimum Eagle's medium (DMEM) containing 10% (v/v) sheep serum and high levels of antibiotics (50 μg/ml gentamycin sulfate, 0.5 mg/ml streptomycin, 0.6 mg/ml penicillin) for the 20-min trip to the laboratory.

We use sterile technique thereafter and all glassware is siliconized. To maintain cell viability, Milli-Q–purified water is necessary in all procedures including the rinsing of glassware and autoclaving. Several cell preparation procedures were compared and the following found optimal for yielding maximum cell numbers and responsiveness. Pituitaries are washed in HEPES dissociating buffer (HDB: 25 mM HEPES, 137 mM NaCl, 5 mM KCl, 0.7 mM Na$_2$HPO$_4 \cdot$ 2H$_2$O, 11 mM glucose, 50 mg gentamycin $\cdot$ SO$_4$/liter, adjusted to pH 7.3 with 0.1 M NaOH). The *pars tuberalis* is removed and the anterior pituitary cut into blocks about 1 mm^3 using a pair of scalpel blades pulled through the tissue in opposition. The blocks are rinsed three times in HDB. Immediately before use collagenase (0.25% w/v), bovine serum albumin (BSA, 0.8% w/v) and DNase (0.002% w/v) are dissolved in HDB and sterile-filtered. Tissue chunks are stirred for 45–70 min at 37°C in a 40-ml tissue-dissociating vial (Bellco Glass, Inc., Vineland, NJ) containing a magnetic spin bar and 25 ml collagenase solution. Dissociation remains incomplete and enzyme exposure is minimized to reduce cell damage. Some batches of collagenase destroyed cell responsiveness—several were tested from different suppliers to select the optimum.

The cell suspension is centrifuged for 8 min at 200g to form a pellet beneath a band of red cells which is removed. The pellet is washed three or four times by resuspending in DMEM containing 10% (v/v) anestrous ewe serum and centrifuged at room temperature (18–22°C) for 6 min at 100g. The washed cells are filtered through two layers of muslin cloth, counted (yield between 20–40 × 10^6 cells/pituitary depending on source of collagenase), and tested for viability by trypan blue exclusion. This is 90% initially, increasing after 2 days of culture to about 100% by removal of nonadhesive cells during medium exchange. We have described the development of these methods (3, 5, 6, 8, 9, 13).

Ovarian Follicles of Xenopus laevis (10, 14)

Toads are anesthetized on ice and their ovarian lobes removed through an incision in the abdominal wall. Follicles are separated with a platinum wire loop in OR-2 medium or modified Barths' solution [88 mM NaCl, 1 mM KCl, 2.4 mM NaHCO$_3$, 0.33 mM Ca(NO$_3$)$_2$, 0.41 mM CaCl$_2$, 0.82 mM MgCl$_2$, 10 mM HEPES, 20 μg penicillin/ml, 20 μg streptomycin/ml, 50 U nystatin/ml, 2 mM sodium pyruvate, pH 7.5] and healthy, mature (stages 5 and 6) ones are selected for experimentation.

Culture of Pituitary Cells

Cells are stabilized for 3 hr after preparation in perifusion medium or cultured for up to 48 hr before stimulation with hormone in perifusion. Culture is on Cytodex beads (Pharmacia, Piscataway, NJ) in DMEM plus 10% anestrous ewe serum, at 37°C in an atmosphere of 96% air/4% CO$_2$.

Packing of Perifusion Columns

Columns of the perifusion apparatus (see below) are packed with 50 μl BioGel P2 (200–400 mesh; Bio-Rad Laboratories, Richmond, CA) and 100 μl Sephadex G-25 (Pharmacia, Piscataway, NJ). The packing materials are preswollen and autoclaved in HDB without glucose. Equal aliquots of pituitary cells (2.5–10 × 10^6 cells/column) are mixed with an extra 50 μl Sephadex G-25 and loaded onto the packing. The column packing type and their volumes were chosen to render negligible the loss of cells during perifusion. Cells on disposable filters (0.45 μm) have been used instead, but we considered that our columns prevented unevenness of flow and allowed us to load cells after culture on Cytodex beads.

At the conclusion of experiments, hormone remaining in the pituitary cells of each column is measured after mixing with a known volume of solution containing 1 mM EDTA, 0.25% ovalbumin, 1 mM bacitracin, and 0.01% sodium azide. Suspensions are frozen and thawed, agitated by sucking in and out of a siliconized Pasteur pipette, and centrifuged for 20 min at 2000g before assay of the supernatant (5, 13).

Testing Cells for Damage to Membranes Caused by Treatment in Vitro

Chromium, as the Cr$_2$O$_4^{2-}$ ion, diffuses across cell membranes and is retained in the cytoplasm (15). The ^{51}Cr-labeled ion has been shown not to be released unless the cell membrane is damaged, and the released material is not then incorporated into undamaged cells. Loaded pituitary cells stimulated with GnRH release LH indistinguishably from unloaded ones and do not leak label. Label (Amersham Corp., Arlington Heights, IL) is diluted to 20–200 μCi/ml in DMEM and added to cells at a final concentration of 3–30 ng/ml (1–10 μCi/ml) for 2 hr or more before being washed with fresh medium three times. Washes are monitored to ensure low background activity. Perifusion medium or cell supernatant is monitored for released ^{51}Cr during procedures. Total releaseable ^{51}Cr is determined after the experiment by cell disruption in hypotonic solution. In static culture, cellular release of ^{51}Cr occurs only when exclusion of trypan blue is also compromised.

Perifusion Apparatus

We constructed our perifusion apparatus (16) as shown in Fig. 2; commercial versions are now available. Tubes from reservoirs holding medium, or medium containing one or more concentrations of stimulatory hormone, are released or pinched by solenoids under microcomputer control, allowing a multichannel peristaltic pump to force liquid through water-jacketed columns

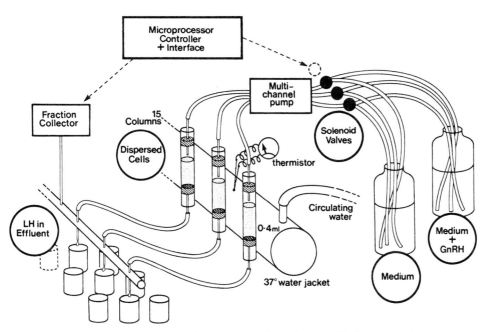

Fig. 2 Diagrammatic representation of our perifusion apparatus.

formed from 1 ml syringe barrels containing dispersed anterior pituitary cells, and into tubes in a modified fraction collector also controlled by the microcomputer. This allows us to perifuse cells for up to about 9 h with a variety of accurately produced trains of approximately square-wave stimulatory pulses of arbitrary complexity, in medium flowing through up to 15 columns simultaneously and which was collected in a fraction collector controlled by the microcomputer and modified to collect as many as 15 fractions at once. (3) Water from an incubator is pumped through a jacket to maintain columns at 37°. Each column is fitted with a fine mesh septum (10 μm) net, #19-0655-01, Pharmacia, Piscataway, NJ) to support and retain the column packing.

Perifusion Procedures

Perifusion medium (Ham's F12 or Hanks' buffered salt solution) contains 2% anestrous ewe serum, and the flow-rate is 0.14 ml/min. Aliquots of about 5×10^6 cells in suspension are loaded onto the column packing and subjected to a variety of patterns of GnRH stimulation. In some experiments, corticotropin-releasing factor (CRF) or arginine vasopressin (AVP) was used as the stimulatory hormone. Any changes in cell properties within an experiment should thus be identical for all cell samples so that differences in response are attributable to differences in the stimulatory signals. LH remaining in cells after experiments is always greater then 40% of the initial amount. Under these conditions the apparatus produces highly reproducible results from replicate columns [typically <10% coefficient of variation (CV)] (4). Columns can be sterilized by flushing for 15 min with an acidified hypochlorite solution and then washed out with sterile water. Effluent is collected into autoanalyzer cups containing 20 mM bacitracin at 5% of the final volume of the fraction. Flow rate changes as tubing becomes worn and must be checked regularly. Rates of 150–200 μl/min are used; release of LH to GnRH stimulation is insensitive to flow rates in this range (4).

Rising linear ramps of GnRH concentration are generated by pumping from mixing vessels which initially contain medium alone and to which are added suitably concentrated solutions of GnRH in medium at half the rate of removal. Different gradients are generated simultaneously using a multiplace magnetic stirrer and multichannel pump. The shape of each gradient can be confirmed by analyzing the column effluents for tritiated water included in the GnRH solutions (4).

Factors Affecting Column Output

We have analyzed mathematically factors affecting column output (17). Particularly relevant in perifusion experiments, where the shape of the stimulatory pulse is important, is that the column may distort the incoming signal at the inlet, thus introducing considerable error into the peak concentration of stimulant.

A Checklist of Potential Spurious Influences on the Outcome of Perifusion Results

In addition to the primary factors being studied, the following can actually or potentially influence perifusion results. To avoid spurious results and conclusions they must be controlled.

Tissue Preparation Method

Responsiveness, yield, and cellular viability depend on the hormonal state and age of the animal from which tissue is taken, the enzyme used for cell dispersion (collagenase, trypsin, hyaluronidase, pancreatin), the batch and supplier of enzymes, the timing of exposure of cells to dispersal agents, the method and vigor of breaking up tissue after enzyme action, the presence or absence of Ca^{2+}, and the loss of cells on nonsiliconized surfaces (1).

Cell Culture

The period of culture; the presence or absence of pulsed or continuous stimulating hormone and other hormones (steroids, etc.) added during culture to simulate the natural hormonal condition from which the tissue is removed; the presence and amount of serum and the hormonal state of the animal from which it is prepared; the type of medium and addition of other hormones such as thyroid-stimulating hormone, ferritin, and insulin; the attachment of cells to a surface and the density of cells in attachment; and the use of preconditioned medium must all be investigated.

Perifusion

Checks are required of the following: column dimensions, the tube type and length of tubing can cause signal distortion (17), as can the amount and type of column packing; the efficiency and constancy of temperature control; the adherence of stimulating or response hormone to tubing or other components; variability in size of small output fractions caused by one collected drop being a significant proportion of the total fraction (4); the preservation of released hormone (4); the baseline perifusion solution differing from stimulant-dissolving medium with respect to salts, pH, osmotic pressure, serum, etc.; a change of pressure on change of stimulating solution, or as columns become partially blocked with cell debris or gas bubbles; the reproducibility of cell loading onto columns and of results from identical multiple columns

(3, 4); loss of cells from death or leakage through the column matrix (loss of ^{51}Cr can be used to detect this); the amount of liquid above the column; gas bubbles forming owing to temperature changes; the solution above the columns running dry; microbial contamination and the effects of antibiotics in the medium; the effects of different media or salt concentrations (particularly Ca^{2+}); the use of medium, preconditioned by culturing cells; degassing or gassing of medium with 95% air or O_2 with 5% CO_2; varying the type and concentration of serum [e.g., horse serum prevented responses from sheep cells (3)]; too slow flow rates or other distortions of stimulation signal and output pattern through the apparatus (adding tritiated water to the stimulatory signal can be used to check this) (4, 17); the preliminary adjustment of cells to changed surrounding solution when perifusion begins; spurious effects arising from the depletion of releasable hormone during the experiment (4); the types and concentrations of substances used to disturb intracellular mechanisms as these may destroy cells and cause nonspecific release [we have measured the loss of ^{51}Cr to detect this (15)]; and a decline in cell responsiveness during perifusion—this can readily be checked using control columns which remain unstimulated until the end of the experiment at which time a pulse identical to that used initially is applied for comparison of cell performance (5–7).

Design of Blood Sampling

The frequency of blood sampling necessary for studying hormone dynamics cannot be guessed in advance. It is determined by the interpeak interval, a clear definition of a secretory episode being obtained only when there are at least four points on the side slowest to rise or fall. To minimize false peaks we assay samples in triplicate in random order and inspect the data for each individual sample. The variation in the measurements on a single sample is arbitrarily required to span less than one-third of the difference between the nadir and peak maximum of the pulse to which it contributes, or reassay is performed. We occasionally reassay sets of samples to confirm assignment of peaks. It should be noted that theoretically the selectivity of the antibody, bioassays, tracers, and standards could prejudice results by reacting disproportionately to the presence of small amounts of less-relevant forms of hormone which may differ from active forms in regard to conditions of secretion and rates of clearance, thus distorting the biological relevance of the measured dynamics. Indeed, without knowing precisely the relative proportions and relevant bioactive forms of hormones, their production in different hormonal states and clearance, and their degree of antibody binding, a comparison of results from one individual in differing hormonal states, or

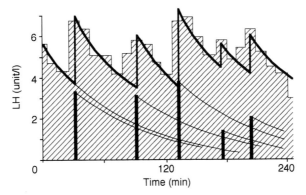

FIG. 3 Analysis by our mathematical model of pulses of LH (stepped curve) in samples of blood serum collected 2 days after the start of menstruation in a normal cycling woman. Output of the model was the estimated amplitude of peaks (vertical bars). Also shown are the decays of individual secretory episodes (thin curves) which when summed give the best fitted description (heavy curves) of the stepped experimental data. [Adapted with permission from Ref. 11.]

between individuals or laboratories, may not accurately reflect the dynamics of the bioactive hormone (11, 12).

Analysis of Peaks in Blood Samples

We assume that GnRH pulses stimulate the pituitary to release LH in discrete episodes which, when observed in blood, are distorted by mixing and clearance. The stimulatory pulses are assumed to be brief relative to the interval of blood sampling. At any time the level of blood LH represents the sum of all previous episodes, each diminished due to clearance by an amount dependent on time since its secretion (Fig. 3) (11).

Estimates of the rates of clearance of LH from blood are made directly by fitting a single exponential decay process to measurements on the descending sides of peaks or by incorporating a clearance coefficient into a more comprehensive mathematical model yielding estimates of the initial amplitude of each episode as observed in blood free of the effects of others (11).

Radioimmunoassay

Samples are analyzed immediately after experiments or stored frozen. All hormones are determined by radioimmunoassay (RIA) with iodinated tracer—sheep LH and FSH using sheep pituitary gonadotropins as both standards and tracers (5, 13); sheep adrenocorticotropic hormone (ACTH), β-lipotropin, and β-endorpin using sheep hormones as standards and tracer (6); and human LH (11) and human growth hormone (GH) (12), using the human hormones as standards and tracers. Most assays were analyzed with a computer program which estimated 95% confidence limits on all results (2, 18).

Release of $^{45}Ca^{2+}$ from Cells on Stimulation with Hormones Binding Receptors Activating Phospholipase C

Measurement of the rate of efflux of $^{45}C^{2+}$ from ovarian follicles of *Xenopus laevis* is used as a sensitive procedure for detecting the presence of receptors activated by Ca^{2+}-mobilizing hormones (10). One hundred follicles are labeled by incubation with 12 μl $^{45}Ca^{2+}$ solution (Amersham Corp., Arlington Heights, IL; 1.8 mCi/ml; 98 μg Ca^{2+}/ml) in a total volume of 500 μl modified Barths' solution for 4–5 hr at room temperature with occasional mixing. After being washed, groups of 10 follicles are transferred to columns of the perifusion apparatus containing a fitted disk of filter paper only and perifused with modified Barths' solution (0.1 ml/min) at room temperature. Stimulatory hormone is added to the medium after baseline release of $^{45}Ca^{2+}$ has been established at about 30 min. Effluent fractions (0.15 ml; 90 sec) are collected, mixed with 1.5 ml Triton X-100 scintillant, and measured for radioactivity in a liquid scintillation counter. All results are calculated as a ratio of (counts in a sample)/(counts in the third fraction of effluent—the last prestimulatory one) and expressed as a percentage, so normalizing the data from each column.

Results and Discussion

In Vitro

Examples of the kinds of information about the dyanmics of hormonal action obtainable by perifusion *in vitro* are illustrated below.

Effect of GnRH Pulse Characteristics on LH Response Pattern (3, 4)

A wide range of patterns of stimulating hormone were applied to sets of identical samples of pituitary cells perifused in columns, and the response dynamics analyzed in terms of pituitary hormone release. Consistent findings such as those illustrated in Figs. 4–6 have led us to the following conclusions.

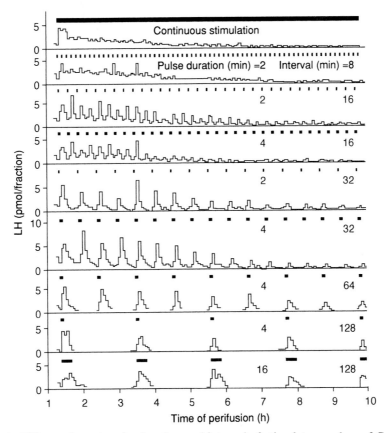

FIG. 4   Effects of varying the duration and interval of stimulatory pulses of GnRH on the release of LH by dispersed pituitary cells in nine columns. The timing and duration of stimulation at a concentration of 0.85 n*M* GnRH (1 ng/ml) is indicated by the bars. The flow rate of perifusion was 0.1 ml/min and the effluent fraction size was 0.4 ml (4-min collection). [Adapted with permission from Ref. 3.]

1. The pulse frequency of stimulant was critical, a recovery time of at least 15 min between pulses being necessary to avoid desensitization of the release response to GnRH in a few hours. Extending the intervals (to a maximum of 2 hr) between identical pulses also increased the amount of LH released at each stimulation. Maximal release of LH over 10 hr occurred with pulse periods of 15–60 min, this period depending on pulse width (3).

2. Wider pulses produced more LH but the efficiency of release (in terms of output per unit of GnRH applied) decreased with time, despite the constant presence of stimulus (3).

3. Above a threshold of 5–10 ng GnRH/ml, pulse amplitude had little influence on LH output or the rate of cellular desensitization, in marked contrast to the strong influence of pulse period (3). Desensitization, therefore, does not result from "swamping" the receptors with excess GnRH, but rather depends on the dynamic factor of too frequent stimulation.

4. Rise rates in the concentration of stimulant slower than 17 pg GnRH/ml · min allowed increased LH response capacity to be activated after initial LH release had occurred (4). This illustrates the sensitivity of the mechanism to changes in stimulatory level. Even with stimulatory concentrations well below those producing maximal LH release, more of the same signal results in a reduction of output, while an increase in stimulation can enhance release if due regard is given to dynamic factors.

5. Low, continuous baselines of stimulatory GnRH within the physiological range as measured in the pituitary portal blood supply decreased proportionally cellular response to superimposed pulses (4). Cells desensitized to continuous levels of GnRH exceeding those causing maximal LH release produced even more LH if stimulated with a much higher concentration of GnRH, even though both levels would have produced the same response prior to desensitization.

Thus, while these cells exhibit high sensitivity to increases in level of stimulation, inherent time lags pace their capacity to respond to too rapid or prolonged signals. There are sensitive phases within the rhythm of their response mechanism during which the delivery of drugs or hormones are most effective (1). Models of molecular mechanisms based on receptor and intracellular events (both spatial and chemical) must be devised which exhibit these qualitative, quantitative, and dynamic characteristics. The implications of this kind of behavior to the delivery of pharmaceuticals affecting other stimulatory systems in general remain to be explored (1).

Effect of GnRH Pulse Characteristics on the Release Patterns of FSH

LH and FSH levels in blood frequently appear to vary independently. We investigated whether the release of LH and FSH from sheep pituitary cells could be controlled differentially by the characteristics of applied signals of stimulatory GnRH alone, free of the effects of steroid feedback or other influences from the whole animal.

When cells were perifused for up to 7 hr with a variety of pulse trains and the effluent assayed for both LH and FSH we found that the outputs of both gonadotropins were significantly correlated in all cases (Figs. 5 and 6) (5). Desensitization of the response of the cells to increasing stimulatory pulse duration was the same for both hormones. Thus, varying the dose, interval,

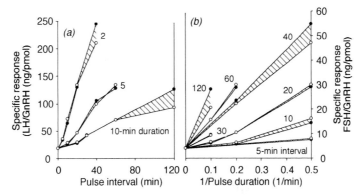

FIG. 5   Effects of different pulse (a) intervals and (b) durations on the specific response of both LH (○) and FSH (●) from freshly dispersed sheep anterior pituitary cells to stimulation in perifusion by a range of pulse trains of 4–23 nM GnRH. In (a) numbers on the graph show the duration of the pulses analyzed, whereas in (b) they indicate the intervals between pulses. The hatching emphasizes that the lines connected represent the results of analyzing for LH and FSH in the same samples. [Adapted with permission from Ref. 5.]

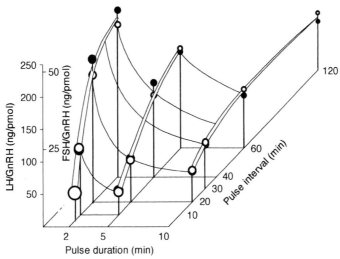

FIG. 6   Specific response of LH (○) and FSH (●) from freshly dispersed sheep anterior pituitary cells to the initial pulses of GnRH before desensitization (second, third, and fourth pulses) as functions of both pulse interval and duration. The smooth curves emphasize the trends. [Adapted with permission from Ref. 5.]

and duration of GnRH pulses did not alter the proportions of LH and FSH released in the short-term from freshly dissociated cells.

However, cells released more LH relative to FSH when treated with maximally stimulating levels of GnRH for 3 hr in the presence of 10% serum from a sheep in the follicular phase of its ovulatory cycle compared with charcoal-treated serum. Because there was no gonadotropin synthesis under the conditions used *in vitro*, this suggested that changes in the LH/ FSH ratio seen in whole animals are more likely to result from differential clearance from the circulation, ovarian feedback at the pituitary, or differential syntheses in intact tissue or another hormone influencing FSH secretion, rather than from differences in the mechanism of acute release controlled by GnRH.

Effects of the Pulse Characteristics of CRF and AVP on Release of ACTH, β-Endorphin, and β-Lipotropin

ACTH, β-endorphin, and β-lipotropin all gave strongly correlated pulsatile responses to each pulse of CRF implying similar mechanisms of release for these hormones.

The conclusions for LH and FSH responses to GnRH in 1 and 2 above are qualitatively the same for ACTH responses to CRF, AVP, or combined CRF/AVP stimuli. That is, the rising edge of the pulse stimulus is the most effective signal for hormone release, and a longer interval between pulses increases the size of the next response. Although the intracellular mechanisms differ (while CRF causes the formation of cAMP, GnRH and AVP produce inositol phosphates) dynamic controls appear to be qualitatively the same. The attributes of the processes controlling patterns of release appear to be similar and unrelated to the process of chemical transduction.

Differences in response to the various stimuli were evidenced in the slower cessation of release after withdrawal of CRF (ACTH took 20 min to fall to baseline), compared with GnRH withdrawal (5 min for LH) or AVP (Fig. 7). When CRF and AVP are used together as stimulant, it is well known that ACTH release exceeds the sum of the responses to the individual hormones. In perifusion this potentiation was seen to be caused by an increased initial height of the response pulse, because the width of the response (the time to fall to baseline) was less with combined AVP/CRF (and with AVP alone) than with CRF alone.

Separate receptors for both AVP and CRF with individual mechanisms of desensitization could be inferred from the observation that while pulse trains of submaximal levels of each produced desensitizing ACTH pulsed output, enhanced ACTH release then occurred to a fresh stimulus of the other hormone (Fig. 7).

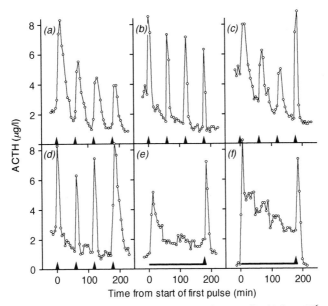

FIG. 7   Release of ACTH by sheep anterior pituitary cells (1.5×10^6 cells) in six perifusion columns receiving the following treatment. (a) Four 10-min pulses of 100 nM CRF with 60 min between pulses; (b) four 10-min pulses of 200 nM AVP with 60 min between pulses; (c) three 10-min pulses of 100 nM CRF, then one 10-min pulse of 200 nM AVP with 60 min between pulses; (d) three 10-min pulses of 200 nM AVP, then one 10-min pulse of 100 nM CRF with 60 min between pulses; (e) continuous perifusion of 20 nM CRF, followed by one 10-min pulse of 2000 nM CRF at 180 min; (f) continuous perifusion of 100 nM AVP, followed by one 10-min pulse of 2000 nM AVP at 180 min. First pulse or continuous perifusion began at 0 min; 5-min fractions were collected. [Adapted with permission from Ref. 7.]

Effects of Intracellular Modifiers and Potential Transduction Chemicals on Release Dynamics (8, 9)

Using the perifusion apparatus, modifiers of intracellular processes have been added to investigate mechanisms controlling the dyanmics of both hormone-stimulated responses, as well as responses stimulated by potential intracellular transduction products themselves.

For example, the transport of cell components by cytoskeletal structures was shown to be unlikely to be a major limitation on the dynamic patterns of LH release. Interference with either microfilaments by cytochalasin or microtubules by colchicine did not alter any aspects of the dynamics of LH release when pituitary cells were stimulated by GnRH binding to receptors, or without receptor mediation by the addition of K^+ or phorbol-12-myristate

13-acetate (PMA). However, intact microfilaments partially inhibited release of LH by all three secretagogues (8).

Stimulation with PMA alone caused an instantaneous and much higher level of LH release than did maximal stimulation with GnRH, indicating that desensitization to GnRH after 10 min is unlikely to be caused by lack of releasable LH. Furthermore, cells already desensitized to GnRH responded strongly to PMA, indicating that desensitization to GnRH occurs at a step before activation of protein kinase C. The presence of lithium in the perifusion medium, which was expected to slow the metabolism of GnRH-stimulated formation of inositol phosphates by the cells, interfered with (retarded) only the rate of desensitization of responses to GnRH (9).

In all these experiments it was important to determine what concentrations of the additives caused cell breakdown and nonspecific hormonal release and only to investigate effects on cell responses well below these levels. Release of radioactive ^{51}Cr previously loaded into the cells is appropriate for determining nonspecific cell breakdown (15).

Calcium Release from Pulsed, Perifused Cells and Tissues (10, 19)

An appropriate use for the dynamic capabilities of the perifusion apparatus has been the rapid, repeatable detection of the presence of naturally or exogenously expressed receptors. It is applicable to multiple samples of cells and can give indications of both dynamic interactions between different receptors as well as likely transduction mechanisms. In particular, we have detected receptors and their interactions and clarified mechanisms giving rise to the release of preloaded radioactive calcium on hormone binding by receptors (Fig. 8). This methodology could be extended to study the presence and dynamics of other transduction events.

Clarifying Intracellular Mechanisms and Their Dynamic Interactions

As an example, acetylcholine has been shown to induce a large increase in the formation of inositol phosphates in ovarian follicles of *X. laevis* which could not be detected on stimulation with angiotensin II under the same conditions (10). However, both hormones caused a similar strong release of $^{45}Ca^{2+}$ from follicles in perifusion which was self- but not cross-desensitizing. Subsequently, very small and more rapid increases in inositol phosphates were shown on stimulation with angiotensin II. This has interesting implications for the similarities and differences between the transduction mechanisms of these two hormone receptors (20).

Detecting Exogenously Expressed Receptors and Studying Their Dynamics

Messenger RNA prepared from sheep pituitaries was microinjected into *X. laevis* follicles which were incubated for 2 days to allow expression to occur

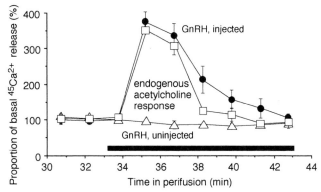

FIG. 8   Detection and desensitization of expressed mammalian GnRH receptors in *Xenopus laevis* follicles after injection of mRNA (●) by analyzing the efflux of $^{45}Ca^{2+}$ in perifusion. The bar shows the duration of hormonal stimulation. Uninjected oocytes (△) do not yield a response. The response to actylcholine (□) comes from endogenous receptors.

(14). Application of the hormones thyrotropin-releasing hormone (TRH) or GnRH in perifusion to groups of mRNA-injected follicles (but not uninjected controls) caused the release of preloaded $^{45}Ca^{2+}$ in a manner similar to that following stimulation of endogenous acetylcholine receptors in uninjected cells (Fig. 8). This allowed the detection of expression of sheep receptors in the follicles more conveniently and rapidly than by means of electrophysiological measurements. Dynamics of desensitization were also shown. Complementary DNA coding for an exogenous serotonin receptor transcribed *in vitro* has also been expressed and detected by us in this way. The dynamics of response and of interactions of these receptors expressed in follicles or other cells could be studied conveniently in perifusion.

Detecting and Studying Dynamics of New Receptors

Using the perifusion system, we have detected receptors for acetylcholine in bovine granulosa cells by measuring the release of $^{45}Ca^{2+}$ on stimulation. Release of $^{45}Ca^{2+}$ by hCG served as a positive control (19). Cells were prepared by the method of McNatty *et al.* (21).

In Vivo

Investigating Hypothalamic Stimulation of the Release of Human LH and Growth Hormone

We have applied our knowledge of the responsiveness of the LH release to rising GnRH levels and desensitization to continuous GnRH stimulation *in vitro* to interpret time series measurements of LH in blood in the normal

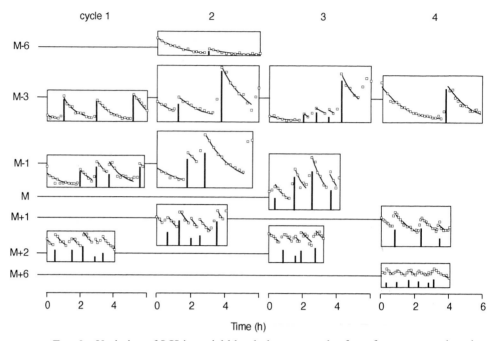

FIG. 9   Variation of LH in serial blood plasma samples from four menstrual cycles of one woman measured around menstruation on selected days during the transition from the luteal to follicular phases and the results of fitting a secretory episode model to the data. M, Day on which menstruation began. □, Measured concentration of LH; smooth curves, results of fitting the model; vertical lines, times and amplitudes of secretory episodes as seen in plasma. [Adapted with permission from Ref. 11.]

human menstrual cycle. We formulated a model incorporating brief, discrete episodic GnRH stimuli causing brief LH secretory responses followed by relatively slower clearance from the general circulation (11). Previously, LH secretion had been described as pulses imposed on a variable LH tonic release. Our model was shown to be physiologically plausible and sufficient, gave a new and detailed description of LH fluctuations in the menstrual cycle, and fitted observed data well (Fig. 9), with no evidence to support tonic release. As with the data obtained *in vitro*, we found a significant correlation between LH pulse amplitude and interval since the preceding pulse ($p < 0.01$), supporting the existence of a recovery time controlling sensitivity of the LH response of the pituitary to stimulation by GnRH.

In contrast to LH, natural secretory episodes of GH measured in the same blood samples increased in concentration much more slowly (38 vs 13 min

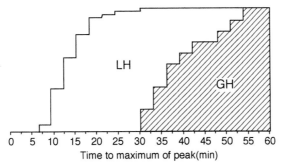

FIG. 10   Illustration of the more rapid rise of LH in comparison with GH expressed as cumulative frequency distributions of the observed times for the concentrations of the hormones to increase from minimum levels in blood to the maxima of peaks. [Adapted with permission from Ref. 12.]

to peak) (Fig. 10). However, because simultaneous intravenous injection of a mixture of GRF and GnRH stimulated indistinguishable dynamics of pituitary release of GH and LH into the blood of these same women, there must be major differences in the natural modes of hypothalamic stimuli of the two hormones. A model of effectively instantaneous pulses of hypothalamic hormone stimulating pituitary release while appropriate for LH cannot explain the secretion of GH.

References

1. R. P. McIntosh, *Trends Pharmacol. Sci.* **5**, 429 (1984).
2. J. E. A. McIntosh and R. P. McIntosh, "Mathematical Modelling and Computers in Endocrinology." Springer-Verlag, New York, 1980.
3. R. P. McIntosh and J. E. A. McIntosh, *J. Endocrinol.* **98**, 411 (1983).
4. R. P. McIntosh and J. E. A. McIntosh, *Endocrinology* **117**, 169 (1985).
5. J. E. A. McIntosh and R. P. McIntosh, *J. Endocrinol.* **109**, 155 (1986).
6. M. J. Evans, J. T. Brett, R. P. McIntosh, J. E. A. McIntosh, H. K. Roud, J. H. Livesey, and R. A. Donald, *Endocrinology (Baltimore)* **117**, 893 (1985).
7. M. J. Evans, J. T. Brett, R. P. McIntosh, J. E. A. McIntosh, H. K. Roud, J. H. Livesey, and R. A. Donald, *J. Endocrinol.* **117**, 387 (1988).
8. L. Starling, R. P. McIntosh, and J. E. A. McIntosh, *J. Endocrinol.* **111**, 167 (1986).
9. R. P. McIntosh, J. E. A. McIntosh, and L. Starling, *J. Endocrinol.* **112**, 289 (1987).
10. R. P. McIntosh and J. E. A. McIntosh, *Arch. Biochem. Biophys.* **283**, 135 (1990).
11. R. P. McIntosh and J. E. A. McIntosh, *J. Endocrinol.* **107**, 231 (1985).
12. R. P. McIntosh, J. E. A. McIntosh, and L. A. Lazarus, *J. Endocrinol.* **118**, 339 (1988).

13. R. P. McIntosh and J. E. A. McIntosh, *Acta Endocrinol.* **102,** 42 (1983).

14. R. P. McIntosh and K. J. Catt, *Proc. Natl. Acad. Sci. U.S.A.* **84,** 9045 (1987).

15. L. Starling, R. P. McIntosh, and J. E. A. McIntosh, in dissertation submitted for Ph.D. degree of L. Starling to University of Otago, New Zealand, 1988.

16. J. E. A. McIntosh, R. P. McIntosh, and R. J. Kean, *Med. Biol. Eng. Comput.* **22,** 259 (1984).

17. W. R. Smith, G. C. Wake, J. E. A. McIntosh, R. P. McIntosh, M. Pettigrew, and R. Kao, *Am. J. Physiol.* **261,** R247 (1991).

18. J. E. A. McIntosh, a program for analyzing the results of protein binding assays on the Macintosh personal computer, 1989.

19. M. P. Lacy, R. P. McIntosh, and J. E. A. McIntosh, in dissertation submitted for Ph.D. degree by M. P. Lacy to University of Otago, New Zealand, 1991.

20. M. P. Lacy, R. P. McIntosh, and J. E. A. McIntosh, *Pfluegers Arch. Eur. J. Physiol.* **420,** 127 (1992).

21. K. P. McNatty, D. A. Heath, K. M. Henderson, S. Lun, P. R. Hurst, L. M. Ellis, G. W. Montgomery, L. Morrison, and D. C. Thurley, *J. Reprod. Fertil.* **72,** 39 (1984).

Section VI

Endocrine Consequences of Pulsatile Hormone Stimulation

[21] Pulsatile Neuropeptide Delivery and Analysis of Hormone Biosynthesis

Margaret A. Shupnik

Introduction

Increasing evidence indicates that pulsatile rather than continuous administration of neuropeptide hormones is critical for appropriate pituitary hormone secretion and biosynthesis (1–3). This method of delivery is particularly crucial for the gonadotropin hormones, but data from other hormone systems have indicated that physiological effects can be maximized by the intermittent versus the continuous presence of hypothalamic factors. Methods have been developed using both *in vivo* and *in vitro* models to measure these effects; however, the *in vivo* systems often suffer from complications in data interpretation due to the presence of many other physiological factors. This review will concentrate on *in vitro* techniques for delivery of hypothalamic hormones to isolated pituitary cells and on methods for detecting those hormonal effects on gene expression.

Many investigators have used perifusion systems to vary patterns of pulsatile hypothalamic peptide administration to modulate pituitary hormone secretion (2–6), but measurements of steady-state mRNA and mRNA synthesis or transcription rates have been more diffiucult to achieve. Rates of mRNA synthesis are not trivial to quantitate accurately, particularly for mRNAs of low abundance in mixed cell populations. Since this situation applies to most pituitary hormones and to many other mRNAs of physiological importance, an assay with the highest possible sensitivity must be used. Methods are described below which combine a continuous perifusion system for neuropeptide delivery with detection of mRNA levels and mRNA synthesis rates by nuclear runoff assays.

Perifusion Systems

The first and chief advantage of continuous perifusion systems is the ability to challenge the cells or tissue with multiple, precise pulses of hormonal treatments for long periods of time. This has special significance when investigating hypothalamic peptide action on pituitary cells, as desensitization of releasing factor receptors can blunt the subsequent or long-term biological responses (1). The gonadotropins appear to be particularly sensitive to the form of gonadotropin-releasing hormone (GnRH) administration, with only pulsatile peptide treatment resulting in meaningful biological effects on two of the three gonadotropin subunits in studies from our laboratory as well as in investigations by Weiss *et al.* (2, 3). Second, medium and any secreted hormone or proteolytic enzymes are constantly being removed from contact with the cells, preventing the harmful action of any accumulated substances or the action of short-loop feedback mechanisms. The system thus represents a more physiological situation. Finally, the use of a solid support to mix with the cells or fragments in most perifusion systems eliminates the need for the cell attachment period and allows the cells to be used immediately. We have found this to be a great advantage in measuring gonadotropin mRNA and mRNA synthesis, which decline continuously in static culture systems, perhaps due to the loss of an important physiological signal.

There are significant limitations to perifusion systems, primarily associated with the need for specialized equipment and the limited number of samples which can be run and analyzed at any one time. The apparatus described below is usually run with 6 chambers, but can be adapted to run with 12—a number which appears to be a usual limit for many such instruments (2–6). This does limit the number of experimental groups which can be included at any one time, and we have found that it is better to run duplicates or triplicates of any one treatment in the same run and to run additional groups in conjunction with additional controls on a subsequent day. This is of vital importance when performing a complicated assay such as transcriptional measurements, in which experimental variation can make comparison of results from different studies complicated and unsatisfactory. A second difficulty is the collection and preparation of samples for analysis, which takes longer and must take into account the presence of the inert cellular support. While not problematic for procedures which destroy the cell and allow for supernatant collection (such as mRNA isolation), this has proven to be more difficult when nuclei must be isolated. In this situation, pituitary fragments instead of dispersed cells may be used in acute experiments to measure changes in transcriptional rates.

Continuous Perifusion of Dispersed Pituitary Cells and Pituitary Fragments

Perifusion experiments involve the preparation of dispersed pituitary cells or fragments, addition of cells to the inert matrix, the perifusion experiment itself, and the measurement of hormone biosynthesis as reflected by changes in mRNA levels or rates of mRNA transcription. Each of these steps is discussed independently, with detailed procedures as well as references to alternate procedures in the literature which have been proven to be valuable in other experimental settings.

Dispersed Pituitary Cells

Dispersed pituitary cells are the best choice for performing many hormonal treatment studies, as they represent a homogeneous population standardized between many experimental animals and can easily and reliably be distributed between many sample wells. Furthermore, isolated cells can be maintained in culture for long periods of time without appreciable cell death and without losing appropriate biological responses to stimuli (4, 7). The accessibility to nutrients and buffer by isolated cells compared to fragments of tissue appears to be responsible for the long-term functionality of monolayer cultures.

Some proposed disadvantages to the use of dispersed cells include the potential loss of pituitary gland architecture which might interfere with cell-to-cell communication and potential damage to cellular membranes and membrane-bound receptors during the isolation procedure. While the importance of the disruption of specific structural contacts between cells remains unknown, several groups have demonstrated that pituitary cells retain or regain their responsivity to stimulatory and inhibitory secretogogues at least as soon as 4 hr after dispersion; GnRH stimulation of luteinizing hormone (LH) secretion can occur normally after various dissociation procedures (4).

Preparation of Dispersed Cells

Mature (200–225 g) female Sprague–Dawley rats (CD strain; Charles River, Wilmington, MA) are used in all protocols. Normal intact females are housed under 14 : 10 hr light : dark cycles. For experiments with ovariectomized (OVX) animals, ovaries are surgically removed by the supplier, and animals are used 18–24 days postovariectomy to allow for maximal increases in gonadotrope cell number and gonadotropin subunit gene transcription rates. For all experiments animals are killed by decapitation, and trunk blood is collected for radioimmunoassay of serum LH, follicle-stimulating hormone (FSH), and estradiol (E_2).

Anterior pituitary glands are removed, separated from the posterior pituitary gland, and collected into Dulbecco's minimal essential medium (DMEM; Gibco/BRL Life Technologies; Gaithersburg, MD) containing streptomycin (2.5 μ/ml) and penicillin (10 U/ml). The time from removal of glands to beginning the cell dispersion or macerating the gland into fragments should be as short as possible, and we usually accomplished this within 30 min.

Collected glands are rinsed several times at room temperature in a petri dish containing HEPES-buffered saline (HBS, 0.15 M NaCl, 0.1 M HEPES, pH 7.2) and then cut with two sterile No. 10 scalpels into approximately 20 pieces per gland. The tissue fragments are then collected into a 15-ml conical tube and rinsed twice with 10 ml HBS, or until all debris and red blood cells are removed. The HBS is then removed and replaced with trypsin solution (0.25% trypsin: Gibco/BRL Life Technologies) at a volume of approximately 1 ml/pituitary gland. The enzyme and tissue are transferred to a water-jacketed (37°C) sterile glass spinner flask (Wheaton Scientific, Millville, NJ), which contains a Teflon stir bar suspended by a metal rod from the top of the chamber. By placing the water-jacketed chamber, connected by rubber tubing to a temperature-controlled circulating water bath such as those available from Lauda (Brinkmann Instruments, Westbury, NY), on top of a mechanical stir plate, the tissue fragments are subjected to continuous stirring while incubating in the trypsin mixture. After 20 min, the flask is removed from the stir plate and circulating water bath, and the fragments are triturated inside the hood with a siliconized, fire-polished Pasteur pipette. If required (that is, if there is no appreciable change in the appearance of the tissue fragments) the incubation can be continued for an additional 10 min. After this treatment, the solution containing the cells and fragments is removed from the chamber and centrifuged in a sterile conical tube at 100 g for 10 min. The pellet and tissue fragments are suspended in an equal volume of pancreatin (Gibco/BRL Life Technologies: final concentration of 2 mg/ml, diluted into HBS) and incubated for an additional 10 min. At this time, an equal volume of calf serum is added to the cell mixture to inhibit further enzyme activity, and the solution is subjected to centrifugation at 100 g for 10 min. Any undigested fragments are removed, and the cells are resuspended in 10 ml HBS and centrifuged again. This process is repeated two to three times, or until all debris and as many as possible red blood cells are removed. A 10-μl aliquot is taken from the cell suspension for cell counting with a hemacytometer. Cell viability, usually >95%, is determined by the exclusion of 0.4% trypan blue (Gibco). While the trypsin protocol results in good yields of viable cells (2–6), other procedures using collagenase digestions (7) have also been used successfully by our laboratory as well as by others.

Cell yields vary between 1.6 and 2.5 × 10^6 cells/pituitary. They do not vary appreciably between intact and OVX animals; in fact, the larger pituitaries from OVX females appear to be more fragile and often require less dispersion time, with lower cell viability than glands from normal intact females. Cells from two glands are routinely used on perifusion columns to provide secretion profiles (4). However, we have found that mRNA isolation is more quantitative and reproducible when $8-10 \times 10^6$ cells per column are used.

Pituitary Fragments

While dispersed pituitary cells are advantageous for many studies, we have not found them to be amenable to the manipulation required for the measurement of gene transcription rates. In particular, in our hands the preparation of nuclei from dispersed cells on an inert support cannot be performed effectively. Trypsin digestion of cells from the column results in low yields and requires a longer time than is optimal for short time points. Homogenization of cell-containing beads does not result in a clean nuclei preparation, as the beads or bed fragments are not separated effectively from nuclei by centrifugation. Nuclei activity, as measured by incorporation of radioactive precursor into nucleic acid, is also low. Thus, pituitary fragments are used as the biological system to measure effects of pulsatile neuropeptide treatment on mRNA synthesis. The fragments can be maintained on columns for up to 6–8 hr, times more than sufficient to measure transcriptional effects, and can easily be separated from the solid support for nuclei isolation.

Preparation of Pituitary Fragments

Animals and anterior pituitary gland collections are as described for dispersed pituitary cells. The gland is separated into hemipituitaries, which are matched for control and treatment groups. Each hemipituitary is placed in a petri dish in HBS and cut with a scalpel into 8–12 fragments. Fragments are removed with fine forceps, rinsed in cold HBS, then transferred to culture wells with DMEM containing 10 U/ml penicillin, 2.5 μg/ml streptomycin, and 2.5% bovine serum albumin (BSA, Fraction V, Sigma Chemical Co., St. Louis, MO), which is also the medium for column perifusion. Fragments are distributed between wells as they are to be distributed between columns, by matching hemipituitaries between control and treatment groups and by randomizing fragments between columns. If possible, fragments from every pituitary are included on each column, and each column contains the tissue equivalent of three to four pituitaries.

Column Matrix

We and many other investigators have followed the methods of Lowry *et al.* (8) in which dispersed cells are mixed with polyacrylamide beads prior to being loaded into the perifusion chamber. Smith and Vale (7) described a similar procedure in which Cytodex beads (Sephadex microcarrier beads) were used, and collagen-coated beads (Cytodex 3; Sigma Chemical Co.) have been successfully utilized to monitor pulsatile effects of hypothalamic peptides on pituitary hormone secretion and mRNA levels (5). Finally, organic substrates such as Matrigel (Collaborative Research, Inc; Bedford, MA) have been used to coat plastic disks as a support for dispersed pituitary cells. These cultures maintain their responsiveness to physiological challenges even after 2 days of perifusion (6). All available data on secretory and biosynthetic responses of the pituitary cells suggest that each of these supports gives satisfactory results and that each would be acceptable in similar experiments.

In our studies, the polyacrylamide gel (BioGel P-2, 200–400 mesh; Bio-Rad, Richmond, CA) is swollen overnight (0.5 g/column) in sterile tubes containing 10 ml autoclaved 0.15 M NaCl. The excess saline is then decanted and the gel mixed in a petri dish with the dispersed cells or with the pituitary fragments. The gel is mixed thoroughly with the cells or tissue and is then introduced into the perifusion columns.

Perifusion Apparatus

The perifusion system used in our laboratory is pictured in Fig. 1 (1) and has successfully been used by others (3, 9). It consists of a bank of up to 12 chambers containing the BioGel and cells. The chambers are 3-ml syringes with hollow barrels (Gilette Surgical, Enfield, Middlesex, England) hung in parallel with clamps in a 37°C water bath. The septum of each syringe is punctured by a 21-gauge needle connected to Tygon tubing ($\frac{1}{32}$-inch inner diameter, VWR Scientific, Philadelphia, PA), which forms the outlet line by which media are transported to a fraction collector. The inflow line is connected to the nozzle of the syringe and medium, hormone treatment, or other solutions are in separate bottles maintained at 37°C in a stationary water bath. Medium or treatment travels through $\frac{3}{32}$-inch diameter Tygon tubing to a peristaltic pump (Brinkmann Instruments, Westbury, NY) and solutions from the pump connect to a T-tube (Acculab, Norwood, NJ) from which a single $\frac{3}{32}$-inch Tygon tubing line carries the mixed solution to the syringe chambers. Treatment is begun when the input line is opened automatically by the three-way stopcock as programmed by a microcomputer.

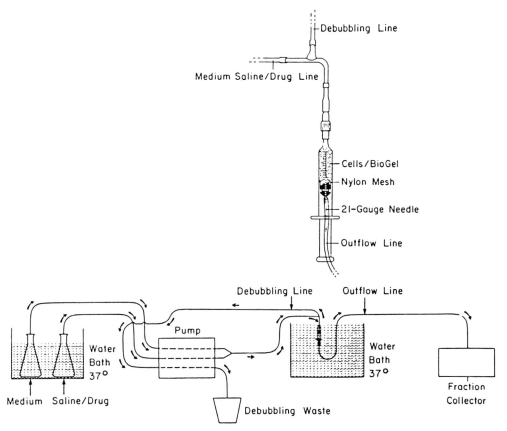

FIG. 1   The perifusion system used for dispersed cells or pituitary fragments. The construction of the perifusion chamber using a hollow-barrel syringe is shown in the upper portion of the figure. [Reproduced with permission from W. S. Evans *et al.* *Endocrinology (Baltimore)* **112,** 535 (1983).]

Perifusion Treatments

BioGel and cells are drawn into the syringe chambers with the output line clamped shut. The cells or fragments and gels are allowed to settle and excess medium is forced out. Final volumes inside the columns are approximately 1.5 ml. Perifusion medium is DMEM containing 2.5% bovine serum albumin (BSA), antibiotics as above, and 10 mM HEPES (Sigma Chemical Co.), pH 7.6. Hormonal treatments are prepared in the same medium. Flow rates are between 0.4 and 0.5 ml/min and may be adjusted by pump speed and tubing diameter. An approximate 1 : 10 dilution of hormonal treatment results with this design, as validated by the measurement of BSA pulses or radioactive tracer. Cells or fragments are equilibrated in the columns for 1–2 hr with perifusion medium prior to the beginning of pulsatile hormone treatment.

Treatment with GnRH (25 ng/ml; Sigma Chemical Co.) is conducted during the final 10 min of the next hour of perifusion. Thus, accounting for the dilution factor, 25 ng of GnRH is delivered over a 10-min interval. Varying doses of GnRH are delivered by varying the concentration of the stock treatment solution, rather than by altering the flow rate or time of delivery. GnRH treatment is usually continued for 3 hr, but we have successfully continued treatment for up to 12 hr for either fragments or cells. Outflow media are collected in 2.5-ml (5 min) fractions and stored at −20°C for radioimmunoassay of secreted peptide hormones using kits from the NIH. After the final GnRH pulse, columns are perfused with control medium for 20 min before tissue or cells are collected for assay. Chambers and lines are washed first with sterile saline and then with 70% ethanol for 2 hr prior to equipment storage.

Other investigators, using similar apparatus, matrix, and cell dispersion methods, have equilibrated the cells for up to 24 hr (3) and have performed GnRH or other hormonal treatments for up to 48 hr (3, 4, 9) with excellent viability and responsiveness. We have found that long-term treatment of fragments (over 12 hr) results in lower nuclei activity and lower amounts of RNA recovery, probability due to necrosis (4). However, as transcriptional effects occur within a few hours, longer treatment periods have not been necessary. The shorter equilibration period (1–2 hr) here compared to some protocols does not appear to have deleterious consequences on cell activity as LH secretory responses to GnRH (Fig. 2) are comparable between this and other protocols. Some custom-made perifusion chambers (0.84 ml total volume), which hold matrigel-coated disks as supports for dispersed pituitary cells (6), appear to be an attractive alternative system for cell maintenance and pulsatile hormone treatments. As the cell-containing matrigel may be processed directly by homogenization or organic solvents, such a system may also be useful for nuclei preparation.

Quantitation of Gonadotropin Subunit mRNA Levels and Gene Transcription Rates

In our experiments to assess the effects of pulsatile GnRH treatment on gonadotropin subunit gene expression, we have concentrated on changes in transcription rates. Direct transcriptional effects occur very rapidly, are usually maximal within 30 min (10), and represent a powerful biosynthetic

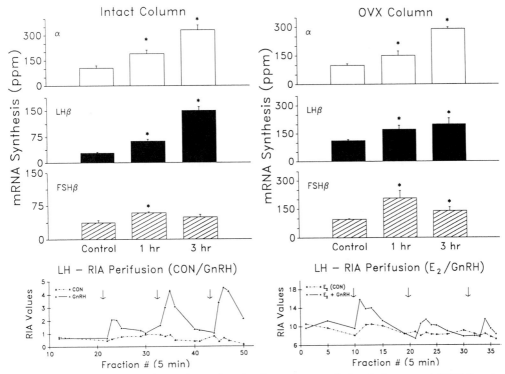

FIG. 2   Rates of gonadotropin subunit gene transcription in intact and OVX female rat pituitary fragments in response to pulsatile GnRH administration. The upper three panels depict the calculated rates of mRNA synthesis in response to 0 (control), 1, or 3 pulses of 25 ng GnRH given during the last 10 min of a 60-min interval. Each bar represents the mean ± SEM of three to four columns/group. *, $p < 0.05$. The lower panel depicts secreted LH (ng/ml) for individual columns from control (dotted lines) and GnRH-treated (solid lines) tissue. The arrows indicate the time of each GnRH pulse. [Reproduced with permission from Shupnik (2).]

response to a given stimulus. We occasionally also measure steady-state mRNA levels. However, since the LHβ and α-subunit mRNAs have very long half-lives (9, 11), only small changes in these levels may be noted during the course of most perifusion experiments. LH secretion measured in all experiments verifies that the pituitary tissue is responding to GnRH under these conditions and that it continues to respond to GnRH at the end of the experiment when mRNA or transcriptional measurements are made. Methods for quantitation of both steady-state mRNA levels and mRNA synthesis rates are given, with emphasis on measurements of gene transcription.

Steady-State mRNA Levels

Isolation of mRNA

Total RNA is isolated by the method of Chirgwin *et al.* (12) in a solution of 4 M guanidinium thiocyanate (Fluka BioChemika Co.; Ronkonkoma, NY), 25 mM sodium citrate, and 0.1 M 2-mercaptoethanol (GTC solution). Unless otherwise noted, all chemicals were from Sigma Chemical Co. Because 2-mercaptoethanol is volatile and is itself a potent ribonuclease inhibitor, the solution is not autoclaved. However, all other solutions, glassware, and nonsterile plasticware are autoclaved or, for sucrose-, Tris-, or HEPES-containing solutions, sterilized by passage through a 0.2-μm filter.

For dispersed cells, the column contents are decanted into a sterile tube containing 3 ml GTC and pipetted up and down several times with a 5-ml pipette, and the BioGel is removed by centrifugation at 100 g for 10 min. This treatment is sufficient to thoroughly disrupt the cells and nuclei. If the solution remains viscous, it is passaged through a 21-gauge needle until the soluton passes easily. Tissue fragments are removed from the gel with forceps, rinsed several times in ice-cold HBS to remove any clinging beads, and sonicated in 3 ml of GTC with a microtip and sonicator (W-225 Heat Systems Ultrasonics, Inc., Farmingdale, NY) with three 5-sec bursts at a 3.5 setting. The homogenate is subjected to centrifugation through a 2 ml cushion of 5.7 M cesium chloride (Gallard-Schlessinger Industries, Inc., Carle Place, NY), 0.1 M EDTA, pH 7.0 (Glisen), in a Beckman ultracentrifuge (Beckman Instruments; Palo Alto, CA) using an SW 55 rotor at 33,000 rpm for 18 hr. The RNA pellet is taken up in 300 μl of sterile 0.3 M sodium acetate and precipitated overnight at $-20°C$ in the presence of three volumes of ethanol. Average RNA yields are 200–250 μg for dispersed cells and 150–200 μg for pituitary fragments. Variations of this technique (3, 6, 13) are in standard use in many laboratories and result in good yields of undegraded mRNA from many sources.

mRNA Quantitation

Because methods to quantitate the gonadotropin subunit mRNAs use common standard protocols discussed at length in many publications (3, 14), they are only outlined briefly here. Aliquots (20 μg in 2 μl) of total RNA from each sample are heated for 5 min in the presence of 2.2 M formaldehyde and subjected to electrophoresis on a 1.4% agarose, 2.2 M formaldehyde-

TABLE I   Comparison of Steady-State Gonadotropin
Subunit mRNA Levels in Several Pituitary
Culture Systems versus Fresh Tissue[a]

	Normalized arbitrary densitometry units		
RNA source	α-Subunit	LHβ	FSHβ
Fresh pituitaries	10.1 ± 1.6	5.7 ± 0.9	3.2 ± 0.7
Monolayer culture	5.0 ± 1.2	3.3 ± 0.9	2.2 ± 0.3
Cell perifusion	5.4 ± 1.1	3.0 ± 0.5	1.3 ± 0.3
Fragment perifusion	4.4 ± 1.7	2.2 ± 0.3	1.5 ± 0.4

[a] Total RNA was isolated from OVX female rat pituitaries, including
fresh tissue, monolayer cell cultures (24 hr), or dispersed cells or
tissue fragments perfused for 6 hr. Aliquots of RNA (20 μg; 4 sam-
ples/group) were run on the same Northern blot and hybridized with
labeled DNA encoding FSHβ, LHβ, α-subunit, and β-actin. Each
sample value was obtained by scanning densitometry and normalization for β-actin mRNA in the same sample. Each value represents
the mean ± SEM for four samples.

containing gel. RNA is transferred by diffusion blotting overnight to a nitrocellulose membrane (Scleicher and Schuell, Keene, NH), and the filter baked
at 70°C for 2 hr to immobilize the RNA. The membrane is hybridized succes-
sively overnight at 42°C in 50% formamide buffer (14) with labeled cDNA
probes for FSHβ, LHβ, α-subunit, and β-actin. Blots are hybridized with
10^6 cpm probe/ml hybridization solution, and probes are labeled by the
random-priming method (15) to a specific activity of 3–8 × 10^7 cpm/μg DNA.
After being washed twice at room temperature for 15 min in 2× SSC (1×
SSC = 0.15 M NaCl, 0.015 M sodium citrate), once at 65°C in 2× SSC, 0.1%
SDS, and twice for 15 min at room temperature in 0.2× SSC, the blots are
exposed to X-ray film (XAR, Eastman Kodak, Rochester, NY) and the
hybridizing bands quantitated by scanning densitometry. Exposure times
(generally 1–5 days) are adjusted so that band intensity falls within 0.5–5
OD units, the linear range of detection. Blots are stripped of bound probe
between hybridizations by incubation with 10 mM Tris, pH 8.0, for 10–15
min at 85°C. Data are corrected for variation in lane loading or transfer by
normalization for β-actin mRNA values.

A comparison of mRNA quantitation in 20 μg of RNA from pituitaries,
monolayer cell cultures, and fragments is shown in Table I. All culture
systems show lower amounts of gonadotropin subunit mRNA compared to
fresh pituitary glands. However, short-term cultures and perifused cells or
fragments have similar amounts of subunit mRNAs and similar ratios between

the subunit mRNAs. Furthermore, the response to pulsatile GnRH appears to be similar in short-term perifusions of fragments and dispersed cells.

Measurement of Gene Transcription Rates

Isolation of Nuclei

After perifusion, pituitary fragments are removed from the BioGel and homogenized on ice in 1 ml of buffer (0.25 M sucrose, 5 mM MgCl$_2$, 0.1% Triton X-100, 20 mM Tris–HCl, pH 7.9). A 2-ml glass hand-held homogenizer (Kontes Co., Vineland, NJ) is used with the tight ''A'' pestle for 10 strokes. This solution and two 1-ml rinses of the homogenizer are layered over 5 ml of sucrose cushion (0.5 M sucrose, 5 mM MgCl$_2$, 20 mM Tris–HCl, pH 7.9) in a 15-ml sterile Corex tube and centrifuged in a Beckman J2-21M centrifuge (JA20 rotor) at 8000 rpm for 10 min at 4°C. Supernatants are decanted and the nuclear pellets dispersed with a sterile 200-μl pipette tip into 70 μl of storage buffer [30% glycerol, 150 mM KCl, 50 mM HEPES, pH 7.4, 5 mM MgCl$_2$, 1 mM dithiothreitol (DTT)] and 1 μl RNasin (Promega Corp., Madison, WI). The nuclei may be stored at −70°C at this point for up to 4 weeks, but we have found that the best results are obained if fresh nuclei are used for the incorporation. Because, however, the processing of the RNA and the hybridization of the RNA must occur immediately after the incorporation, time constraints on the investigator will determine if nuclei storage is required. The nuclei preparation step is the single most important determinant in the success of a transcription experiment, and gentle treatment is essential. It may be possible to obtain higher yields of nuclei with more rigorous homogenization, but we have found that this results in lower nucleotide incorporation. The pelleting of the nuclei through the sucrose cushion results in a cleaner preparation and appears to remove substances which lower nuclei activity.

Preparation of Labeled RNA Transcripts

Methods for the measurement of pituitary gonadotropin subunit gene transcription are largely based on those of McKnight and Palmiter (10) and have proved successful in many laboratories to measure many gene transcription rates. Isolated nuclei (68 μl) are incubated in 1.5-ml sterile microfuge tubes with O-ring screwtops (Sarstedt Co., Newton, NC) with 250 μCi [α-^{32}P]UTP (800 Ci/millimol; New England Nuclear, DuPont, Boston, MA) in a 100-μl volume containing final concentrations of 150 mM KCl, 5 mM MgCl$_2$, 20% glycerol (from nuclei), 2 mM DTT, 9 μM creatine phosphate, 16 μg/ml creatine phosphokinase, and 0.4 mM each of rATP, rGTP, and rCTP (Promega Corp.). We have found that the inclusion of the enzymatic energy-regenerating system increases the amount of newly labeled RNA two-fold, and we add the enzyme, creatine phosphate, and nucleotides separately from stock solutions to the incorporation reaction. Incubations proceed at room temperature in a radiation hood for 30 min. Longer incubation times result in lower levels of acid-insoluble radioactivity, presumably because of endogenous RNase activity. Because these reactions contain large amounts of radioactivity and require several manipulations, we have found it is best to use screwtop tubes and to parafilm the tops tightly for each incubation and centrifugation. We also designate a specific microfuge for transcription reactions if possible. The need for large amounts of radioactivity may be alleviated by a method which measures steady-state levels of unlabeled intronic mRNA in the primary transcripts by RNase protection assays (16). This method assumes that levels of transcribed RNA are directly proportional to the rate of gene transcription, not independently regulated, and of sufficient mass to be detected by liquid hybridization techniques. While this is true for the proopiomelanocortin gene (16), we have been unsuccessful in applying this method to the gonoadotropin subunits, possibly because of the low levels of mRNA transcribed.

After the incorporation, carrier RNA [10 μl containing 30 μg rat liver poly(A)$^-$ RNA] is added with an equal volume (10 μl) of 2× DNase buffer [20 mM HEPES, pH 7.4, 5 mM MgCl$_2$, 2 mM CaCl$_2$, 2 mM MnCl$_2$ and freshly added 100 μg/ml RQ DNase (RNase-free Dnase, Promega Corp.)] and incubated at 37°C for 15 min. After DNase digestion, an equal volume (220 μl) of freshly made 2× proteinase K solution [20 mM HEPES, pH 7.4, 10 mM EDTA, 2.0% w/v sodium dodecyl sulfate (SDS), and 400 μg/ml proteinase K (Boehringer-Mannheim Biochemicals, Indianapolis, IN)] is added and the reaction incubated at 60°C for 45 min. This solution is then extracted with an equal volume of PIC (phenol : isoamyl alcohol : chloroform at 24 : 2 : 25 v : v : v), and the aqueous upper phase is transferred to another sterile screwtop microfuge tube. At this point, a small aliquot (2 μl) may be taken to spot on glass fiber filters to determine trichloroacetic acid-precipitable radioactivity, if desired. Nucleic acids are precipitated from the aqueous solution by the addition of 1/10 volume (40 μl) 3 M sodium acetate, pH 5.5, and 2 volumes of cold absolute ethanol. The tubes are then incubated overnight at −20°C, or for 1 hr on dry ice, and spun in a microfuge at 15,000 g for 20 min at 4°C to precipitate the nucleic acids. The pellet is lyophilized to just dryness and then resuspended in 100 μl of 1× DNase buffer (without enzyme) by vortexing and heating at 60°C if necessary. An additional 100 μl of 1× DNase buffer containing 100 μg/ml DNase is added and the reactions are incubated at 37°C for 15 min as above. The proteinase K incubation and PIC extraction are repeated exactly as above.

After the second PIC extraction, the aqueous phase is transferred to another clean sterile tube, and 5 μg of yeast tRNA and 40 μl of 100% trichloroacetic acid (TCA) (w/v) are added. The tubes are incubated on ice for 10 min, and the precipitate is collected by centrifugation for 10 min in a microfuge. The supernatant is decanted, the tubes swabbed with a cotton tip, and the hard, marble-like pellets air-dried for 10 min. The pellets are then dissolved in elution buffer (20 mM Tris–HCl, pH 8.0, 1 mM EDTA, 0.5% SDS, 50 μg/ml yeast tRNA) by heating to 65°C for 10 min and vortexing. The pure RNA is collected by ethanol precipitation, centrifugation, and lyophilization as above, and the pellet hydrated in 23 μl sterile water overnight at 4°C. A 1-μl aliquot of hydrated ^{32}P-labeled RNA is then counted by scintillation spectroscopy to determine the yield of labeled RNA, which is required to calculate the final rate of transcription, below.

We have also prepared labeled RNA by combining the proteinase K solution with GTC buffer and centrifugation over CsCl as described for total RNA above (12). However, the yields of RNA are sometimes quite low with this procedure and large volumes of radioactive solution which must be spun overnight in an ultracentrifuge. Thus, the ability to contain the radioactivity in a smaller volume, and in a procedure which does not contaminate expensive equipment, coupled with the greater consistency of the McKnight and Palmiter method have combined to make us favor this technique. The TCA precipitation does result in partial hydrolysis of the RNA and must not be allowed to continue for more than the 10 min incubation time. However, these somewhat smaller RNA chains hybridize more efficiently than the long primary transcripts, and a higher percentage hybridization results.

Hybridization of Labeled RNA

Specific mRNA sequences are detected by hybridization to cDNAs or gene fragments immobilized on 7-mm nitrocellulose disks (BA85, Scleicher and Schuell). The filters are prepared by the method of Kafatos (17). Plasmids containing the cDNA coding sequence for α-subunit (18) or FSHβ (14) or the LHβ gene (19) are enzymatically linearized and denatured by the addition of 1/10 volume of 4 M NaOH and incubation for 15 min. The solution is neutralized by the addition of an equal volume of sterile 2 M ammonium acetate (1 M final concentration). The denatured DNA is then applied to nitrocellulose filters which have been equilibrated with 1 M ammonium acetate. DNA (2 μg) is applied to each filter in a 20-μl volume to each disk sitting on a prewet nitrocellulose sheet. After the DNA is adsorbed by the filter, the disk is washed with an additional 20-μl aliquot of 1 M ammonium acetate. The disks are then air-dried, baked at 70°C under vacuum for 2 hr, and stored at −70°C if not used immediately. Separate filters containing the cloning vector, usually the plasmids pGEM or pBR322, are also prepared and used in the hybridization reactions to measure background binding. When multiple mRNAs are to be measured simultaneously, the filters are cut or notched after baking so they may be distinguished after hybridization and washing.

Each hybridization reaction contains 22 μl of ^{32}P-RNA and approximately 1000 cpm of sense ^{3}H-RNA for each gonadotropin subunit synthesized from pGEM vectors by an *in vitro* transcription kit (Promega Corp.) for a total aqueous volume of 25 μl. To the labeled RNA is added 2 volumes (50 μl) of hybridization buffer (50% deionized formamide; 75 mM PIPES, pH 7.0; 3 mM EDTA; 0.75% SDS: 0.75 M NaCl; 200 μg/ml yeast tRNA) and separate filters each containing immobilized cloning vector or gonadotropin subunit cDNAs or genes. Prior to use, filters are prehybridized in batches at 42°C for a minimum of 4 hr in hybridization buffer diluted one-third with sterile water. We routinely use round-bottom 12 × 75-mm polypropylene tubes (Sarstedt) for hybridizations, but small sealed pouches as used for Northern or Southern blotting may also be used. The filter-containing hybridizations are incubated at 42°C for 48–72 hr with constant shaking.

After hybridization, each filter is washed independently in plastic tubes with 1 ml of Buffer A (0.3 M NaCl; 2 mM EDTA; 10 mM Tris, pH 7.4) once at room temperature for 30 min and once at 45°C for 30 min, followed by a wash at 37°C in Buffer A containing 1 μg/ml RNase A (Sigma Chemical Co.) and 10 U/ml RNase T1 (Gibco/BRL Life Technologies) and a final wash at 60°C for 30–45 min in buffer A containing 0.1% SDS.

After being washed, filters are transferred to individual scintillation vials and incubated for 30 min at room temperature in 250 μl of 0.04 M NaOH to remove bound RNA for more efficient counting. After neutralization with 100 μl of 0.1 M acetic acid, 10 ml of ReadySafe scintillation fluid (Beckman) is added, and samples are counted for 20 min with a dual-channel program for ^{3}H and ^{32}P in a LKB Wallac 1214 Rackbeta scintillation counter (Turku, Finland). Efficiency of counting is 35% for tritium and 98% for phosphorus-32, and spillover between channels is calculated and corrected automatically.

Calculation of Transcription Rates and Assay Validation

Once filters have been counted, the rates of gene transcription or mRNA synthesis may be calculated. For each gonadotropin subunit filter, the number of bound ^{3}H- and ^{32}P-RNA counts is corrected for counts hybridizing to the cloning vector filter. With this protocol background hybridization is almost nondetectable for tritium and usually less than 0.0001% (10 parts per million) for phosphorus-32. The percentage hybridization of each ^{3}H-RNA is calculated to determine the percentage efficiency of binding and usually ranges between 25 and 60%. There is no cross-hybridization between the ^{3}H-RNAs and the other cDNA filters (e.g., between ^{3}H-FSHβ mRNA and the α-subunit

TABLE II   Analysis of Gonadotropin Subunit mRNA Synthesis in Isolated Pituitary Nuclei[a]

	Input RNA	[32P]RNA bound				[3H]RNA bound			mRNA synthesis		
		α	LHβ	FSHβ	pGEM	α	LHβ	FSHβ	α	LHβ	FSHβ
Experiment I		cpm $\times$ 10^6				%			ppm		
Control	5.0	358	333	196	18	30	33	22	227	191	164
	6.3	414	491	210	30	29	35	20	209	210	142
α-Amanitin	1.9	23	23	18	10	28	30	24	22	21	17
	2.4	30	26	21	11	31	33	25	26	19	17
Experiment II											
Control	7.0	635	616	353	45	35	38	26	240	215	169
+10 μg RNA	7.0	516	569	312	47	28	33	22	239	226	172
+50 μg RNA	7.0	122	259	202	36	5	15	15	245	212	158

[a] Nuclei were isolated from 21-day OVX female rats and incubated in nuclear runoff reactions. Transcription rates were calculated after hybridizing labeled mRNA to filter-bound unlabeled DNA encoding the gonadotropin subunits. In Experiment I, the RNA polymerase II inhibitor α-amanitin (2 μg/ml) was included in the incubation reaction. In Experiment II, competitor total pituitary RNA was included in three separate hybridization reactions from a single incorporation.

or LHβ filters) as tested in individual separate hybridizations. Although the efficiency of binding of a particular subunit mRNA is usually identical among many samples within a given experiment, efficiency values vary between experiments and are often different when the subunit mRNAs are compared (Table II). For each filter, the specifically bound ^{32}P-RNA counts in a given sample are then corrected for the efficiency of subunit mRNA binding, and the amount of input ^{32}P-RNA, in millions of counts. The larger the amount of input ^{32}P-RNA, the better the results, and less than one million cpm of input RNA is insufficient to obtain values of transcriptional rates with any confidence. While we have used 1–2 $\times$ 10^6 cpm, we generally use 4–20 $\times$ 10^6 cpm of input RNA in the hybridizations. Some investigators prefer to standardize the hybridizations by using only a common amount of input RNA and to use autoradiography of the filters to determine transcription rate (20). This less laborious method is particularly attractive if only one subunit mRNA or other mRNA is to be measured, and relative changes in transcription rates are all that is desired. Specificity of transcriptional effects are then determined by normalization for transcription rate changes of a housekeeping gene such as β-actin. We prefer to use all newly synthesized RNA and to determine the absolute rate of mRNA synthesis so that the rates of gene transcription between subunits can be compared. The final calculated value for mRNA synthesis, as shown in Eq. (1), is expressed in parts per million, or ppm.

$$\text{mRNA synthesis} = \frac{\text{Specific }^{32}\text{P-RNA bound}}{(\text{Binding efficiency})\,(\text{Input }^{32}\text{P-RNA} \times 10^6)} \quad (1)$$
$$= \text{parts per million (ppm)}$$

Sample calculations are shown in Table II in which the assay was validated by the inclusion of the inhibitor α-amanitin in the nuclear incorporation reaction. OVX female rats were used as a source of pituitary nuclei. At the concentration used (2 μg/ml) α-amanitin specifically inhibits the action of RNA polymerase II and thus the incorporation of radioactive precursor into mRNA. This is reflected in the lower amount of ^{32}P-RNA obtained and the severely diminished calculated rate of mRNA synthesis for all three gonadotropin subunit mRNAs. Note that the efficiency of hybridization is quite similar between the four hybridization reactions using control and inhibitor-treated nuclei.

In Table II, the specificity of the hybridization reaction was tested by the addition of unlabeled competitor pituitary RNA to the hybridization reactions. As increasing amounts of pituitary RNA are added, the amounts of hybridizing ^{3}H- and ^{32}P-RNA decrease in parallel; however, the calculated rates of mRNA synthesis for all the subunits are the same. Thus, any contaminating cytoplasmic mRNA from the nuclear preparations will not bias the calculation of transcription rates.

Determination of Gonadotropin Subunit Gene Transcription Rates in Response to Pulsatile GnRH

Static GnRH treatment of pituitary cells *in vitro* can stimulate α-subunit gene expression, but has little effect on the transcription rate of the LHβ or FSHβ genes (2). Because pulsatile GnRH treatment *in vivo* can stimulate the transcription rate of all the gonadotropin subunit genes in a frequency-dependent manner (21), pulsatile GnRH administration *in vitro* would more effectively mimic the physiological situation and provide a true test of direct GnRH effects on gene transcription. Pituitary fragments from either intact or 21-day postovariectomy female rats were mounted in the columns of the perifusion apparatus in Fig. 1. After a 2-hr preincubation period, the pituitary fragments were treated with a 25 ng GnRH pulse administered over the last 10 min of a 60-min interval for 1 or 3 hr (Fig. 2). A single GnRH pulse stimulated the transcription rate of all three subunit genes approximately 2-fold. The levels of mRNA synthesis for α-subunit and LHβ were stimulated 3- to 5-fold over untreated levels after 3 hr of treatment, and no additional

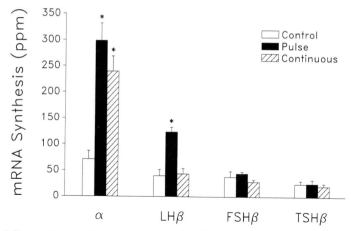

FIG. 3   Effects of pulsatile or continuous GnRH treatment on gonadotropin subunit gene transcription. Pituitary fragments from intact female rats were mounted on perifusion columns and treated for 6 hr with media alone (control), pulses of GnRH (25 ng over 10 min/hr), or continuous GnRH (2.5 ng/min). Transcription assays were performed immediately after treatment and tissue collection. Each bar represents the mean ± SEM for four determinations. *, $p < 0.05$. [Reproduced with permission from Shupnik (2).]

stimulation was noted after 6 hr of GnRH (not shown). The FSHβ response to GnRH treatment is less consistent, with a single pulse of GnRH nearly always increasing mRNA synthesis, averaging 180% of control values, but longer treatments have little effect. In separate experiments, we have occasionally noted an increase in FSHβ mRNA synthesis after 3 hr of GnRH (three/eight experiments), but the response is insignificant when results from all eight experiments are averaged. Similar transcriptional responses were noted in tissue from either intact or OVX animals, and secreted LH was stimulated 4- to 10-fold over control values for the duration of the experiment.

To determine if intermittent, rather than continuous, GnRH is truly necessary for stimulation of LHβ gene transcription, an experiment in which GnRH is administered to pituitary fragments in either a pulsatile or a continuous manner was performed (Fig. 3). Four hours of either pulsatile or continuous GnRH stimulate α-subunit gene transcription; however, only pulsatile GnRH is capable of stimulating LHβ mRNA synthesis. No effect on FSHβ or TSHβ mRNA synthesis is seen. Thus, pulsatile GnRH can specifically stimulate the LHβ gene and is capable of stimulating the α-subunit gene as well. Measurement of steady-state levels of gonadotropin subunit mRNA

TABLE III   Effects of Short-Term Pulsatile
GnRH Treatment on Steady-State
Levels of Gonadotropin
Subunit mRNA[a]

	mRNA (normalized arbitrary densitometry units)		
	α-Subunit	LHβ	FSHβ
Control	6.4 ± 0.6	3.4 ± 0.5	2.6 ± 0.2
6-hr GnRH	10.1 ± 2.3	4.2 ± 0.3	4.8 ± 0.3*

[a] Pituitary fragments from intact female rats were mounted on perifusion columns and treated for 6 hr with medium alone (control) or GnRH (25 ng once/hr). Total RNA from each column was analyzed on Northern blots and values normalized for β-actin mRNA in each sample. Each value represents the mean ± SEM for three samples.

(Table III) show that 6 hr of pulsatile or continuous GnRH can slightly increase α-subunit mRNA, while having little effect on LHβ mRNA. Only pulsatile GnRH increases the levels of FSHβ mRNA (2, 3). Effects on the steady-state levels of α-subunit and LHβ mRNA often take many hours or days to observe, as their half-lives are quite long (11) and thus are not very dramatic during this perifusion period. Pulsatile GnRH administered for 48 hr or longer *in vivo* has been demonstrated to increase all three gonadotropin subunit mRNAs in a frequency-dependent manner (11, 21). When direct effects of GnRH are to be measured *in vitro*, it is often impractical to treat cells for long periods of time. However, changes in mRNA synthesis are easily measured after 1 to 3 hr of treatment and are a powerful indication of the ability of any stimulus to alter mRNA levels and thus protein synthesis, and the runoff assay has been used with great success by several investigators to measure changes in pitutiary hormone gene transcription rates (22, 23).

Summary

The disadvantages of coupling perifusion of pituitary tissue to mRNA quantitation or nuclear runoff assays are clearly the laborious nature of the procedure, the requirement for specialized equipment, and the high levels of radioactivity involved for transcriptional measurements. Commercial instruments are available and can certainly be used for these experiments; we have found that the relatively simple and less costly apparatus described here is also sufficient. We and others have found that pulsatile administration of hypothalamic hormones, mimicking physiological conditions, is absolutely critical to detect appropriate biosynthetic responses of pituitary hormones. The ability to measure the rates of mRNA synthesis for the gonadotropins *in situ* is a powerful and sensitive technique to measure biosynthetic changes in response to physiological signals. We have found that the measurement of mRNA synthesis changes in this manner is a useful guide to planning future experiments on the identification of gene regulatory regions, or protocols involving transgenic animals, as well as providing critical information on physiological regulation of gene transcription.

Acknowledgments

The author expresses sincere appreciation for the technical assistance of Barry A. Rosenzweig in the performance of some of these studies and acknowledges the support of the National Institutes of Health (RO1-HD 25719).

References

1. P. E. Beltchez, T. M. Plant, Y. Nakai, E. G. Keough, and E. Knobil, *Science* **202,** 631 (1978).
2. M. A. Shupnik, *Mol. Endocrinol.* **4,** 1444 (1990).
3. J. Weiss, J. L. Jameson, J. M. Burrin, and W. F. Crowley, Jr., *Mol. Endocrinol.* **4,** 597 (1990).
4. W. S. Evans, M. J. Cronin, and M. O. Thorner, *in* "Methods in Enzymology" (P. M. Conn, ed.), Vol. 103, p. 294. Academic Press, San Diego, 1983.
5. D. J. Haisenleder, G. A. Ortolano, A. C. Dalkin, M. Yasin, and J. C. Marshall, *Endocrinology (Baltimore)* **130,** 2917 (1992).
6. D. J. Haisenleder, M. Yasin, and J. C. Marshall. *Endocrinology (Baltimore)* **131,** 3027 (1992).
7. M. A. Smith and W. W. Vale, *Endocrinology (Baltimore)* **107,** 1425 (1980).
8. P. J. Lowry, C. Martin, and J. Peters, *J. Endocrinol.* **59,** 43 (1973).
9. J. Weiss, W. F. Crowley, Jr., and J. L. Jameson, *Endocrinology (Baltimore)* **130,** 415 (1992).
10. G. S. McKnight and R. D. Palmiter, *J. Biol. Chem.* **254,** 9050 (1979).
11. S. J. Paul, G. A. Ortolano, D. J. Haisenleder, J. M. Stewart, M. A. Shupnik, and J. C. Marshall, *Mol. Endocrinol.* **4,** 1943 (1990).
12. J. M. Chirgwin, A. E. Przybla, R. J. MacDonald, and W. J. Rutter, *Biochemistry* **18,** 5294 (1980).
13. P. Chomczynsk and N. Sacchi, *Anal. Biochem.* **162,** 156 (1987).
14. S. D. Gharib, M. E. Wierman, T. M. Badger, and W. W. Chin, *J. Clin. Invest.* **80,** 294 (1987).

15. A. P. Feinberg and B. Vogelstein, *Anal. Biochem.* **132,** 6 (1983).
16. D. J. A. Autelitano, M. Blum, M. Lopingco, R. G. Allen, and J. L. Roberts, *Neuroendocrinology* **51,** 123 (1990).
17. F. C. Kafatos, C. W. Jones, and A. Efstadiatis, *Nucleic Acids Res.* **7,** 1541 (1979).
18. J. E. Godine, W. W. Chin, and J. F. Habener, *J. Biol. Chem.* **257,** 8368 (1982).
19. J. L. Jameson, W. W. Chin, A. H. Hollenberg, A. S. Chang, and J. F. Habener, *J. Biol. Chem.* **259,** 15,474 (1983).
20. M. E. Greenberg and E. B. Ziff, *Nature (London)* **331,** 433 (1984).
21. D. J. Haisenleder, A. C. Dalkin, G. A. Ortolano, J. C. Marshall, and M. A. Shupnik, *Endocrinology (Baltimore)* **128,** 509 (1991).
22. R. A. Maurer *J. Biol. Chem.* **257,** 2133 (1981).
23. J. H. Eberwine and J. L. Roberts, *J. Biol. Chem.* **259,** 2166 (1984).

[22] Use of an *in Vitro* Perifusion System to Study the Effects of Pulsatile Hormone Administration on the Control of the Hypothalamic–Pituitary–Ovarian Axis

Jacqueline F. Ackland, Kerry L. Knox, Adria A. Elskus, Patricia C. Fallest, Eve S. Hiatt, and Neena B. Schwartz

Introduction

Pulsatile hormone release is essential for the functional maintenance of the reproductive axis. Pulsatile release of gonadotropin-releasing hormone (GnRH) from the hypothalamus is required to stimulate the synthesis and release of the gonadotropins, luteinizing hormone (LH), and follicle-stimulating hormone (FSH) from the pituitary. LH and FSH in turn are released in pulses and act on the gonads to stimulate steroidogenesis and gametogenesis.

Static cultures of pituitary and ovarian granulosa cells, and to a lesser extent hypothalamic cells, have been widely used to study factors affecting hormone release from these tissues (1–3). However, pulsatile administration of stimulatory factors cannot easily be achieved using static cell cultures. Frequent sampling of hormonal output is more difficult to perform with static cultures than with perifusion systems and the use of static cultures can result in an accumulation of secreted products which may affect hormonal output. Thus many investigators have used perifusion techniques to study hormone release from endocrine tissue (4, 5).

In this chapter we describe the use of an automated perifusion system, the Acusyst, to study the output of GnRH from hypothalamic tissue, the effects of pulsatile GnRH administration on pituitary LH and FSH release, and the effects of both continuous and pulsatile LH and FSH administration on inhibin and progesterone release from ovarian tissue.

Description of the Acusyst

We have used two different Acusyst models (Endotronics, Inc., Coon Rapids, MN), the 1501 and the APS 10. The main difference between them is that the 1501 is computer controlled, rather than microprocessor controlled. The

Methods in Neurosciences, Volume 20

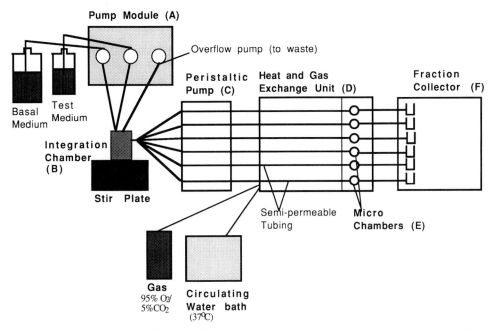

FIG. 1 Schematic diagram of the Acusyst perifusion system. Basal and stimulation media are pumped through the pump module (A) into the integration chamber (B) where they are mixed. They are then pumped through the multichannel peristaltic pump (C) and the heat- and gas-exchange unit (D) and into the microchambers (E) containing the tissue. Effluent from the microchambers is collected in the fraction collector (F).

computer allows for more flexibility in designing pulses, so that during one run each pulse can be different if desired. Also the computer-controlled pumps can be programmed to run at different speeds during the run, thus enabling a rapid washout and hence a more rapid falling phase at the end of each pulse. This is required for programming short, sharp pulses which we have found to be required for GnRH administration to pituitaries. A schematic diagram of the Acusyst is shown in Fig. 1. Each model has the following components (upper case letters refer to labeling on Fig. 1):

i. An Acusyst pump module (A) consisting of three pumps on the APS 10 and up to 10 pumps on the 1501, although we never use more than three pumps at any one time. Of the three pumps one is used to deliver basal medium, a second to deliver the concentrated test substances (e.g., GnRH) used for pulses, and a third to siphon off overflow waste from the integration chamber.

ii. Multiple microchamber module (MMCM) perifusion system, consisting of a 1-ml integration chamber (B) with micro stir bar which is placed on top of a stir plate for mixing the chemical signal with the basal perifusion medium; a multichannel peristaltic pump (C) for delivering medium to the microchambers; a heat- and gas-exchange unit (D) filled with circulating warmed water and gas outlets through which the Silastic gas-permeable tubing passes en route to the microchambers; and six microchambers (E) containing micropore (5 μm) filters and O-ring assemblies at the top and bottom in which the tissue is placed.

iii. A fraction collector (F), capable of collecting fractions from all six microchambers simultaneously.

iv. A microprocessor (Model APS 10) or microcomputer (Model 1501) not shown in Fig. 1) which is programmed to deliver pulses. With the 1501 all pulse variables, i.e., frequency, duration of rising phase, duration of plateau phase (if required), and duration of washout phase can be specified as required; these variables can be altered for each pulse during a run. With the APS 10 model only the pulse duration and interval between pulses can be entered, and every pulse and pulse interval has to be the same throughout the run. The computer on the 1501 can also be programmed to set the gassing schedule, fraction collector schedule, and pump rate on the multichannel peristaltic pump, while on the APS 10 these have to be set manually.

Running the Acusyst

Prior to each run all pumps including the multichannel peristaltic pump are calibrated; the microchambers are assembled with filters and O-rings; the microchambers, integration chamber, all glassware, connective tubing, and fittings are sterilized by autoclaving; the computer or microprocessor is programmed for required run conditions. Although sterilization is not absolutely required for the short experiments that we usually perform (maximum 10 hr) it does prevent buildup of contamination in the tubing and chambers which cannot be removed by washing with bleach. Immediately prior to each run the tubing and microchambers are pumped full of basal medium and all connections are checked to ensure that they are air-tight.

Tissue Collection

Adult male and female Sprague–Dawley CD rats (Charles River, Portage, MI) are used for all experiments. In females estrous-stage cycle is assessed by vaginal cytology and presence of intraluminal water in the uterus. For each perifusion run the appropriate number of animals are killed by decapitation. Trunk blood is collected and the serum assayed for relevant hormone levels. The required tissue is removed from the animals immediately after decapitation. Usually only one tissue type is perifused in any one experiment. Preoptic area/mediobasal hypothalamic tissue blocks are dissected by sectioning along the following boundaries: laterally, 1 mm lateral to the median eminence on each side; posteriorly, anterior to the mammillary bodies; anteriorly, anterior border of the optic chiasm; dorsally, 1 mm in depth. For pituitaries the posterior and intermediate lobes are discarded, and the anterior pituitary is cut into eighths. Ovaries are dissected free from fat and cut into quarters. Each tissue is placed in a beaker of warmed gassed basal medium until all tissue has been collected. Tissue fragments from each animal are then washed twice in warmed, gassed basal medium. We have found this washing to be a very important step, particularly with pituitary fragments. If thorough washing is not carried out, the time taken *in vitro* for LH and FSH secretion to reach a steady-state "baseline" is extended. After being washed, tissue is placed in the microchambers for perifusion. Two hundred-microliter chambers are used for pituitary fragments and 500-μl chambers are used for hypothalamic blocks and ovarian pieces.

Perifusion

The microchambers are placed in the Acusyst and the tissue is initially perifused with basal medium. Basal medium is pumped from the reservoir into the integration chamber; it is then pumped from the integration chamber through the multichannel peristaltic pump, through the heat and gas exchange, and into the microchambers where it flows over the tissue. The outflow from each microchamber is collected in the fraction collector. An equilibrium period (typically 30 min) is included at the beginning of each run before pulses are administered. When pulses are required, concentrated treatment medium is pumped into the integration chamber where it is mixed with basal medium before being pumped onto the tissue. The Acusyst can also be used to deliver basal treatment only or continuous (tonic) treatment with required factors. In these cases the integration chamber is not used and medium (plus treatment) is pumped directly through the multichannel peristaltic pump. The lag time between the integration chamber and the microchambers obviously depends on the flow rate; for a flow rate of 10 ml/hr it is approximately 10 min.

The time of the equilibration period before the first pulse, the duration and peak dose of each pulse, the pulse frequency, the medium flow rate, and the fraction size vary depending on the type of tissue under study. Details are given in each section below. At the end of each run tissue is removed from the chambers. Tissue can be frozen for subsequent hormone extraction and measurement or can be placed in a suitable preservative such as Bouin's solution for subsequent histology. The whole system is then washed out with approximately 200 ml bleach (Clorox, 0.1% v/v in H_2O) followed by approximately 400 ml H_2O. The tubing is then pumped dry.

Culture Medium

Basal medium for most experiments is Medium 199 with 25 mM HEPES, Earle's salts, and L-glutamine, without phenol red (Gibco Laboratories, Grand Island, NY) containing 0.5% bovine serum albumin (BSA; Bovuminar Cohn fraction V powder, Armour Pharmaceutical, Kankakee IL), 90 U/liter bacitracin (Sigma Chemical Co., St. Louis, MO), and 25 μg/ml gentamicin (Garamycin, Schering Corp., Kenilworth, NJ). Phenol red is omitted from the medium as it has been shown to have weak estrogenic activity which could interfere with our experiments (6).

Hormone Assays

All fractions collected are stored at $-20°C$ until assay for the appropriate hormone levels by radioimmunoassay [i.e., GnRH for hypothalamic tissue, LH and FSH for pituitaries, and immunoreactive inhibin alpha (IrIα) and progesterone (P_4) for ovarian tissue].

GnRH measurements use synthetic GnRH [luteinizing hormone-releasing hormone (LHRH) acetate salt, Sigma, St. Louis, MO] for iodination and standards and EL-14 antibody (W. E. Ellinwood). Intra- and interassay coefficients of variation (CVs) are 7.0 and 15.0%, respectively. This radioimmunoassay (RIA) has been validated by Ellinwood and colleagues (7).

FSH is measured using the rat–rat RIA reagents with FSH-RP1 as standard and S11 antibody. Intra- and interassay CVs are 3.5 and 6.7%, respectively. LH is measured with an ovine–rat RIA using NIH LH S25 as standard and S10 LH antibody. Intra- and interassay CVs are 5.3 and 10.7%, respectively. These reagents are supplied by NIDDK.

IrIα is measured using an antiserum raised against synthetic porcine inhibin alpha (1-26)-Gly-Tyr. The same synthetic peptide is used for standards and for the preparation of tracer. This assay is based on a previously described method (8, 9) and has been described in detail elsewhere (10). Results are expressed as pg/ml (picograms per milliliter) of synthetic peptide standard. Intra- and interassay CVs are 9.8 and 10.4%, respectively.

Progesterone is measured using the coated tube assay from ICN Biomedicals (Costa Mesa, CA). Intra- and interassay CVs are 4.2 and 12.4%, respectively.

Data Analysis

The first 30 min of each run (equilibrium period) is usually excluded from calculations as baseline secretion levels are not achieved for at least 30 min. Results either are plotted as amounts of hormone per milliliter of medium in each fraction or are summed to give hourly secretion rates of hormone, usually for 1 hr following the start of each treatment pulse, or for the corresponding times in basal runs. Group means ± SEM are calculated for each fraction and for the hourly secretion rates. These calculations are performed using a spreadsheet such as Lotus or Excel. Statistical differences between treatment groups are analyzed using hourly secretion rate data by analysis of variance (ANOVA) with repeated measures. Post hoc analysis is performed with Tukey's HSD or Scheffe's test. Statistical calculations are performed with either SYSTAT (Systat, Inc., Evanston, IL) or CRISP, Crunch Interactive Statistical Package (Crunch Software, Oakland, CA).

Validation of the Acusyst

In order to determine whether pulses of test factors reaching the tissues were exactly the same as computed pulses, samples of dye, iodinated GnRH, and GnRH peptide were administered through the system in separate runs. The resulting fractions were measured for absorbance or radioactivity or assayed by RIA. Results from these experiments showed that there was a good recovery of added factors and that the actual pulse patterns closely paralleled the calculated patterns (11).

Use of the Acusyst with Hypothalamic Fragments

For hypothalamic fragments the Acusyst is run with a flow rate of 2.4 ml/hr, run time is 6 hr, and 5-min fractions are collected. Fractions are heated to 80–90°C for 5 min to inactivate proteases that can destroy GnRH.

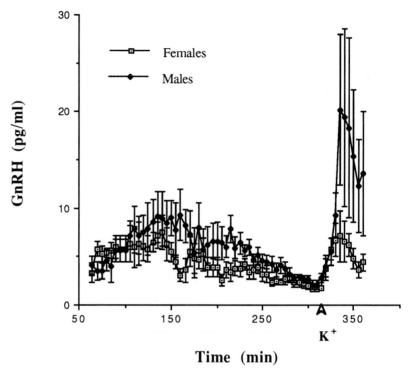

FIG. 2   *In vitro* secretion of GnRH from perifused hypothalamic tissue removed from intact female rats (open symbols) and male rats (solid symbols). Medium containing 60 mM K$^+$ was administered from 315 to 360 min. There was no significant difference in the mean basal or K$^+$-stimulated secretion rates between males and females. All values are mean ± SEM ($n = 4$).

Figure 2 shows mean basal GnRH secretion patterns from hypothalami removed from male and metestrous female rats. GnRH secretion was significantly increased in response to 60 mM K$^+$ stimulation ($p < 0.0005$). There was no significant sex difference between either basal or K$^+$-stimulated GnRH secretion rates (12).

Use of the Acusyst with Pituitary Fragments

We have used the Acusyst most extensively with pituitary fragments. In this section we describe the effects of varying the GnRH pulse duration and frequency, the effects of prior *in vivo* treatments and physiological status, and the effects of various *in vitro* treatments on the pituitary responsiveness to GnRH in terms of LH and FSH release. The usual conditions for pituitary runs are as follows: flow rate is 10 ml/hr, pulses of GnRH are administered 1/hr, the peak dose is 50 ng/ml; and 5-min fractions are collected. A total of 60 mM K$^+$ is included in the perifusion medium for the final 30 min of each run in order to assess tissue viability. If the tissue shows no response to K$^+$ by increased hormone release the data from that channel are discarded.

Effect of GnRH Pulse Duration on Pituitary LH and FSH Release

In early experiments we used a 3-hr equilibrium period and square wave pulses of GnRH consisting of a 5-min rising phase, a 10- to 15-min plateau phase, and a 5-min washout phase (11, 13). However, this pulse pattern did not reliably stimulate FSH and LH secretion from pituitaries removed from male rats. In fact, because basal FSH secretion was so high from male pituitaries, there was either no net increase or a net decrease in FSH secretion after GnRH treatment. In current experiments we use a 30- or 60-min equilibrium period and sharp pulses of GnRH consisting of a 30-sec rising phase followed immediately by a washout period which is 50% complete after 1.5 min (14, 15). Representative results from the two types of pulses are shown in Fig. 3. The short sharp pulses were more effective in eliciting LH and FSH responses to GnRH, particularly from pituitaries removed from male rats. Using this type of pulse we have not observed any desensitization in the LH and FSH responses to GnRH with repetitive pulses.

Effect of GnRH Pulse Frequency on Pituitary LH and FSH Release

In order to determine the effect of GnRH pulse frequency on pituitary LH and FSH secretion, pituitaries were removed from female rats on the morning of metestrus and perifused for 8 hr with a flow rate of 10 ml/hr. Brief GnRH pulses (50 ng/ml) were delivered (30-sec rising phase, 2-min duration, 30-sec falling phase) once per hour (1/hr), twice per hour (2/hr), or once every hour and a half (1/1.5 hr). Between-pulse differences in gonadotropin release were examined by ANOVA. The within-group variable was total gonadotropin released for each half hour (2/hr), each hour (1/hr), and each hour and a half (1/1.5 hr) of perifusion using 14, 7, and 5 levels (i.e., pulses), respectively.

For pituitaries receiving two pulses of GnRH per hour the LH response to consecutive GnRH pulses remained consistent over the 8-hr perifusion period (Fig. 4a). Despite declining basal LH secretion rates over time of perifusion (data not shown), LH responsivity to two pulses per hour remains

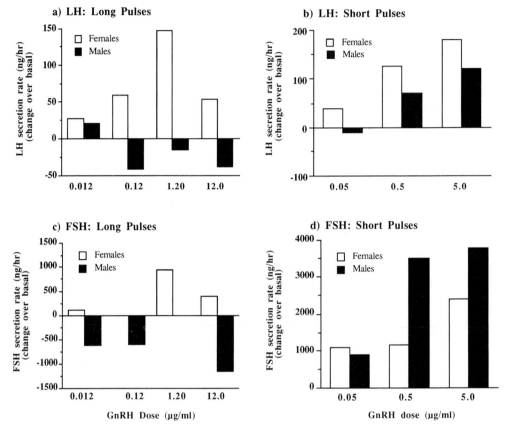

FIG. 3   Comparison of two different GnRH pulse patterns on FSH secretion from pituitaries removed from intact female rats (open bars) and male rats (filled bars). Data are shown as mean GnRH-stimulated secretion rate (ng/hr) expressed as secretion rate above or below mean basal secretion rate. Long pulses were square wave pulses with 5-min rising phase, 10-min plateau phase, and 5-min falling phase. Short pulses were sharp pulses with a 30-sec rising phase and approximately 1.5-min falling phase. All pulses were administered at 1/hr. Where no bar is apparent, GnRH-stimulated hormone secretion was not significantly different from basal hormone secretion. Short pulses were more effective at eliciting both LH and FSH responses to GnRH, especially from male pituitaries.

consistently strong throughout the perifusion. This suggests either that pituitary stores of LH are large or that LH is continuously synthesized under these *in vitro* conditions.

Female pituitaries released distinct LH pulses in response to GnRH pulses

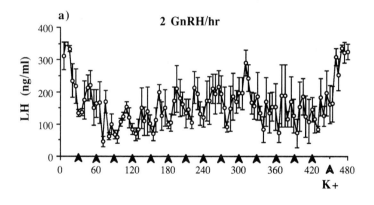

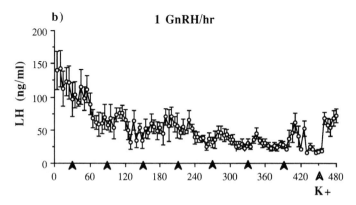

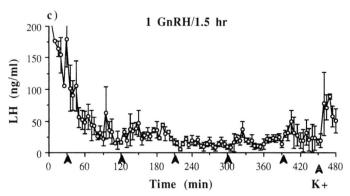

FIG. 4 *In vitro* release of luteinizing hormone (LH) by pituitaries from metestrous females in response to exogenous administration of three different pulse frequencies of GnRH: (a) 2/hr; (b) 1/hr; (c) 1/1.5 hr. Values represent ng/ml LH for each 5-min fraction (mean ± SEM) for individual pituitaries (*n* = 3 or 4). Arrows represent time of GnRH pulses. Note scale differences.

delivered once per hour (Fig. 4b). LH response to the first two GnRH pulses was greater than that to succeeding pulses. The remaining LH pulses were not significantly different from one another, indicating consistent responsivity over time. Pituitaries receiving one pulse of GnRH every 1.5 hr, the slowest pulse frequency tested, released LH pulses which were smaller and less discrete than those produced in response to the other, faster GnRH frequencies (Fig. 4c). There was a direct relationship between GnRH pulse frequency and LH release, total nanograms of LH released per GnRH pulse being highest in response to 2 GnRH pulses/hr and least in response to 1 pulse/1.5 hr. This agrees with *in vitro* studies with rat pituitaries demonstrating that transcription of LHβ-mRNA is favored by faster GnRH pulse frequencies (16), but is contrary to *in vivo* studies in monkeys in which LH release was optimal at 1 GnRH pulse/hr and declined at frequencies higher or lower than this (17), suggesting possible species differences. In all Acusyst runs pituitaries responded strongly to a 60 mM K$^+$ delivered during the last half-hour of perifusion, confirming viability of the tissue.

Effect of Estrous Cycle Stage on Pituitary LH and FSH Release

This study was undertaken to determine the role of GnRH pulses in driving the secondary surge of FSH which takes place on the late evening of the proestrus and the early morning of estrus. Anterior pituitaries were obtained from female rats at 0900 and 2400 hr on each day of the estrous cycle and perifused for 8 hr with either basal medium only or with hourly pulses of GnRH starting at 30 min. Analysis of the hourly secretion rates of LH and FSH following GnRH pulses showed that the secretion of LH dropped from a maximum for pituitaries removed at 0900 hr on proestrus to a minimum for pituitaries removed at 2400 hr on proestrus, whereas FSH secretion remained elevated at 2400 hr. Therefore the ratio of FSH to LH secreted in response to GnRH was highest during the secondary FSH surge and lowest on the morning of proestrus (Fig. 5). There was a significant effect of cycle stage on LH release ($p < 0.001$), FSH ($p < 0.001$), and FSH:LH ratios ($p < 0.05$). Under basal conditions the secretion of LH decreased during perifusion, whereas the secretion of FSH increased with perifusion time, presumably due to removal of inhibin negative feedback. Initial basal FSH secretion was higher on the morning of proestrus than on the evening of proestrus (basal results not shown). From these results we concluded that both increased basal FSH release and maintained FSH responsiveness, but not LH responsiveness, to GnRH pulses contribute to the generation of the secondary FSH surge (14).

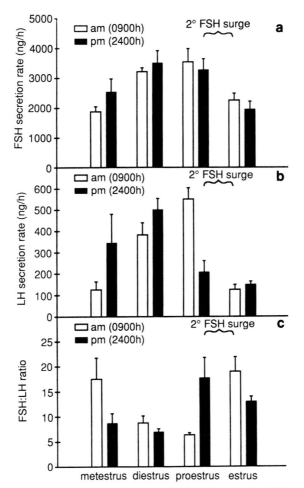

FIG. 5   GnRH-stimulated secretion rates of (a) LH and (b) FSH throughout the 4-day rat estrous cycle. Mean hourly secretion rates are shown for pituitaries removed at 0900 hr (open bars) or 2400 hr (filled bars) on each day of the cycle. (c) Ratios of FSH : LH secretion. There were significant differences between cycle stages for FSH secretion ($p < 0.001$), LH secretion ($p < 0.001$), and FSH : LH ratios ($p < 0.05$). All values are means ± SEM ($n = 3$). [Reproduced with permission from Fallest and Schwartz (14).]

Effect of in Vivo Administration of GnRH Antagonist on Pituitary LH and FSH Release

When administered *in vivo* to cycling rats on the day of proestrus, antagonist to GnRH prevents the normal rise in serum levels of LH and FSH on the evening of proestrus and blocks the secondary FSH surge on the morning of estrus (18). To determine whether these effects of GnRH antagonist *in vivo* could be observed directly at the pituitary level *in vitro* we used the Acusyst to perifuse pituitaries from animals treated on proestrus. On the day of proestrus, female rats were injected sc at 1230 hr with either sesame oil as control or 100 μg GnRH antagonist (WY45760, ([Ac-βNAL(2)^1, 4FD-Phe^2, D-Trp^3, D-Arg^6]-LHRH), Wyeth Laboratories, Philadelphia, PA) in 0.25 ml sesame oil. Rats were sacrificed the next day on the morning of estrus and the pituitaries were removed as described previously. Pituitaries were then perifused for 8 hr with Medium 199 without GnRH stimulation.

Figure 6 shows hourly basal secretion rates (BSRs) from pituitaries of rats treated with either oil or GnRH antagonist *in vivo*. Treatment with GnRH antagonist significantly reduced BSRs for both LH and FSH ($p < 0.01$ and $p < 0.001$, respectively). These results show that use of a dynamic perifusion system can confirm, directly at the level of the pituitary, the pattern of LH and FSH secretion observed *in vivo* under experimental conditions. We interpret the suppression of basal LH and FSH secretion *in vitro* to reflect the absence of normal GnRH occupancy of its receptors for 20 hr on proestrus and estrus, thus blocking gonadotropin synthesis.

Effect of in Vitro Activin Antibody on LH and FSH Release

Activin is a gonadal hormone which stimulates the release of FSH from the pituitary. However activin is also present in the pituitary and is thought to have an autocrine or paracrine effect on pituitary FSH release which is probably more important than the endocrine effects of gonadal activin (19). Basal secretion of FSH is much higher from male than from female pituitaries. In order to investigate the possible role of activin in the sex differences of FSH we treated pituitary fragments from male and female rats in the Acusyst with medium containing 20 μg/ml of a monoclonal antibody (Mab) to activin (No. 2A5.2C7, provided by R. Schwall, Genentech, South San Francisco, CA). The perifusion protocol is as follows: the pituitary fragments were perifused for 1.5 hr without Mab, 4 hr with Mab, 4 hr without Mab, then 30 min with 60 mM K$^+$. GnRH pulses (peak dose 50 ng/ml) were administered 1/hr starting at 30 min, flow rate was 6 ml/hr, and 10-min fractions were

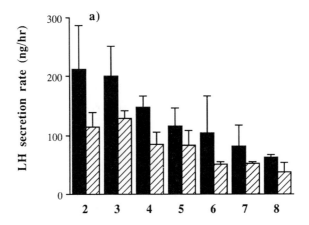

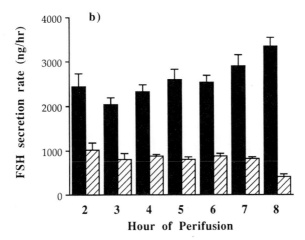

FIG. 6   Effects of *in vivo* treatment with GnRH antagonist on *in vitro* LH and FSH secretion: (a) basal LH secretion rate and (b) basal FSH secretion rate from pituitaries removed from female rats treated *in vivo* with oil (solid bars) or GnRH antagonist (cross-hatched bars). GnRH antagonist treatment was given at 1230 hr on proestrus and the rats were sacrificed at 0800 hr on estrus. GnRH antagonist treatment *in vivo* significantly decreased both LH and FSH secretion *in vitro* ($p < 0.01$ and $p < 0.001$, respectively). All values are means ± SEM ($n = 4$).

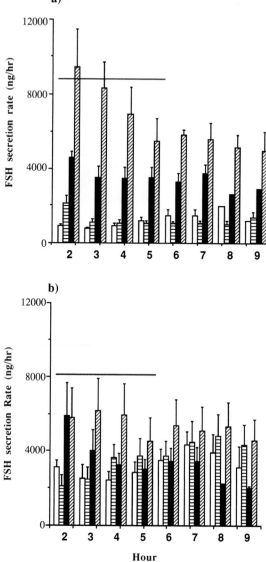

a)

b)

FIG. 7   Effects of *in vitro* treatment with a monoclonal antibody to activin (Mab) on pituitary FSH secretion: (a) basal secretion rates and (b) GnRH-stimulated secretion rates of FSH from female and male rat pituitaries during and after treatment with activin Mab. Duration of Mab treatment is shown by the horizontal line. Open bars, females no Mab treatment; horizontally hatched bars, females with Mab treatment; filled bars, males no Mab treatment; cross-hatched bars, males with Mab treatment. Activin Mab significantly increased basal and GnRH-stimulated FSH release from male pituitaries ($p < 0.0001$ and $p < 0.005$, respectively), but had no effect on FSH release from female pituitaries. All values are means ± SEM ($n = 4$ or 5).

collected. The slower than usual flow rate was used to conserve the Mab and resulted in broader GnRH pulses than normal with a 1-min rising phase and washout was 75% complete after 20 min. Using this pulse pattern we oberved significant increases in FSH secretion in response to GnRH with female pituitaries ($p < 0.0001$) but not with male pituitaries.

Activin Mab significantly increased FSH release from male, but not female, pituitaries. Basal FSH release increased by 79% over control ($p < 0.0001$) and GnRH-stimulated FSH release increased by 46% ($p < 0.005$) (Fig. 7). This is in contrast to what was observed when activin Mab was administered to static cultures of rat pituitary cells (20), where activin Mab inhibited FSH release. Thus there are important differences in tissue responses to certain factors which depend on the type of system used to study them. It has also been shown that activin itself has a much greater stimulatory effect on FSHβ mRNA when administered in a perifusion system than in static cultures (21).

Effect of in Vitro Estradiol on Pituitary LH and FSH Release

Attempts to demonstrate a direct inhibitory effect of estradiol (E_2) on LH release from the pituitary have been inconsistent (22, 23). The aim of this study was to determine if E_2 can suppress either basal or GnRH-stimulated gonadotropin release directly at the level of the pituitary, using rats at different stages of the estrous cycle (15).

Pituitaries were removed from female rats on the morning of proestrus or metestrus and perifused for 8 hr with 1 nM E_2 or ethanol as vehicle included in the perifusion medium. Both basal and GnRH-stimulated runs were carried out. GnRH pulses with a peak dose of 50 ng/ml were administered 1/hr starting at 60 min. Five-minute fractions were collected and assayed for LH and FSH. Blood was collected from donor rats and serum assayed for LH, FSH, E_2, and progesterone (P_4).

Both basal and GnRH-stimulated LH and FSH secretion was higher from pituitaries removed from proestrous than from metestrous rats. Basal LH secretion from metestrous pituitaries was unchanged by E_2, while FSH secretion was significantly suppressed ($p < 0.005$) (data not shown). Basal secretion of LH from proestrous pituitaries was reduced during Hours 2–4 of perifusion, but was not significantly changed overall; basal FSH secretion from these pituitaries was unaffected by E_2. GnRH-stimulated LH release from metestrous pituitaries was significantly suppressed by E_2 ($p < 0.05$), but there was no overall effect on GnRH-stimulated FSH secretion (Fig. 8a). There was no significant effect of E_2 on GnRH-stimulated LH or FSH release from pituitaries removed on proestrus (Fig. 8b).

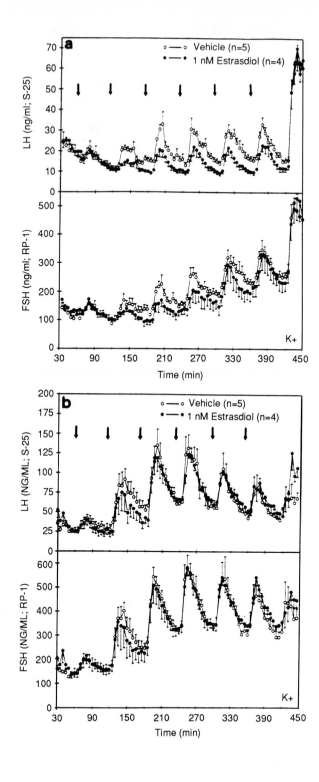

Thus a negative effect of E_2 on LH secretion was only observed on pituitaries taken at metestrus when serum levels of E_2 are low and serum levels of P_4 are high, but not on proestrus when serum E_2 levels are high and serum P_4 levels are low. Thus the *in vivo* steroid environment can determine the pituitary response to *in vitro* steroid treatments (15). This type of effect is much harder to demonstrate with static cultures of pituitary cells as the cells have to be in culture for 2–3 days before treatments can be applied.

Use of the Acusyst with Ovary Fragments

Pituitary gonadotropins act on the granulosa cells of the ovaries to stimulate synthesis and production of both steroid hormones, such as progesterone, and peptide hormones, such as inhibin. However the differential regulation of the secretion of peptide and steroid hormones by LH and FSH is not well understood.

Ovaries were removed from adult female rats on the morning of metestrus or proestrus and collected into basal medium containing 0.2 U/liter insulin (Lente Ilentin I, Eli Lilly, Indianapolis, IN) and 0.33 U/liter heparin (Elkins-Sinn, Cherry Hill, NC). Insulin (0.2 U/liter) is also included in the perifusion medium. The methods are based on those of Peluso *et al.* (24). For all ovary experiments one ovary from each rat is perifused with basal medium only and the contralateral ovary is perifused with treatment medium. LH and FSH are administered either continuously or in pulses. For continuous (tonic) treatment LH and FSH doses are 10 ng/ml and 40 ng/ml, respectively. For pulsatile treatment pulses are administered 1/hr with peak doses of 60 ng/ml LH and 240 ng/ml FSH. The rising phase of each pulse is 5 min and washout is 95% completed after a further 20 min. The total amount of LH and FSH administered is approximately the same for both treatments. Flow rate is 6 ml/hr and 10-min (1 ml) fractions are collected and stored frozen until assay for irIα and P_4 by RIA.

FIG. 8   Effects of *in vitro* estradiol treatment on GnRH-stimulated LH (top) and FSH (bottom) secretion from female rat pituitaries removed on the mornings of (a) metestrus and (b) proestrus. Pituitaries which received vehicle treatment are shown in open symbols, pituitaries which received estradiol are shown in filled symbols. Arrows indicate the times of GnRH pulses. Estradiol significantly decreased LH secretion from metestrous pituitaries ($p < 0.05$), but had no effect on FSH secretion from metestrous pituitaries or LH or FSH secretion from proestrous pituitaries. All values are means $\pm$ SEM ($n = 4$ or 5). [Reproduced with permission from Fallest and Schwartz (15).]

For ovaries removed on the morning of metestrus tonic LH and FSH had no effect on P_4 release but significantly stimulated irIα release by 30% ($p < 0.05$). However, pulsatile LH and FSH did not significantly alter irIα release but significantly stimulated P_4 release by 32% ($p < 0.05$) (Figs. 9a and 9c). For ovaries removed on the morning of proestrus tonic LH and FSH had no significant effect on either irIα or P_4 release. However, pulsatile LH and FSH significantly decreased irIα release by 25% ($p < 0.005$) and significantly increased P_4 release by 44% ($p < 0.005$) (Figs. 9b and 9d).

These results indicate that continuous gonadotropin treatment appears to favor irIα release, while pulsatile gonadotropins favor the release of P_4. Thus the differential regulation of ovarian steroid and peptide hormones during the estrous cycle may be achieved by altering gonadotropin secretion patterns.

Discussion

This chapter describes the use of the Acusyst perifusion system to study extensively all aspects of the hypothalamic–pituitary–ovarian axis. Hormone secretion can be successfully measured from all three tissue types. The system is excellent both for administering pulses of stimulatory factors and for measuring pulsatile output of hormones. In particular the utility of dynamic perifusion for examining the differential effects of GnRH pulse frequency on gonadotropin secretion by isolated pituitaries has been demonstrated. Such studies cannot be duplicated by static systems due to the necessity for rapid washout of GnRH signal after each pulse. This type of signal design is essential in order to mimic the brief and discrete GnRH pulses known to occur *in vivo* (25). This system has also allowed us to directly compare the effects of continuous and pulsatile hormone treatment on the differential regulation of steroid and peptide ovarian hormone release.

We have carried out experiments to manipulate hormonal inputs to a given tissue and to determine how a fixed input can result in varying outputs depending on the prior physiological state of the donor animal. The fact that we are not dispersing cells is important when animals of different physiological states are used since this means that there are no alterations in cell-surface receptors. Additionally the use of tissue pieces ensures that cell–cell

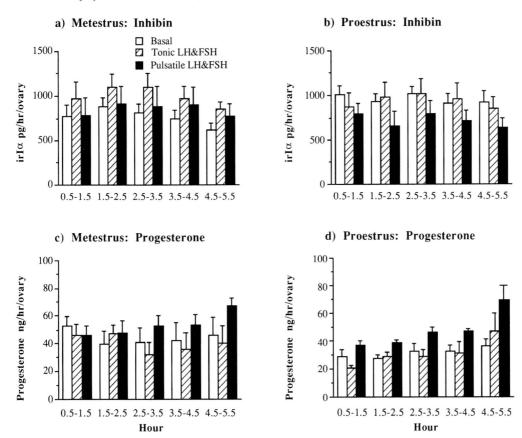

Fig. 9 Effects of tonic and pulsatile LH and FSH treatment on the hourly secretion rates of irIα (a,c) and progesterone (b,d) from ovaries removed from rats on the morning of metestrus (a,c) or proestrus (b,d). For ovaries removed on metestrus, tonic LH and FSH significantly stimulated irIα release ($p < 0.05$) while pulsatile LH and FSH significantly stimulated progesterone release ($p < 0.05$). For ovaries removed on proestrus, pulsatile LH and FSH significantly decreased irIα release ($p < 0.005$) and significantly increased progesterone release ($p < 0.005$). All values are means ± SEM ($n = 4$ or 5).

communications (e.g., gap junctions, synapses) are maintained. These connections are critical for hypothalamic and ovarian tissue and appear also to be important with pituitary tissue as suggested by the potential paracrine actions of activin and inhibin.

Acknowledgment

This work was supported in part by NIH Grants RO1 HD 07504, PO1 HD 07068, P30 HD 28048, T32 HD 07068, F32 DK 08513 (to K.L.K.), and F32 HD 07657 (to A.A.E.).

References

1. A. Tixier-Vidal and A. Faivre-Bauman, *in* "Methods in Neuroscience" (P. M. Conn, ed.), Vol. 2, p. 355. Academic Press, New York, 1990.
2. W. Vale, J. Vaughan, G. Yamamoto, T. Bruhn, C. Douglas, D. Dalton, C. Rivier, and J. Rivier, *in* "Methods in Enzymology" (P. M. Conn, ed.), Vol. 103, p. 565. Academic Press, New York, 1983.
3. A. J. W. Hsueh, E. Y. Adashi, P. B. C. Jones, and T. H. Welsh Jr., *Endocr. Rev.* **5,** 79 (1984).
4. J. R. Hansen, and P. M. Conn, *in* "Methods in Neuroscience" (P. M. Conn, ed.), Vol. 2, p. 181. Academic Press, New York, 1990.
5. H. F. Urbanski and S. R. Ojeda, *Endocrinology (Baltimore)* **117,** 638 (1985).
6. J.-F. Hubert, A. Vincent, and F. Labrie, *Biochem. Biophys. Res. Commun.* **141,** 885 (1986).
7. W. E. Ellinwood, O. K. Ronnekleiv, M. J. Kelly, and J. A. Resko, *Peptides* **6,** 45 (1985).
8. J. M. Vaughan, J. Rivier, A. Z. Corrigan, R. McClintock, C. A. Campen, D. Jolley, J. K. Voglmayr, C. W. Bardin, C. Rivier, and W. Vale, *in* "Methods in Enzymology" (P. M. Conn, ed.), Vol. 168, p. 588. Academic Press, New York, 1989.
9. C. Rivier, S. Cajander, J. Vaughan, A. Hsueh, and W. Vale, *Endocrinology (Baltimore)* **123,** 120 (1988).
10. J. F. Ackland, J. B. D'Agostino, S. J. Ringstrom, J. P. Hostetler, B. G. Mann, and N. B. Schwartz, *Biol. Reprod.* **43,** 347 (1990).
11. E. S. Hiatt, Doctoral dissertation, Northwestern University, Evanston, IL, 1987.
12. P. C. Fallest, Doctoral dissertation, Northwestern University, Evanston, IL, 1990.
13. E. S. Hiatt and N. B. Schwartz, *Neuroendocrinology* **50,** 158 (1989).
14. P. C. Fallest and N. B. Schwartz, *Biol. Reprod.* **43,** 977 (1990).
15. P. C. Fallest and N. B. Schwartz, *Endocrinology (Baltimore)* **128,** 273 (1991).
16. D. J. Haisenleder, A. C. Dalkin, G. A. Ortolano, J. C. Marshall, and M. A. Shupnik, *Endocrinology (Baltimore)* **128,** 509 (1991).
17. L. A. Wildt, G. Hansler, J. S. Marshall, J. S. Hutchinson, T. M. Plant, P. E. Belchetz, and E. Knobil, *Endocrinology (Baltimore)* **109,** 376 (1981).
18. T. K. Woodruff, J. D'Agostino, N. B. Schwartz, and K. E. Mayo, *Endocrinology (Baltimore)* **124,** 2193 (1989).
19. J. Schwartz and R. Cherny, *Endoc. Rev.* **13,** 453 (1992).

20. A. Z. Corrigan, L. M. Bilezikjian, R. S. Carroll, C. H. Schmelzer, B. M. Fendly, A. J. Mason, W. W. Chin, R. H. Schwall, and W. Vale, *Endocrinology* (*Baltimore*) **128,** 1682 (1991).
21. J. Weiss, P. E. Harris, L. M. Halvorson, W. F. Crowley, Jr., and J. L. Jameson, *Endocrinology* (*Baltimore*) **131,** 1403 (1992).
22. L. S. Frawley, and J. D. Neill, *Endocrinology* (*Baltimore*) **114,** 659 (1984).
23. J. L. Turgeon and D. W. Waring, *Endocrinology* **108,** 413 (1981).
24. J. J. Peluso, M. C. Downey, and M. L. Gruenberg, *J. Reprod. Fertil.* **71,** 107 (1984).
25. J. Meredith and J. E. Levine, *Brain Res.* **571,** 181 (1992).

[23] Pulsatile Administration of Insulin and Glucagon in Man

Pierre J. Lefèbvre, Giuseppe Paolisso, and André J. Scheen

Introduction

As reviewed elsewhere (1, 2), numerous *in vitro* and *in vivo* studies have shown that insulin and glucagon are released in a pulsatile manner: oscillations in insulin and glucagon plasma levels have been demonstrated in peripheral and portal blood in man and in animals, sustained oscillations in the release of insulin and glucagon from the isolated perfused dog pancreas have been reported repeatedly, while pulsatility of hormone release by isolated islets has been strongly suggested. These *in vitro* observations have led to the proposal that the pulsatility of pancreatic hormone release depends on a pacemaker system present in the gland itself (reviewed in 2) while *in vivo* analysis suggests that feedback control loops may generate oscillations of longer duration and greater amplitude (3). *In vitro* systems permit precise modeling of the response of target tissues to glucagon and insulin; such studies have been analyzed by Goodner in Chapter 11 in this volume (4). In this chapter, we review the effects of pulsatile administration of insulin, glucagon, or both hormones together on carbohydrate metabolism and islet-cell function. We have restricted our analysis to studies performed *in vivo* in healthy man or in diabetic patients.

Pulsatile Administration of Insulin

Studies in Normal Man

Effects on Carbohydrate Metabolism

Matthews *et al.* (5) were the first to suggest that pulsatile insulin may have greater biologic effects than continuous delivery; in six normal men, in whom pancreatic insulin output was suppressed by somatostatin, the researchers showed that intermittently delivered insulin (2-min pulses separated by 11-min gaps) had a greater hypoglycemic effect than the same total amount of insulin delivered continuously. In subsequent studies, various authors at first failed to confirm such a superior effect of pulsatile insulin. Using the

Methods in Neurosciences, Volume 20

euglycemic hyperinsulinemic clamp procedure, Verdin *et al.* (6) reported similar metabolic effects of pulsatile versus continuous insulin delivery in normal man; however, in that study, the amounts of insulin infused with both modes of administration resulted in peripheral plasma levels ranging between 10 and 45 μU/ml, sufficient to induce complete suppression of hepatic glucose output; therefore such a protocol was not appropriate to demonstrate the possibly greater metabolic effect of pulsatile insulin if that effect occurred at the liver site. In a subsequent study, Paolisso *et al.* (7) used a similar protocol, but suppressed insulin and glucagon by a somatostatin infusion, replaced glucagon by an exogenous infusion (7.5 μg/hr), and compared the effects of continuously administered insulin to insulin infused in a pulsatile manner (2/11 on/off) at identical doses in both protocols and low enough so that hepatic glucose production was not completely inhibited. Here, again, the results were negative, in the sense that the greater metabolic effect of insulin described by Matthews *et al.* (5) was not confirmed. In that study, glucagon replacement during somatostatin infusion resulted in circulatory plasma glucagon levels between 180 and 200 pg/ml, while basal plasma glucagon levels were 110–120 pg/ml. In fact, we demonstrated in a subsequent study that indeed such slight hyperglucagonemia is sufficient to abolish the higher efficacy of pulsatile insulin (8). Finally, Paolisso *et al.* (9) were able to design the experimental protocol that confirmed the superior metabolic effect of pulsatile insulin: six healthy volunteers were submitted to a 325-min glucose-controlled glucose intravenous infusion using the Biostator; the endogenous secretion of pancreatic hormones was inhibited by somatostatin (2 μg/min); glucagon was replaced at a continuous infusion rate of 67 ng/min resulting in peripheral plasma glucagon levels similar to the preinfusion basal levels; insulin was infused either continuously or in identical total amounts in 2-min pulses separated by 11-min intervals during which no insulin was infused; the dose of insulin was selected so that hepatic glucose output was not completely inhibited; glucose turnover parameters were studied using D-[3-^{3}H]glucose infusion. Under these conditions, it was clearly demonstrated that pulsatile insulin exerts an inhibitory effect on hepatic glucose output greater than that of the same amount of the hormone infused continuously. No effect was observed on glucose utilization or metabolic clearance rate. Using a similar protocol, but a higher dose of insulin, Schmitz *et al.* (10) completely inhibited hepatic glucose output with both pulsatile and continuous insulin; under these conditions, a greater effect of pulsatile insulin on glucose uptake, expressed as metabolic clearance rate, was observed; this effect however was not found consistently until after 210 min of pulsatile insulin administration.

In all the preceding studies, the investigators used 10- to 13-min pulse frequencies, close to those reported for spontaneous oscillations in plasma insulin as observed in various experimental conditions *in vivo* and *in vitro*, in animals and in man (reviewed in 1). Finally Paolisso *et al.* (11) studied whether the greater inhibitory effect of insulin on hepatic glucose output when insulin is given in 13-min pulses remains when the same amount of insulin is delivered using pulses delivered every 26 min. The study was performed on nine healthy male volunteers submitted to a 325-min glucose-controlled glucose intravenous infusion again using the Biostator. The endogenous secretion of pancreatic hormones was inhibited by somatostatin. Three experiments were performed in each subject on different days and in random order. In all cases, glucagon was replaced at a rate of 58 ng/min resulting in plasma glucagon levels averaging 100 ng/liter. The total amounts of insulin infused were identical in all three experiments but the hormone was given either continuously or as 2-min pulses separated by periods of 11 or 24 min during which no insulin was infused. As reported previously, when compared with continuous insulin delivery, insulin pulses every 13 min induced a significantly greater inhibition of endogenous glucose production. Interestingly this effect disappeared when insulin pulses were delivered every 26 min. It was therefore concluded that a pulse frequency close to that reported for spontaneous oscillations is required to allow the greater inhibition of endogenous glucose production by pulsatile insulin to appear. Finally, Ward *et al.* (12) showed that prolonged pulsatile hyperinsulinemia (pulses every 13 min), using a 20-hr glucose clamp, resulted in a better insulin sensitivity index than an identical-dose steady infusion.

Effects on Pancreatic Islet-Cell Function

Asplin *et al.* (13) reported that hyperinsulinemia, within the physiological range and achieved by continuous insulin infusion, inhibited the endogenous insulin response to arginine and potentiated the glucagon release. This last finding was attributed to suppression of the inhibitory effect exerted by locally released insulin on A-cell function through a paracrine mechanism. This observation was entirely confirmed by Paolisso *et al.* (14). Furthermore, these authors demonstrated that the same dose of insulin administered in 2-min pulses every 11 min had greater effects than continuous delivery in (i) decreasing basal plasma glucagon and C-peptide levels, (ii) enhancing the arginine-induced glucagon release, and (iii) reducing, although not significantly, the arginine-induced C-peptide response. These data support the concept that insulin per se is a potent physiologic modulator of pancreatic A- and B-cells (15–17) and that these effects of insulin are reinforced when the hormone is administered in an intermittent manner in an attempt to reproduce the intraislet pulsatility of physiologically released insulin. The greater effect of pulsatile insulin on endogenous insulin secretion in man was confirmed by Ward *et al.* (18) who also showed that pulsatile insulin has a longer-lasting suppressive effect on glucagon secretion.

Studies in Diabetic Patients

Effects on Carbohydrate Metabolism

Bratusch-Marrain *et al.* (19) compared the effects of continuous and pulsatile insulin administration on hepatic glucose production and glucose utilization in *type 1 diabetic patients* submitted to a euglycemic insulin clamp procedure. The total amount of insulin infused in the pulsatile manner was 40% less than when it was infused continuously. Despite this reduction, insulin given in the pulsatile manner was equally potent in reducing hepatic glucose output and stimulating glucose utilization. It has been suggested that intravenous pulsatile administration of insulin might reduce systemic hyperinsulinemia and, in the long run, attenuate insulin resistance (19). Paolisso *et al.* (8) confirmed the greater efficacy of pulsatile insulin in reducing plasma glucose levels in *type 1 diabetic patients* but demonstrated that this effect was critically dependent on plasma glucagon levels; while completely absent at plasma concentrations averaging 200 ng/ml, it was observed at glucagon levels averaging 130 ng/ml but occurred earlier, and was more pronounced, when plasma glucagon concentrations were only 75 ng/ml. In contrast, Heinemann *et al.* (20) did not find any beneficial effect of pulsatile insulin (10 pulses of 20 sec duration with intervals of 6 min, three times a day) on oral glucose tolerance in 9 *type 1 diabetic patients*.

In *type 2 diabetic patients*, intermittent administration of insulin also had a greater hypoglycemic effect than the same amount of insulin infused continuously (21). This effect was recently confirmed in relatively aged subjects (mean 67.5 years) with non-insulin-dependent diabetes and secondary failure to hypoglycemic agents (22). It was entirely due to a greater inhibition of hepatic glucose output; interestingly, pulsatile insulin delivery exerted metabolic effects identical to those of a 33% greater dose infused continuously.

Effects on Pancreatic Islet-Cell Function

Nine patients with *type 1 diabetes mellitus* and no residual insulin secretion were investigated (14). They were infused, in random order and on different days, with either saline or a small amount of insulin delivered continuously (0.5 mU/kg × min) or in a pulsatile manner (0.97 mU/kg × min for 2 min followed by 11 min during which no insulin was infused). In all experiments, 5 g arginine was given iv as a bolus 30 min before the end of the study. While the glucagon response to arginine was not modified by the small amount of insulin infused continuously, it was significantly reduced when the same amount of insulin was delivered intermittently. These data support the concept that insulin per se is a potent physiological modulator of A-cells and demonstrate that the effect of insulin is reinforced when the hormone is administered in an intermittent manner in an attempt to reproduce the intraislet pulsatility of physiologically released insulin. We have suggested (14, 23) that the hyperglucagonemia of type 2 diabetes, a universally recognized but still poorly explained finding (23), may result from the loss in these patients of the normal oscillatory pattern of insulin release, as described by Lang *et al.* (24).

Subcutaneous Intermittent Insulin Administration

Attempts to achieve better control of type 1 diabetes by pulsed insulin given subcutaneously have failed. In the study performed by Levy-Marchal *et al.* (25) in six *type 1 diabetic patients*, overnight metabolic control was similar when a given amount of insulin was delivered subcutaneously either in a continuous manner or intermittently as pulses spaced at 30-, 60-, and 120-min intervals. It should be noted, however, that under these conditions no oscillations in plasma insulin were achieved. In contrast to what has been reported above with intravenous insulin administration (26), a reduction of the dose of insulin infused subcutaneously induces a metabolic deterioration that is not compensated for by the intermittent (every 30 min) administration of the same total amount of the hormone. Here again, intermittent subcutaneous insulin administration did not induce any clear oscillations in peripheral plasma insulin levels.

Pulsatile Administration of Glucagon

Studies in Normal Man

In vitro studies, reviewed in detail in Chapter 11 of this book (4) have shown convincingly that glucagon given as a series of brief pulses induces a greater glucose output from both perfused rat hepatocytes and isolated perfused rat liver.

The first study investigating the respective effects of continuous and intermittent glucagon administration in man has been negative in the sense that no greater effect of pulsatile glucagon administration has been identified (27). In that study however, relatively high plasma glucagon concentration had been achieved: 189 ± 38 ng/liter in the continuous infusions and oscillations between 95 and 101 ng/liter in the intermittent mode of glucagon administration. It is likely that such high plasma levels were out of the "window" of glucagon concentrations for which the glucagon enhancement effect on liver glucose output had been observed *in vitro* (28–30). Indeed, in a subsequent study (9), lower glucagon doses were administered (under pancreatic hormone secretion inhibition by somatostatin and continuous insulin infusion to replace basal insulin levels); in this setting, pulsatile glucagon administration induced a greater stimulation of hepatic glucose output than an identical dose of the hormone infused continuously for 325 min. Finally, in the presence of somatostatin-induced insulin deficiency (with no insulin replacement), pulsatile glucagon induced greater rises in blood glucose, plasma nonesterified fatty acid, glycerol, and β-hydroxybutyrate levels than did its continuous delivery (31). Interestingly, in the elderly (69.4 $\pm$ 2.0 years), the lipolytic and ketogenic, but not the hyperglycemic, responses to pulsatile glucagon were significantly reduced when compared to the effects observed in healthy young volunteers (24.2 $\pm$ 1.2 years), an observation that may be relevant for the understanding of the pathophysiology of hyperosmolar nonketotic coma in elderly people (31). Finally, Attvall *et al.* (32) investigated the insulin-antagonistic effects of pulsatile (3-min pulses every 20 min) and continuous glucagon over 4 hr with the euglycemic clamp technique in healthy subjects. Glucose production and utilization were evaluated with D-[3-^{3}H]glucose while, again, somatostatin was used in all studies to inhibit endogenous insulin and glucagon release. In this setting, the amount of glucagon given during the pulsatile infusion (27% of that during continuous infusion) was adjusted so that the peak glucagon levels (371 $\pm$ 22 ng/liter) were similar to those used during the continuous infusion (365 $\pm$ 20 ng/liter). The insulin-antagonistic effects of pulsatile and continuous glucagon infusions on glucose production were similar during the first hour and impaired the insulin effect 44 $\pm$ 8 and 47 $\pm$ 6%, respectively. However, the effect of glucagon when infused continuously declined rapidly, whereas the effect of the pulsatile infusion decreased more slowly and was evident for 3 hr. Raising the glucagon level four-fold restored the insulin-antgonistic effect again, suggesting that the liver had become desensitized.

Studies in Diabetic Patients

To our knowledge, one study only has investigated the respective effects of continuous and pulsatile intravenous glucagon delivery in type 1 diabetic patients (33). The study was performed in seven *insulin-dependent (type 1) diabetic subjects* proved to have no residual insulin secretion. In random order and on different days, each subject was submitted to glucagon delivery given continuously for 325 min (58 ng/min) or in a pulsatile manner (same total dose but given in 2-min pulses separated by 11-min periods during which no glucagon was infused). Endogenous pancreatic hormone secretion was inhibited by somatostatin. Insulin was infused overnight and continued until 120 min before the experiment. In the continuous glucagon infusion protocol, plasma glucagon averaged 109 ± 13 ng/liter. In the intermittent glucagon administration, plasma glucagon levels oscillated between 28 and 197 ng/liter. Pulsatile glucagon delivery resulted in higher plasma glucose, glycerol, β-hydroxybutyrate, and triglyceride levels than did continuous delivery.

Combined Pulsatile Administration of Insulin and Glucagon

One study, which we reported in 1989 (9), investigated the respective effects of continuous intravenous delivery of both insulin and glucagon compared with those of pulsatile insulin (and continuous glucagon), pulsatile glucagon (and continuous insulin), and both hormones administered in a pulsatile manner (but out of phase) on various parameters of glucose turnover. The study was performed on six healthy male volunteers submitted to a 325-min glucose-controlled glucose intravenous infusion using the Biostator. The endogenous secretion of pancreatic hormones was inhibited by somatostatin ($2 \mu g$/min). Four combinations of continuous and pulsatile infusions of insulin and glucagon were performed on different days and in random order. The amounts of hormone infused were identical in all instances. In the case of pulsatile administration of both hormones, the pulses of insulin and glucagon were given out of phase with a 6-min interval (Figs. 1 and 2). Blood glucose levels and glucose infusion rate were monitored continuously by the Biostator, and classic methodology using a D-[3-^{3}H]glucose infusion allowed glucose turnover to be studied (Fig. 3). When compared with pulsatile insulin and continuous glucagon, pulsatile glucagon and continuous insulin were characterized by significantly higher endogenous (hepatic) glucose production. When both insulin and glucagon were delivered in a pulsatile manner, the effect of pulsatile glucagon was predominant, maintaining a high endogenous glucose production. In no circumstance was an effect on glucose utilization or clearance detected. This study demonstrated that pulsatile delivery of insulin or glucagon in humans has greater effects in modulating endogenous glucose production than continuous infusion. Furthermore, when both insulin and glucagon were delivered intermittently and out of phase, the stimulatory effect of glucagon on endogenous glucose production clearly prevailed over the inhibitory effect of insulin.

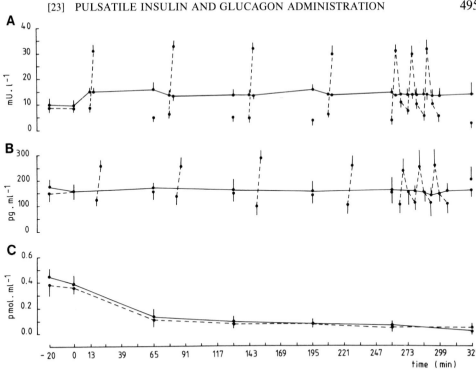

FIG. 1   Plasma insulin (A), glucagon (B), and C-peptide (C) levels during continuous (solid line) or pulsatile (dashed line) insulin and glucagon infusion. Multiple collections of blood permitting demonstration of oscillations in plasma insulin and glucagon were performed from 260 to 305 min only. Results are expressed as means ± SE ($n = 6$). [Reproduced with permission from Paolisso *et al.* (9).]

Conclusions

A number of studies performed in man over the past 10 years have clearly established that insulin and glucagon administered intravenously exert greater effects when given intermittently rather than continuously. Greater effects of pulsatile insulin have been observed in normal man and in diabetic subjects. In healthy volunteers, pulsatile intravenous delivery of insulin is more efficient than an identical amount of insulin infused continuously in reducing blood glucose and inhibiting liver glucose production. Such greater effects of pulsatile insulin are observed at a pulse frequency of 11–13 min (not 26 min) and are abolished by high circulating levels of glucagon. Furthermore, pulsatile insulin is more efficient than its continuous delivery in reducing basal

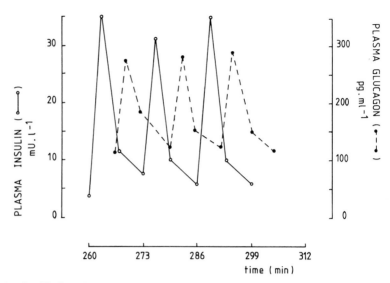

FIG. 2   Oscillations in plasma insulin and glucagon levels during pulsatile infusion of both hormones. Insulin was infused during first 2 min and glucagon from 6 to 8 min of each cycle of 13 min, leading to a 6-min phase displacement between insulin and glucagon pulses. Results are expressed as means ± SE ($n = 6$). [Reproduced with permission from Paolisso *et al.* (9).]

glucagon release, inhibiting endogenous insulin release, and, consequently, enhancing arginine-induced glucagon release.

In both type 1 and type 2 diabetic patients, insulin delivered intravenously in a pulsatile manner is more efficient than identical doses infused continuously in reducing blood glucose, endogenous glucose production, and, according to one report, increasing glucose uptake. In contrast, no beneficial effect of intermittent subcutaneous insulin administration has been reported.

Providing that it is delivered in an appropriate window, glucagon also exerts greater effects on blood glucose, endogenous glucose production, lipolysis, and ketogenesis when it is administered in 11- to 13-min pulses rather than continuously. These greater effects of pulsatile glucagon have been observed both in heatlhy subjects and in diabetic patients.

When both insulin and glucagon are delivered in pulses so that plasma levels of both hormones oscillate out of phase, the greater effect of glucagon in stimulating endogenous glucose production prevails over the greater effect of insulin in inhibiting this parameter.

Finally, it must be emphasized that the fluctuations in plasma insulin and glucagon concentrations generated by the intermittent intravenous adminis-

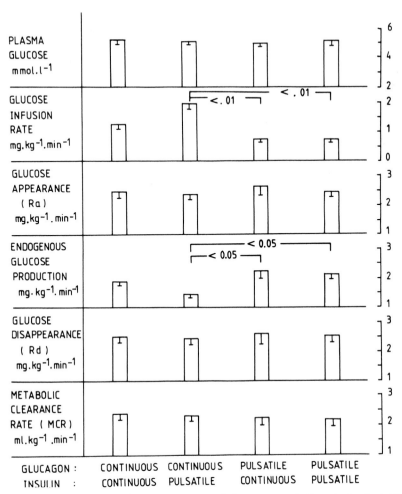

FIG. 3 Comparison of various parameters of glucose metabolism during last 65 min of each test under four experimental conditions: continuous glucagon–continuous insulin, continuous glucagon–pulsatile insulin, pulsatile glucagon–continuous insulin, and pulsatile glucagon–pulsatile insulin infusions. For each subject, mean values of five measurements carried out during last 65 min of study were calculated. Results are expressed as means ± SE ($n = 6$). [Reproduced with permission from Paolisso et al. (9).]

tration of these two hormones are much greater than those spontaneously observed in the peripheral plasma (see review in 1, 2); however, they are not far from those reported by others in the portal plasma of dogs, baboons, and even humans (34, 35), an observation that is of interest since most of the effects observed appear to be at the liver site.

Acknowledgments

We acknowledge the expert secretarial help of E. Vaessen-Petit. Our own studies in the field were performed in the framework of a collaboration between the Universities of Liège (Belgium) and Naples (Italy). Generous support was provided by the Fonds de la Recherche Scientifique Médicale of Belgium and the Fonds de la Recherche Facultaire of the Faculty of Medicine, University of Liège (Belgium).

References

1. P. J. Lefèbvre, G. Paolisso, A. J. Scheen, and J. C. Henquin, *Diabetologia* **30,** 443 (1987).
2. J. I. Stagner, *in* "The Endocrine Pancreas" (E. Samols, ed.), p. 283. Raven Press, New York, 1991.
3. C. Simon, G. Brandenberger, and M. Follenius, *J. Clin. Endocrinol. Metab.* **64,** 669 (1987).
4. C. Goodner, Chapter 11, this volume.
5. D. R. Matthews, B. A. Naylor, R. G. Jones, G. M. Ward, and R. C. Turner, *Diabetes* **32,** 617 (1983).
6. E. Verdin, M. Castillo, A. S. Luyckx, and P. J. Lefèbvre, *Diabetes* **33,** 1169 (1984).
7. G. Paolisso, A. J. Scheen, E. M. Verdin, A. S. Luyckx, and P. J. Lefèbvre, *J. Clin. Endocrinol. Metab.* **63,** 520 (1986).
8. G. Paolisso, S. Sgambato, N. Passariello, A. Scheen, F. D'Onofrio, and P. J. Lefèbvre, *Diabetes* **36,** 566 (1987).
9. G. Paolisso, A. J. Scheen, A. Albert, and P. J. Lefèbvre, *Am. J. Physiol.* **257** (*Endocrinol. Metab.* **20**), E686 (1989).
10. O. Schmitz, J. Arnfred, O. Hother Nielsen, H. Beck-Nielsen, and H. Ørskov, *Acta Endocrinol. (Copenhagen)* **113,** 559 (1986).
11. G. Paolisso, A. J. Scheen, D. Giugliano, S. Sgambato, A. Albert, M. Varricchio, F. D'Onofrio, and P. J. Lefèbvre, *J. Clin. Endocrinol. Metab.* **72,** 607 (1991).
12. G. M. Ward, J. M. Walters, P. M. Aitken, J. D. Best, and F. P. Alford, *Diabetes* **39,** 501 (1990).
13. C. M. Asplin, T. L. Paquette, and J. P. Palmer, *J. Clin. Invest.* **68,** 314 (1981).
14. G. Paolisso, S. Sgambato, R. Torella, M. Varricchio, A. Scheen, F. D'Onofrio, and P. J. Lefèbvre, *J. Clin. Endocrinol. Metab.* **66,** 1220 (1988).

15. E. Samols, G. C. Weir, and S. Bonner-Weir, *in* "Glucagon: Handbook of Experimental Pharmacology" (P. J. Lefèbvre, ed.), Part 2, Vol. 66, p. 133. Springer, Berlin/Heidelberg/New York/Tokyo, 1983.

16. E. Samols, *in* "Glucagon: Handbook of Experimental Pharmacology" (P. J. Lefèbvre, ed.), Part 1, Vol. 66, p. 485. Springer, Berlin/Heidelberg/New York/Tokyo, 1983.

17. B. Draznin, M. Goodman, and K. Sussman, *Endocrinology (Baltimore)* **118,** 1054 (1986).

18. G. M. Ward, A. G. Marangou, J. D. Best, P. M. Aitken, and F. P. Alford, *Metabolism* **38,** 297 (1989).

19. P. R. Bratusch-Marrain, M. Komjati, and W. K. Waldhäusel, *Diabetes* **35,** 922 (1986).

20. L. Heinemann, G. E. Sonnenberg, A. Hohmann, A. Ritzenhoff, M. Berger, J. Benn, P. Sönksen, D. Kelley, J. Gerich, T. Aoki, and J. Sorensen, *J. Intern. Med.* **226,** 325 (1989).

21. G. Paolisso, S. Sgambato, S. Gentile, P. Memoli, D. Giugliano, M. Varricchio, and F. D'Onofrio, *J. Clin. Endocrinol. Metab.* **67,** 1005 (1988).

22. G. Paolisso, S. Sgambato, M. Varricchio, A. J. Scheen, F. D'Onofrio, and P. Lefèbvre, *Eur. J. Med.* **1,** 261 (1992).

23. P. Lefèbvre, G. Paolisso, and A. Scheen, *in* "New Directions in Research and Clinical Works for Obesity and Diabetes Mellitus" (N. Sakamoto, A. Angel, and N. Hotta, eds.), p. 25. Elsevier Sciences, Amsterdam, 1991.

24. D. A. Lang, D. R. Matthews, M. Burnett, and R. C. Turner, *Diabetes* **30,** 435 (1981).

25. C. Levy-Marchal, M. Albisser, and B. Zinman, *Diabetes Care* **6,** 356 (1983).

26. H. Lilet, G. Krzentowski, A. Bodson, A. J. Scheen, and P. J. Lefèbvre, *Diabete Metab. (Paris)* **17,** 372 (1991).

27. G. Paolisso, A. J. Scheen, A. S. Luyckx, and P. J. Lefèbvre, *Am. J. Physiol.* **251** (*Endocrinol. Metab.* **15**), El (1987).

28. D. S. Weigle and C. J. Goodner, *Endocrinology (Baltimore)* **118,** 1606 (1986).

29. D. S. Weigle, D. J. Koerker, and C. J. Goodner, *Am. J. Physiol.* **247** (*Endocrinol. Metab.* **10**), E564 (1984).

30. D. S. Weigle, D. J. Koerker, and C. J. Goodner, *Am. J. Physiol.* **248** (*Endocrinol. Metab.* **11**), E681 (1985).

31. G. Paolisso, S. Buonocore, S. Gentile, S. Sgambato, M. Varricchio, A. Scheen, F. D'Onofrio, and P. J. Lefèbvre, *Diabetologia* **33,** 272 (1990).

32. S. Attvall, J. Fowelin, H. Von Schenck, U. Smith, and I. Lager, *J. Clin. Endocrinol. Metab.* **74,** 1110 (1992).

33. G. Paolisso, S. Sgambato, R. Giunta, M. Varricchio, and F. D'Onofrio, *Diabete Metab. (Paris)* **16,** 42 (1990).

34. B. C. Hansen, K-L. C. Jen, D. J. Koerker, C. J. Goodner, and R. A. Wolfe, *Am. J. Physiol.* **242,** R255 (1982).

35. J. B. Jaspan, E. Lever, K. S. Polonsky, and E. Van Cauter, *Am. J. Physiol.* **251,** E215 (1986).

Index